The Heinemann
New Family Medical
Encyclopaedia

By the same authors

By David Rubenstein and David Wayne
Lecture Notes on Clinical Medicine
Multiple Choice Questions on Lecture Notes on Clinical Medicine
Aids to Prescribing (with Nicholas Coni)

By David Rubenstein
The Human Body (with Paul Lewis)

THE HEINEMANN
NEW FAMILY MEDICAL
ENCYCLOPAEDIA

Paul Paxton MBBS MRCGP DRCOG
General Practitioner, Cambridge

David Rubenstein MA MD FRCP
Consultant Physician, Addenbrooke's Hospital,
Cambridge

Andrew Smith BSc MBBS DRCOG
General Practitioner, Saffron Waldron

David Wayne MA BM FRCP (Lond) FRCP (Edin)
Consultant Physician, District General Hospital,
Gorleston, Great Yarmouth

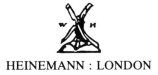

HEINEMANN : LONDON

William Heinemann Ltd
10 Upper Grosvenor Street, London W1X 9PA
LONDON   MELBOURNE   TORONTO
JOHANNESBURG   AUCKLAND

First published 1983
© David Rubenstein and David Wayne 1983
434 65410 8

Printed in West Germany

CONTENTS

Preface

This book describes the structure and function of the human body and its common disorders. The causes of the common symptoms are explained in detail, their significance analysed and a recommended course of action suggested. Other medical terms commonly encountered are also included in the A – Z section.

We have tried to relieve unnecessary anxiety about medical matters with simple direct explanations of the facts. When dealing with serious disease we have not obscured the simple, if unpleasant, truth with universal reassurance, but given a course of action to follow and some guidance about what to expect. Many people are worried about the unfamiliar so we have written special sections on topics such as Going into hospital, Home care of the elderly, Child development, Accidents in the home and Commonly used drugs.

We give advice on when to consult your doctor, and a star indicates a situation which is urgent. If you remain uncertain or your anxiety continues, always seek medical advice so that the worries can be relieved and important diseases detected and treated early. We hope that you will use this book not only as a reference when in need of authoritative medical advice, but also as a source of interesting information about how the body works in health and disease.

Acknowledgements

Sir Edward Wayne, lately Regius Professor of Practice of Medicine in the University of Glasgow, kindly read the entire text critically and made many helpful suggestions about the medical content.

It was a pleasure to work with Gillian Clarke, who edited the text.

We wish to thank the following colleagues and friends for the loan of photographic illustrations: Peter Black, John Keats-Butler, Adrian Dixon, Stephen Roberts, Paul Siklos, Trevor Wheatley, Phillip Wraight, and the Department of Medical Illustration, Addenbrooke's Hospital, Cambridge.

The authors and publisher would like to thank the Institute of Ophthalmology, London, for permission to use the photographs illustrating colour defective vision; Parke-Davis Research Laboratories for the photographs illustrating the use of eye drops and ointment; and Novo Laboratories for the photographs illustrating insulin injections.

The illustrations and diagrams in this book were conceived, designed and produced by The Paul Press, 22 Bruton Street, London W1X 7DA.

They were drawn by the following artists and studios: Claire Belfield, Nigel Fradgely, Cathy Hargreaves, Haywood and Martin, Cindy Scott.

Part 1

A – Z of Common Terms and Problems

A

Abdomen

Contains the stomach and intestines, the pancreas, liver, spleen and kidneys, and the organs within the pelvis—i.e. the bladder, the uterus and ovaries in women, and the prostate in men. These are enclosed by the diaphragm above, the muscles and bones of the pelvis below, and by the abdominal muscles. The relationship of these structures is shown below.

Abdominal pain
IN ADULTS

The most common causes of abdominal pain are gastritis, peptic ulcer, constipation, gastro-enteritis, appendicitis, and oesophagitis due to acid regurgitation (reflux) with or without a hiatus hernia.

Gastritis and peptic ulcers
The pain is felt at the top of the abdomen, where the stomach lies, and is usually burning or sore in character. It is caused by acute inflammation of the delicate inner lining of the stomach wall which may even develop small superficial ulcers. The pain may be altered by food and drink: hot, spicy foods and

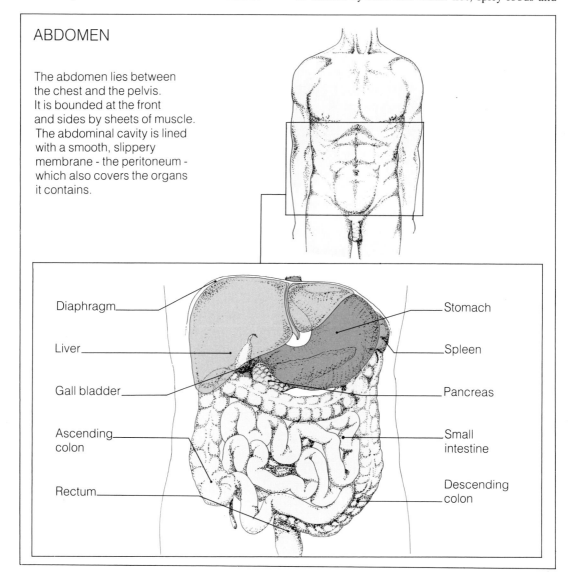

ABDOMEN

The abdomen lies between the chest and the pelvis. It is bounded at the front and sides by sheets of muscle. The abdominal cavity is lined with a smooth, slippery membrane - the peritoneum - which also covers the organs it contains.

Diaphragm — Stomach
Liver — Spleen
Gall bladder — Pancreas
Ascending colon — Small intestine
Rectum — Descending colon

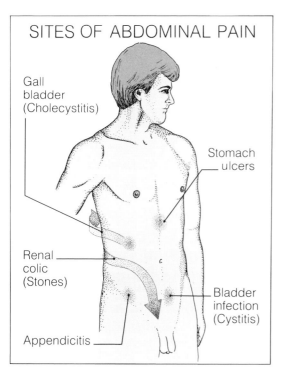

SITES OF ABDOMINAL PAIN

Gall bladder (Cholecystitis)

Stomach ulcers

Renal colic (Stones)

Bladder infection (Cystitis)

Appendicitis

towards the rectum. Every so often these muscles relax and the pain disappears, only to return in a few minutes. Constipation may be extremely uncomfortable but is virtually never serious. (It is discussed in detail on page 64.)

The elderly are prone to chronic constipation, and often require regular bran and laxatives (aperients) to empty the bowel. If the pain changes character and particularly if it becomes griping or colicky, it may suggest early obstruction in the intestines—and medical advice should be sought.

Gastro-enteritis

The pain is griping or colicky (see Colic), coming and going in waves and making the sufferer roll about in agony. It is usually felt in the middle of the abdomen near the navel (umbilicus), but is frequently felt over the entire abdomen. A bout of pain may be followed by diarrhoea and there is often associated vomiting. The abdomen may rumble continuously.

Gastro-enteritis is usually infectious, and may follow food poisoning. Acute gastro-enteritis is rarely serious except in young children, and the vomiting, diarrhoea and pain settle within 48–72 hours. (For treatment, see Gastro-enteritis.)

Appendicitis see page 25

Gall stones and cholecystitis (inflammation of the gall bladder)

The pain is felt in the upper half of the abdomen, usually on the right-hand side just below the ribs. It may be worse after meals, especially fatty ones, and be accompanied by belching. The pain may be 'colicky' (see Colic) if a gall stone leaves the gall bladder and passes down the narrow bile duct leading to the bowel.

Abdominal pain accompanied by jaundice usually indicates gall bladder disease, although hepatitis also produces similar symptoms.

Colitis

Inflammation or infection of the colon. The pain varies from a mild dragging discomfort felt on both sides of the lower abdomen to a constant searing pain in the abdomen, which is very tender to touch. It is likely to be accompanied by watery diarrhoea and the motions may contain blood and slime. It usually improves after defecation. Colitis results from infection by viruses or bacteria following food poisoning, and settles within 5–7 days. Ulcerative colitis (page 232) may begin in a similar way.

alcohol tend to exacerbate it, while bland food and alkalis (e.g. milk or Milk of Magnesia) relieve it. Worry, stress, over-eating or irregular meals may also make the pain worse, whereas small regular meals help to relieve it. Aspirin-containing drugs are best avoided because aspirin directly irritates the stomach lining. Many of the proprietary pain killers available at a chemist's contain aspirin (e.g. Alka-Seltzer, Beecham's Powders, Anadin), so if in doubt ask the pharmacist's advice.

Gastritis and peptic ulcers also cause belching and vomiting, which may relieve the pain. Smoking prevents ulcer healing.

Constipation

A common cause of abdominal discomfort and pain felt in the middle of the abdomen near the navel (umbilicus) or low down on the left-hand side. It causes a dragging discomfort relieved by defecation. Often referred to as 'wind pain', the description of the pain as 'cramp-like' is a good one, as it is produced by the powerful contraction and spasm of the bowel muscles which push the hard motion

Tension or depression

May cause persistent abdominal discomfort rather than severe pain. It may be difficult to localize in the abdomen, and tends to be worse during acute episodes of stress or depression. Psychological upset is a frequent cause of recurrent abdominal pain, and is common in children just starting a new school.

Hiatus hernia

The pain is felt in the mid-line in the lower chest or at the top of the abdomen. It is induced by eating or drinking hot food, bending over, straining, lying down flat or by tight corsets. There may also be heartburn—a sensation of burning behind the breastbone (sternum) and a bitter acid taste in the back of the mouth, produced by the gastric acid as it regurgitates (refluxes) up the oesophagus. The stomach has a specialized lining which is resistant to the acid it produces, but the oesophagus has not. A valve mechanism normally prevents acid in the stomach from passing upwards into the lower end of the oesophagus but, if this is incompetent, acid leaks up and inflames its delicate lining.

Treatment involves avoiding all the precipitating factors mentioned above. In addition, antacids and milk can help by neutralizing the acid. Sleeping propped up in bed may be the only way to prevent acid reflux and allow a reasonable night's sleep. If the symptoms persist or if there is loss of weight, medical advice should be obtained.

Cancer of the stomach

The pain is a dull or gnawing ache and, like the pain of gastritis or ulcers, is felt in the top of the abdomen. Instead of periods of days or weeks with relief, cancer of the stomach usually produces pain which gets steadily worse. There is also loss of appetite, lack of energy and weight loss.

Cystitis

The pain is felt low down in the abdomen, over the bladder just above the pelvic bone. There may be tenderness to pressure at the same place. It is a continuous aching discomfort normally accompanied by frequency of micturition (page 105) and burning pain on passing urine (dysuria), sometimes with blood in the urine and a fever. The phrase 'honeymoon cystitis' underlines the association of cystitis in the female with sexual activity. Cystitis in men is uncommon. (*See also* Cystitis.)

Kidney infections and kidney stones

Kidney infections (pyelonephritis) produce pain in the loin and are accompanied by frequency of micturition (page 105) and burning pain on passing urine, blood in the urine and fever.

Kidney stones (page 141) cause severe 'colicky' pain (*see* Colic) which may start in the flank and radiate round the side of the abdomen to the groin, and into the testis in the male.

Pelvic infections in women (salpingitis—infection of the Fallopian tubes)

The pain is low down in the abdomen. It is a continual 'gnawing' discomfort and may be accompanied by a smelly brown discharge from the vagina, backache and a fever. The abdomen is tender to touch overlying the site of pain.

Abdominal pain
IN CHILDREN

Abdominal pain in children is caused by emotional factors in 9 out of 10 cases. All children get 'stomach ache' at some time, and it is rare for any precipitating emotional upset to be serious.

Typically, pain comes on just before the child is due to do something which he does not wish—such as going to school. Not surprisingly, it disappears when the unwanted activity has passed or been avoided. The child remains well and there is no fever, vomiting or diarrhoea.

If vomiting, fever or diarrhoea is present, medical advice should be obtained because these features strongly suggest food poisoning, viral gastro-enteritis or appendicitis.

The periodic syndrome (abdominal migraine)

Occurs in 'highly strung' or excitable children. There are recurrent episodes of abdominal pain with vomiting, fever and a headache. Usually everything subsides in 2–3 hours. The child should be put to bed and, if vomiting, given only water or fruit squashes to drink. Between acute attacks such children are perfectly well.

The cause is uncertain but probably is the result of an emotional upset to which all children are prone. It is helpful to determine the cause of the emotional problem but children are often reluctant to tell of their deepest fears and it is probably best to veer on the side of playing things down. Some authorities consider that children who get easily tired are the most susceptible to these attacks and should go to bed early at night and even have an afternoon sleep. Most children grow out of the attacks in 2 or 3 years. However, when adults, they may suffer from migraine, which often affects their parents.

Other causes

The physical causes of abdominal pain in children include constipation, gastro-enteritis, appendicitis and infections in the throat, ear or urine. (For further details, *see under* Abdominal pain: in adults.) Children tend to be more susceptible than adults to unusual or rich food, which may produce abdominal pain, with or without vomiting; it settles rapidly after 4–6 hours.

Note If any doubt exists about the cause of a child's abdominal pain, it is always best to seek ★ medical advice, particularly if the child is not prone to stomach aches. Appendicitis can sometimes be very difficult to diagnose, and children known to have 'abdominal migraine' have the same chance of developing appendicitis as have the others.

Abortion
(LATIN: *ABORIRI*, TO MISCARRY)

The expulsion or removal from the uterus of the developing, and frequently malformed, fetus. Abortion may be spontaneous, or therapeutic if performed electively for the mother's health (*see* Pregnancy: bleeding *and* Pregnancy: termination).

★ Spontaneous abortion is common and usually occurs within the first 2–3 months of pregnancy. It is understandably disturbing for the mother, and the father's distress should not be forgotten. The cause is usually unknown but is probably the result of intra-uterine infection, or inadequate attachment of the developing fetus to the inner lining wall of the womb (uterus). In such situations the fetus, if it develops further, could be abnormal.

Therapeutic abortion is performed on the advice of two medical practitioners when continuation of the pregnancy would be detrimental to the mother's health. This decision cannot be taken lightly by the mother, for whom it can be a very disturbing experience, and can be arrived at only after very careful consideration of her physical and psychological health. The operation is technically straightforward and safe but, following it, strong yet gentle support is needed from the patient's close friends, family and family physician. (*See* Pregnancy: termination.)

Abscess

A collection of pus, anywhere in the body. The most common example is a boil, which reaches a head and drains spontaneously. Abscesses in other parts of the body such as the lung, liver, kidney and brain, produce features of infection, with high fever, night sweat and weight loss. There is usually pain over the site. To prevent further spread of infection, the abscess must be drained surgically and this results in rapid improvement.

Accidents

Accidents in the home and on the road are the commonest cause of illness and death in children and in the 15- to 25-year age group, respectively. Simple preventive measures such as fire and cooker guards, locking chemicals and drugs out of the reach of young children, safety helmets for motorcyclists and safety belts for car drivers and passengers would dramatically reduce the number of injuries.

Emergency treatment is discussed in the section on First aid (page 269).

Acetabulum

The cup formed by the pelvic bone to take the head of the femur. Together these form the hip joint (page 126).

Acetylsalicylic acid
SEE ASPIRIN

Acne

A common skin complaint, usually affecting teenagers, who develop greasy skin and unsightly spots over the face, shoulders, back and chest. It disappears after adolescence. Hormonal changes which occur at puberty produce greasy skin which blocks the small sweat ducts where they open at the surface of the skin. Initially only a few blackheads are produced, but if the blockage persists, greasy secretions build up underneath the surface and become infected by bacteria. This infected material spreads into the surrounding skin to cause inflammation and irritation.

Acne is most unsightly and can cause great distress. Adolescents can be reassured that it will almost certainly disappear within a few years, but in the meantime the skin must be kept scrupulously clean and make-up avoided because this also blocks the sweat ducts. Squeezing and picking the skin increases the risk of disseminating infection or may cause permanent scarring.

Some skin specialists advise that chocolate be

avoided and that vitamin C tablets or citrus fruits be taken regularly. If these measures are ineffective, a degreasing lotion should be tried—e.g. benzoyl peroxide (Benoxyl, Panoxyl, Quinoderm), coal tar (Polytar). Sunlight is beneficial and acne sufferers usually find that the skin improves during the summer. Ultraviolet treatment may be equally effective.

If simple remedies fail, antibiotics such as tetracycline may be used in a course lasting several weeks, or months. They are usually very effective, but, as with all potent drugs, should be taken only with medical supervision.

Acromegaly
(GREEK: *AKRON,* EXTREMITY; *MEGAS*, GREAT)

A disease caused by a tumour of the pituitary gland, which secretes excess 'growth hormone' and results in over-growth of bone. The typical features are tall stature, large skull and jaw, and large hands and feet. If the disease becomes progressive, the pituitary may have to be removed surgically.

Acupuncture

Has been used widely in China for many centuries; the practice dates back to at least 7000 BC and is used to cure disease, and for pain relief and anaesthesia.

Acupuncture and disease
The ancient Chinese had a relatively simple explanation for how acupuncture relieved illness. They believed that every internal organ was represented on the surface of the body. When the organ was functioning normally, its two polarized forces—Yin, the feminine negative passive force, and Yang, the masculine positive active force—were in balance. The forces within the organ could be modified by stimulation of the appropriate areas of the skin. Thus, if the liver was diseased because Yin and Yang were out of balance, stimulation of the 'liver points' on the skin would restore equilibrium to these forces and effect a cure. The Chinese still use acupuncture to cure disease in this way. It is believed by acupuncturists that when the needles are inserted into the skin they stimulate the nerve fibres running just underneath the surface. Stimulation is produced either by rotating the needles gently between the fingers or by passing a small electric current through them.

There are two types of nerve fibre carrying pain information from the skin, classified as large or small fibres. The large ones conduct impulses rapidly to the spinal cord and brain, while the smaller ones conduct their impulses at a slightly slower rate. The object is to stimulate the larger fibres, whose information then reaches the brain first, and blocks any pain impulse which arrives slightly later along the small fibres. This is the 'gate control' theory of pain.

Recently, it has been claimed that acupuncture triggers the production of a chemical within the brain which is itself a pain killer. There is now considerable evidence to suggest that this substance is synthesized in the body, probably in the brain, and is chemically related to the morphine group of drugs, the most potent analgesics in use. Scientific evaluation of acupuncture by Western doctors was severely hampered during the cultural revolution in China, as a result of the banning of all scientific journals until 1973. Since then it has come under close scrutiny, with encouraging results.

Although the potential uses of acupuncture appear enormous, insufficient scientific research has been done to evaluate its role in Western medical practice.

In China over half a million surgical operations have been carried out using acupuncture anaesthesia with successful pain relief in over 90 per cent. The Chinese state that not everyone is suitable for acupuncture and this high success rate was achieved only by careful selection of the patients. It has been used to relieve pain during operations on the chest, brain and abdomen and also during tooth extractions. It is not appropriate to use acupuncture in people of a nervous or anxious disposition.

Acute illness

An illness which begins suddenly and is usually severe for a short period of time and sometimes up to a few weeks (e.g. acute meningitis, pneumonia, appendicitis, acute bronchitis). Strictly speaking it does not necessarily mean that the illness is severe.

Acute rheumatism
(FIBROSITIS; MUSCULAR RHEUMATISM)

Rheumatism denotes pain in joints, muscles and tendons and is usually the result of a minor strain, tear or bruise which settles after 4–6 weeks without treatment (*see* Fibrositis). Persistent or recurrent pain occurs in osteoarthritis (page 163), rheumatoid arthritis (page 197), gout (page 114) and, rarely, in rheumatic fever (page 195).

Addiction

All addictive drugs are potentially dangerous, and a psychological need for them develops if taken regularly. The drugs which fall into this category are those producing a pleasurable mental state; alcohol, heroin and morphine, barbiturates and amphetamines are all potentially addictive for this reason. Once they are taken regularly, tolerance develops and larger quantities must be taken to produce the same effect. It then becomes harder to 'kick the habit'. The drug user becomes dependent on regular supplies, and if they suddenly run out, he feels either physically ill or mentally extremely low (dependence). Alcoholism is the commonest form of drug addiction world wide, and is dealt with separately (*see* Alcoholism).

Heroin and morphine addiction is an increasing problem, and is more prevalent in the United States than Europe. When injected intravenously the addict experiences a rapid physical and psychological uplift or 'high'. Very soon life becomes directed towards the acquisition of further supplies. Nothing else matters to an addict; many live in appalling squalor, ceasing to eat or to care about their personal hygiene, and beg or steal.

Death from infection or hepatitis is the usual outcome.

Many experts believe that the only way to get people off heroin is under close medical supervision. The heroin or morphine intake is slowly reduced, avoiding the worst of the withdrawal symptoms of irritability, extreme restlessness, catarrh and diarrhoea, which tend to follow any sudden withdrawal of the drug. Sedative drugs are also given to reduce these symptoms. Though stopping taking addictive drugs is very difficult, it is even more difficult to remain off them, and many addicts relapse within months or years.

Certain personalities are more susceptible to drug addiction than others and they remain very much at risk of relapse. Both they and their friends must exert constant vigilance, and former addicts should never be tempted to try even a single further dose. (*See also* Alcoholism; *and* Heroin.)

Addison's disease

A disease caused by under-activity of the adrenal gland (*see below*).

Adenoids

The adenoids are sited at the back of the upper pharynx, and, with the tonsils, constitute the drainage glands for infections in the mouth and throat. They are usually removed with the tonsils at tonsillectomy (page 226).

Adhesions

Bands of thick fibrous tissue commonly found in the abdomen in the healing tissues which follow infection or surgery. Rarely, loops of bowel twist round the bands and obstruct the intestines. They may unwind spontaneously, but surgery is often necessary to divide the adhesions.

Adrenal glands

Also termed suprarenal glands because they sit on top of the kidneys. The adrenals secrete steroid hormones, which control growth and metabolism, water and salt balance, and also contribute to normal sexual and reproductive function.

Tumours of the adrenal gland cause Cushing's disease (page 71), characterized by weight gain and swelling of the tissues from water retention, raised blood pressure (hypertension, page 41) and bone pain due to deficiency of bone structure. The tumour can be removed surgically.

Under-activity causes Addison's disease (see above), with weakness, skin pigmentation and a fall in blood pressure. This is reversed by replacing the hormone deficiency with steroid drugs (page 216) which are taken by mouth.

AIDS (Acquired Immunodeficiency Syndrome)

This 'new' and increasingly common disease, first recognized in the US, causes a markedly reduced defence response to infections. The features include fever, marked lethargy and weight loss, diarrhoea, lymph node enlargement, and disseminated tuberculosis, virus and fungal infections. Most sufferers are male homosexuals (75 per cent) often with many partners, and drug addicts (15 per cent). The cause is unknown and death occurs in over half despite intensive treatment.

Air swallowing

Everyone swallows air into the stomach during normal eating and drinking, but some swallow to excess. The stomach becomes distended with gas and the abdomen swells, sometimes very dramatically, with associated discomfort relieved by breaking wind (belching or burping). Air swallowing may be very uncomfortable but is never dangerous.

Albinism
(LATIN: *ALBUS,* WHITE)

A rare disorder, present from birth, in which there is absence of melanin—the pigment which darkens the skin. Albinos have white hair, thin white skin and pink eyes.

Alcoholism

A large medical and social problem: an estimated 400,000 people in the United Kingdom are alcoholics. In the United States this number is nearer 5 million, and it is estimated that 15 billion dollars are spent every year to pay for the damage to health, accidents and absenteeism caused by alcohol. In France, which has the highest per head consumption of alcohol in the world, about 50 per cent of all hospital beds are occupied because of alcohol-related disorders.

In an average size adult 100 millilitres (4 fluid ounces) of absolute (100%) alcohol taken daily is enough to produce cirrhosis. This amount of absolute alcohol is contained in:

1/3 bottle spirits (9 fluid ounces)
1/2 bottle sherry (13 fluid ounces)
1 bottle of table wine
5 pints of beer

Women appear to be more susceptible in this respect although the reason remains obscure.

Definition of alcoholism
The World Health Organization defines alcoholism as 'those excessive drinkers whose dependence on alcohol has attained a degree that shows a noticeable mental disturbance or interference with their mental or bodily health, their inter-personal relations and their smooth social and economic functioning...they therefore require treatment'.

Dependence on alcohol takes two forms—mental and physical. Many regular social drinkers are dependent on alcohol, and use it as a drug to make stressful situations more tolerable. Provided this happens only occasionally and they are able to control their intake, they cannot be considered alcoholics. The true alcoholic finds it difficult to control consumption and also feels physically and mentally ill if he does not drink. As a result, his whole existence becomes directed to securing further supplies.

The stages of alcoholism
Stage 1—the pre-alcoholic phase
Begins with social drinking only, but the individual soon realizes that alcohol helps him in stressful situations. He therefore turns to it when he is unable to cope, at first only from time to time. He then becomes less able to handle the normal trivial stresses of life and turns to the bottle more frequently, especially in the evenings. At this stage, even close friends may not notice anything abnormal.

Stage 2—the prodromal phase
The consumption of alcohol is rising and the drinker begins to have feelings of guilt and to drink secretly. Although able to carry on a normal day-to-day routine, drinking bouts may become bad enough to cause periods of amnesia. At this stage, addiction is beginning and the drinker becomes preoccupied with making sure where the next drink is coming from.

Stage 3—the crucial phase
As the intake of alcohol rises, the body steadily becomes resistant to its effects. This is known as 'tolerance' and means that the regular drinker has to take more alcohol to achieve the same effect. In the crucial phase even a small drink creates an overwhelming physical desire to have another. The drinker has lost control of his consumption and continues to drink until too intoxicated to continue. By now it is obvious to his family and friends that he is drinking to excess. He is liable to invent excuses to cover this up and may respond aggressively if warned about the dangers. By now he may have lost his job, his friends and his family. His morale is shattered and physically he is broken.

Stage 4—the chronic phase
The alcoholic is intoxicated for much of the time. One bout of drinking follows another and he may remain drunk for days on end. Although likely to have had a slightly unstable personality before, he is now obviously mentally ill.

Physical effects of alcohol
Alcohol is eliminated from the body in its original state by the kidneys and by the lungs in the breath. About 90 per cent is broken down by the liver. In the body, alcohol exerts its main effects on the following organs.

Liver
Excessive alcohol taken regularly damages the liver, to cause cirrhosis. Persistent poisoning will cause progressive damage, resulting in liver failure.

Heart
Small amounts of alcohol increase the pulse rate, and dilate blood vessels in general. This accounts for the warm, red flush. Chronic alcoholism damages the heart muscle, which eventually fails.

Kidneys
The kidneys remove alcohol from the blood into the urine. The alcohol increases the volume of urine produced by the kidneys, so that for every pint of beer that is drunk, slightly more than one pint of urine is produced. This results in dehydration, which is in part responsible for the 'hangover'. The headache can be avoided if, immediately before going to bed, a glass of water is drunk for every two or three alcoholic drinks consumed.

Stomach
Alcohol increases the quantity of acid produced by the stomach and therefore is toxic to the inner lining of the stomach. Acute gastritis (irritation of the stomach lining) with pain high in the middle of the abdomen and vomiting may occur. Gastric ulcers are more common in alcoholics.

Sex organs
Alcohol 'provokes the desire, but it takes away the performance.' (*Macbeth*.)

Nervous system
Small amounts of alcohol slow reactions and impair concentration (*see also* Alcohol and the law). Alcohol appears to stimulate the brain but is actually

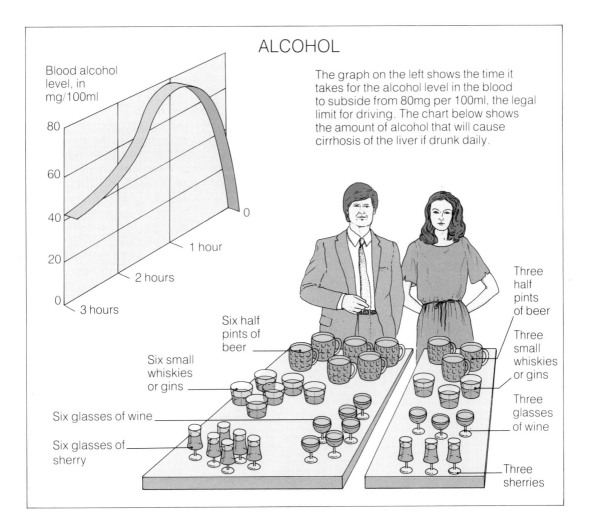

ALCOHOL

Blood alcohol level, in mg/100ml

The graph on the left shows the time it takes for the alcohol level in the blood to subside from 80mg per 100ml, the legal limit for driving. The chart below shows the amount of alcohol that will cause cirrhosis of the liver if drunk daily.

1 hour
2 hours
3 hours

Six half pints of beer
Six small whiskies or gins
Six glasses of wine
Six glasses of sherry

Three half pints of beer
Three small whiskies or gins
Three glasses of wine
Three sherries

a sedative. Behaviour may become less restrained. It is the sedative effect of alcohol which makes it such a potent drug in relieving mild anxiety and tension.

When taken in excess, its effects on the nervous system produce slurring of speech, inability to stand or walk, followed by confusion and finally unconsciousness.

Death occasionally occurs after a session of determined drinking. This is usually from aspiration of vomit into the lungs due to loss of the cough reflex depressed by the excess alcohol. The unconscious alcoholic should be laid on his side, with the head slightly lower than the body—the coma position.

Alcohol and the law

The law is remarkably tolerant to people who drink, provided they are not being a nuisance or endangering safety. This is not the case with drinking and driving. Small amounts of alcohol impair judgement and slow reactions, and many authorities consider the legal limit of 80 milligrams of alcohol per 100 millilitres of blood too generous.

The chart on page 15 sets down the approximate blood levels of alcohol produced by different alcoholic drinks taken on an empty stomach. This is only a rough guide, and the level of alcohol produced in any individual varies depending on when he last ate, his size and weight, and whether drinking has been spread over a few minutes or several hours.

Once alcohol enters the body, the process of elimination starts immediately. It is broken down by the liver, and also removed by the kidneys (in the urine) and the lungs (in the breath)—hence the use of the Breathalyser. If the liver is not accustomed to alcohol or if it is damaged, the breakdown will be slower and the level of alcohol in the blood will not fall as rapidly as expected. The body usually eliminates alcohol at a fairly constant rate, and once drinking has stopped the blood level can be expected to fall by a steady 10 milligrams per 100 millilitres per hour.

The amount of alcohol removed from the body by the lungs is small but increases as the level in the blood rises. The Breathalyser measures how much alcohol is present in the breath and indicates whether the driver is likely to have a blood level over the legal limit. The only way of being absolutely sure is to measure the concentration of alcohol in the blood.

Treatment

Dependence on alcohol usually indicates an underlying psychiatric disorder, and medical advice—usually from psychiatrists with special experience—is required. If the wish to give up drinking is sufficiently strong, Alcoholics Anonymous are successful in helping the drinker through the phases of withdrawal.

Allergy

A state of increased sensitivity to some specific external stimuli (allergens) occurring in susceptible individuals. Common allergic responses include asthma (page 31), hay fever from pollen allergy (page 119) and acute urticaria (page 233) from nettles, and allergy to certain foods such as shellfish and strawberries which causes vomiting, diarrhoea, and sometimes urticaria. Allergy tends to run in families.

Alopecia

(GREEK: *ALOPEKIA*, A DISEASE LIKE FOX MANGE) *SEE* HAIR LOSS

Amenorrhoea

(GREEK: *A*, WITHOUT; *MEN*, MONTH; *RHOIA*, FLOW)

Monthly periods may not begin at the expected time (menarche) in adolescence (primary amenorrhoea) or may cease after years of normal periods (secondary amenorrhoea)—usually due to pregnancy. Women with amenorrhoea require careful medical assessment and investigation (*see* Periods).

Amniocentesis

Removal of a small quantity of the amniotic fluid which surrounds the growing fetus, and is then examined to determine whether there is a risk of Mongolism or spina bifida. An ultrasound scan is performed (page 199) to determine the position of the placenta and the optimal site to insert a small needle through the anterior abdominal wall. A small quantity of fluid is removed, and the risk in skilled hands is very small (*see* Pregnancy).

Amoebiasis

This is caused by *Entamoeba histolytica*, an organism which is ingested in contaminated food and infects the large intestine. The result varies from slight looseness of the stool to full-blown dysentery—a severe illness with fever, exhaustion, profuse diarrhoea and rectal bleeding. The diagnosis is made by seeing amoebic cysts in the stool specimens under a microscope. Treatment consists of carefully ensuring that the patient does not become dehydrated from the severe diarrhoea, and destroying the organism with metronidazole (Flagyl) taken by mouth.

Occasionally the infection results in localized abscesses of amoebic pus within the wall of the intestine or in the liver. Successful treatment usually follows a full course of metronidazole, which is given in a larger dose for a longer period. In all cases, scrupulous precautions must be taken to prevent transmission to other members of the family; everyone infected must be meticulous with washing after defecation, and they should not cook or serve food until the infection is cleared.

Amphetamines

Used to be prescribed to suppress appetite (page 25), but have been withdrawn because the side-effects of elation and excitement led to addiction.

Ampicillin

One of the penicillins, commonly prescribed for acute infections of the lung, urinary tract and middle ear of children. As with all penicillins (page 169), ampicillin used correctly is a safe drug, but skin rashes are a common side-effect.

Amputation

Surgical removal of a limb or part of a limb, either because it is no longer viable because of infection or obstruction to its blood supply, or to remove a tumour.

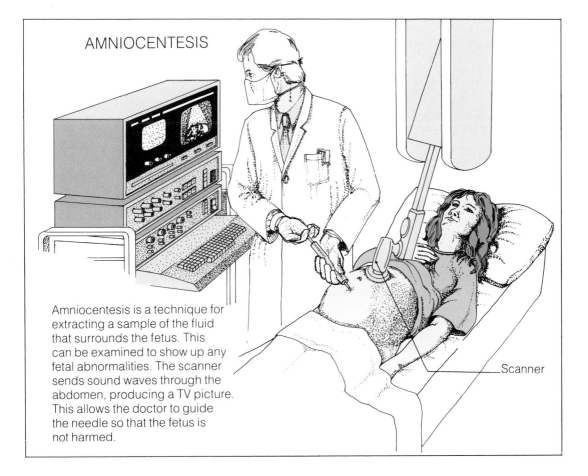

AMNIOCENTESIS

Amniocentesis is a technique for extracting a sample of the fluid that surrounds the fetus. This can be examined to show up any fetal abnormalities. The scanner sends sound waves through the abdomen, producing a TV picture. This allows the doctor to guide the needle so that the fetus is not harmed.

Scanner

Anaemia

Results from a deficiency of haemoglobin, the chemical constituent of red blood cells which carries oxygen from the lungs to the rest of the body. Anaemia is very common, and in Western Europe 15–20 per cent of adult women are anaemic to some degree during reproductive years when they are menstruating. There may be no symptoms if the anaemia is mild unless heavy work or athletic activity is performed. Severe anaemia causes lethargy, weakness, shortness of breath and faintness. These symptoms of anaemia can develop insidiously and may be ignored, particularly in the elderly.

Causes of anaemia

Young children: during rapid growth, especially between 3 and 6 months of age. Children fed solely on milk for more than a few months may become anaemic if supplements of iron-rich foods are not given.

Adolescent children: during the phase of rapid growth at puberty (page 190), especially in girls.

Adults: bleeding from peptic ulcers or haemorrhoids.

Adult women: in their reproductive years if menstruation is heavy.

Pregnant women: demands for iron are increased by the growing fetus; it is usual to take iron tablets, usually combined with folic acid (e.g. Fefol tablets), during pregnancy.

Breast-feeding mothers: there is a constant drain on iron reserves in the milk.

Old people: often have low-iron diets based on bread, cakes and tea, and without meat.

Heavy periods

The haemoglobin lost in the blood during normal menstruation is replaced by the bone marrow from the normal dietary intake of iron and protein. If the periods become abnormally heavy or prolonged, the loss cannot be recovered from the diet alone. If the diet is deficient in meat—the main source of iron—the resulting anaemia is more severe. The average monthly blood loss is about 30 millilitres (1 fluid ounce), or two-thirds of an eggcup. Many women lose two or three times this amount and do not become anaemic, but greater loss eventually results in anaemia.

Dietary deficiency

Iron is essential for the production of haemoglobin, and meat is the main dietary source; other sources are liver, eggs, wholemeal cereals, oatmeal, beans, peas and lentils.

Aspirin

Long-term aspirin ingestion causes minute but persistent loss of blood from the stomach. The blood loss is not obvious and not dangerous in itself, but if it persists over many years, anaemia results. This responds to oral iron.

Most anti-rheumatic drugs carry a similar risk.

Pernicious anaemia

Vitamin B_{12} is essential for normal blood production. In pernicious anaemia the stomach lacks 'intrinsic factor', a chemical produced in the stomach which modifies dietary vitamin B_{12} and facilitates its absorption from the small intestine. Treatment involves regular monthly injections of vitamin B_{12} for life, which produces complete cure. (*See also* Pernicious anaemia.)

Tropical diseases

The normal life span of a red blood cell is about 4 months, but if large numbers are destroyed or lost before this, the bone marrow is unable to replace them. This occurs in malaria (world-wide), in sickle cell anaemia (West Africa) and with intestinal parasite diseases such as hookworm.

Debilitating illnesses

Anaemia may be an early feature of rheumatoid arthritis, liver disease, kidney disease, chronic infections and, rarely, cancer and leukaemia.

Drugs

Drugs may directly poison the bone marrow—where the blood cells are produced—or destroy blood cells in the circulation faster than they can be produced (haemolysis). The drug must be stopped immediately, and the anaemia usually disappears rapidly.

Abnormal haemoglobin

Haemoglobin is the oxygen-binding chemical within the red blood cells. Abnormal haemoglobins are inherited and, if present, induce destruction of the red cells (haemolysis) and anaemia. Sickle cell anaemia occurs mainly in Negroes from West Africa, and thalassaemia in people from the Mediterranean.

Anaesthetics

Drugs used to prevent pain during surgery. They may be given locally; that is, into one or two pain-sensitive nerves to block pain from one site, such as a finger or toe. During such operations the patient remains fully conscious.

Normally, general anaesthetics are used. They are given by injection or as a gas, and cause complete loss of consciousness in addition to total prevention of pain.

Pain relief during childbirth is described on page 183.

Anal fissure

A small split in the skin at the entrance to the rectum. Fissures are caused by the passage of a hard stool which scratches and tears the skin. Unlike small scratches elsewhere, healing is very slow because the fissure is repeatedly damaged during defecation. Fissures may make defecation very painful and any tendency to constipation is liable to make them worse. They frequently bleed.

Creams such as Anusol or Proctosedyl often relieve the pain and it is important to ensure that constipation is avoided. Healing often takes weeks or months and a minor operation may be needed if other measures fail to bring relief. Fissures are extremely painful, though in no way dangerous.

Analgesia
(PAIN RELIEF)

The removal and prevention of pain is a major consideration in all forms of medical management.

The pain of mild headaches, backache and similar short-term disorders can usually be helped by simple remedies—e.g. warmth from a hot-water bottle and drugs such as aspirin (page 29) or paracetamol (page 166). More severe pain may require more powerful analgesics, and occasionally potent drugs such as pethidine (page 173) and morphine (page 154). Anaesthesia is the art of prevention of pain and anxiety during surgery; this may be achieved by general anaesthesia, where the patient is kept completely unconscious, or local anaesthesia (or analgesia) when an injection of an analgesic drug is made into the appropriate pain-receptive nerves.

Acupuncture (page 12) is widely practised in China for pain relief and anaesthesia, with great success.

★ Angina

Heart pain, recognized by its tight constricting character. It usually occurs in the front of the chest over the sternum or breast bone. Sometimes the pain passes into the arms, the jaw and the neck. It is brought on by exercise, emotion, heavy meals and cold weather. The pain is usually sufficiently severe to stop activity, and with rest the pain settles. Angina varies from mild pain occurring infrequently and only on severe exertion, to frequent severe pain occurring many times a day on the slightest exertion. The pain is caused by lack of blood and oxygen to the heart muscle and is comparable to cramp in the legs. The decreased supply of blood is almost invariably due to narrowing of the arteries to the heart (see diagram, page 20; also Heart attack), resulting from infiltration of the delicate inner lining of the arteries with fats (page 100) and cholesterol (page 61). This is known as atherosclerosis, commonly referred to as 'hardening of the arteries' (see Arterial disease).

Prevention of angina
Cigarette smoking is the greatest known risk factor, and smokers have a three times greater chance of angina and heart attacks than non-smokers. Regular exercise—this need not be very energetic—and maintaining a reasonable weight are strongly recommended (see Ideal weight charts, page 292). Elevated blood pressure also is a major risk factor. If you are of normal weight, the level of cholesterol in the blood (tested on blood taken after an overnight fast) is probably normal; weight reduction usually brings marginally raised blood levels of cholesterol down to normal. Rarely is it necessary to restrict cholesterol-containing foods.

Treatment
Most people with angina respond rapidly to simple measures such as weight reduction and regular non-strenuous exercise such as walking or cycling. Strenuous exercise such as competitive games or digging is not advised (see Exercise).

Smoking should be stopped.

Drugs may be required. The most common in use is glyceryl trinitrate, which is held under the tongue before or during an attack of angina. Other commonly used drugs include isosorbide (Sorbitrate) and 'beta-blocking' agents (page 38) such as propranolol (Inderal).

If angina is severe and not controlled by drugs, the obstructed coronary arteries can be bypassed using a vein taken from the leg. The operation (coronary artery bypass) is rarely necessary but is very successful.

Ankle joint

This is a hinge joint between the lower end of the tibia and fibula, and the foot (see diagram, page 267). The joint is very stable and the bone held firmly by powerful ligaments and surrounding muscle tendons.

Ankle swelling

Usually caused by the accumulation of water in the tissues around the ankles. It tends to collect here simply because the ankles and feet are dependent when standing or sitting. The swelling (oedema) decreases during the night on lying down, only to return during the course of the day.

Many find that their ankles swell after a long journey in a car or plane, particularly if they have not been able to move their legs. The swelling, which is usually mild, develops because of the inactivity of the calf muscles which squeeze blood in the deep veins up towards the heart during activity. This is made possible by a system of non-return valves in the deep veins which prevent back-flow. If the muscles are inactive or the valves leak (varicose veins), swelling develops. Swelling due to a combination of posture and inactivity can be reduced or prevented by taking a walk during long plane journeys, regularly contracting the calf muscles during car journeys and, if possible, keeping the legs straight when sitting by supporting the heels on a cushion so that the calves are not compressed. This is especially important in the elderly and in those with varicose veins, in pregnancy, and following childbirth or an abdominal operation.

Other causes of ankle swelling

1   Varicose veins—if sufficiently severe to cause swelling, they are usually prominent (page 239).
2   Acute trauma—with torn ligaments or fractures.
3   Acute infection of the ankle or surrounding skin.

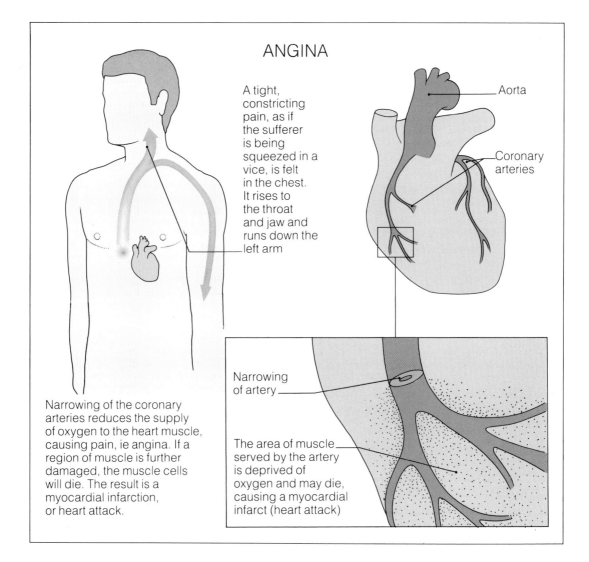

ANGINA

A tight, constricting pain, as if the sufferer is being squeezed in a vice, is felt in the chest. It rises to the throat and jaw and runs down the left arm

Aorta

Coronary arteries

Narrowing of artery

Narrowing of the coronary arteries reduces the supply of oxygen to the heart muscle, causing pain, ie angina. If a region of muscle is further damaged, the muscle cells will die. The result is a myocardial infarction, or heart attack.

The area of muscle served by the artery is deprived of oxygen and may die, causing a myocardial infarct (heart attack)

4   Heart disease. The efficiency of the heart as a pump diminishes in the elderly and back-pressure results in ankle swelling. This may be accompanied by shortness of breath on exercise, or on lying flat. As with postural ankle oedema, it tends to get worse during the course of the day and improves when lying down at night. It is relieved by diuretic drugs, which increase the urine loss of excess water.

5   Thrombosis. Thrombosis in the veins of the leg produces swelling, usually of one leg, accompanied by pain and tenderness in the calf muscles. The overlying skin may be hot and red.

Ankle swelling is often due to a combination of factors; for example, immobility in the elderly patient who has mild heart disease and varicose veins. Medical advice should always be sought to ensure that there are no treatable underlying problems and to prevent later complications of infection and skin ulceration.

Ankylosing spondylitis

A painful disease, mainly of young men, which affects the spine. The spine tends to become fixed (or ankylosed) to some degree and this diminishes the normal range of movement required for bending and stretching (*see* Spondylosis). The pain is progressive and eventually persists through the day and night.

The diagnosis is made on the x-ray appearance of the spine, and treatment with expert physiotherapy and analgesic drugs is usually very successful if started early.

Anorexia nervosa
(GREEK: *A*, WITHOUT; *OREXIS*, APPETITE)

A disease caused by nervous or psychological factors. The typical patient with anorexia nervosa is a girl in her teens, often from a family at the upper end of the socio-economic scale and of above average intelligence. At school she is likely to be hard working, serious and quiet. She may be slightly overweight, until a chance remark by a relative or friend, or something she reads or sees, starts her dieting furiously. Sometimes the dieting is short-lived, and normal eating and adolescent development are quickly re-established. Nevertheless, even a short period of dieting, if it results in significant weight loss (about 25 per cent of the total), may lead to a temporary cessation of monthly periods.

Anorexia nervosa is not a new disease but it has only been recognized as a separate condition since World War II, and has also become more common in the last 20 years. In recent years adolescents of both sexes, but particularly girls, have been under bombardment from the media. Everywhere they look, the virtues of being thin are extolled and the most attractive girls are projected as being the skinniest. Many girls become obsessed by the idea of losing weight and staying thin. To a small number the idea of being fat becomes horrifying and they develop a real fear of food and of eating. If this fear becomes overwhelming, they eat very little or induce vomiting after eating, and become extremely undernourished. Some experts believe that a few months' anorexia and amenorrhoea (absence of periods) calls a temporary halt in physical development and allows emotional development to catch up.

Sometimes the problem goes far deeper and may represent a complete rejection by the anorexic girl of her own sexuality. Dieting achieves this by making her thin, with loss of her 'female' shape and depriving her of her periods. The problem can be precipitated by a sexual adventure which goes wrong, ending in intercourse before being emotionally ready and perhaps even abortion.

Management
The parents of an anorexic invariably find it impossible to grasp why their daughter is deliberately damaging her health and appearance by seemingly pointless dieting, and they must be helped to understand the compulsive fear of eating and getting fat. The anorexic also develops a warped idea of what constitutes a 'normal' size or weight and will usually place herself at an unrealistically high point on this scale, even when she may be excessively thin.

In many instances, understanding parents with the assistance of their doctor are able to help the girl through this difficult phase of adolescence.

So much weight may be lost that admission to hospital may be necessary. In the initial stages, tranquillizers are used to alleviate the fear of eating, and bed rest is advised so that the minimum of calories is expended. A target is agreed of a minimum weight (usually based on height and weight tables) which must be achieved before physical symptoms such as absence of monthly periods (amenorrhoea) are likely to resolve. Initially meals are taken alone or possibly with a sympathetic member of staff until the patient feels able to eat with others.

Often underlying strains in the anorexic's relations with her parents will come to light in the course of treatment.

The sign that recovery is well on the way is a slow

steady weight gain, although the return of normal periods may take 6–12 months. Slowly the anorexic will begin to mix more easily and develop social confidence.

Most girls want to be thin and a few develop a mild dislike of food which may last for 3–6 months. Usually this resolves but very occasionally anorexia nervosa develops—a serious sign is if the periods cease. If so, medical advice should be sought. Severe anorexia nervosa is very rare and requires expert guidance.

Girls with anorexia nervosa require long-term expert care, and sometimes need periods of hospital admission if other methods fail to help them to gain weight. In a few the loss of weight is progressive and they become malnourished and susceptible to severe infections—particularly pneumonia.

Antacid

Antacids are drugs given to relieve the pain of gastritis or peptic ulcer (*see* Gastritis; *and* Stomach ulcer). They act by partially neutralizing the acid in the stomach. Antacids also relieve ulcer pain by covering the stomach lining with a protective layer which prevents the acid attacking the ulcer surface.

There are many antacids available—for example, magnesium trisilicate mixture, Milk of Magnesia, Bisodol, Rennie, Asilone, Aludrox, Kolanticon, Altacite—and they all relieve pain though it will probably recur after 1–2 hours. If pain is not relieved, or if doses in excess of two teaspoonfuls four or five times a day are needed, then you should seek medical advice.

Aspirin (acetylsalicylic acid) and drugs containing aspirin irritate the stomach and are not recommended to relieve the pain of peptic ulcers or gastritis.

Ante-partum haemorrhage

Bleeding from the uterus and vagina before term—the time of fetal maturity, when it is usually delivered—may denote a threatened spontaneous abortion (page 11), or placenta praevia when the placenta lies across the cervix. If the bleed is small, the pregnant mother should rest quietly and medical advice be sought immediately. If the bleeding is excessive, and particularly if the woman is shocked (pale and sweaty with a fast, faint pulse), she should be transferred immediately to the nearest maternity hospital for blood transfusion and expert obstetric management (*see also* Pregnancy: bleeding).

Anthrax

A bacterial disease transmitted from the hair of animals, and usually seen in sheep-workers and butchers. The disease begins as a small red pimple on the face or hand, and this enlarges over the next few days and finally discharges pus, leaving a black scar. Anthrax can be prevented by damping animal skins before handling, and the infection responds well to penicillin.

Very rarely, anthrax is inhaled and causes a severe, and often fatal, pneumonia.

Antibiotics

Used to treat infections caused by bacteria. Antibiotics are the most misused drugs in medicine and are often given unnecessarily. They have an important part to play in the treatment of illnesses caused by bacteria (such as pneumonia, urinary infections, ear infections, tuberculosis or meningitis) but are of no value in infections due to viruses, such as the common cold, simple 'flu and most sore throats. General practitioners are often pressured into giving penicillin for a sore throat, though about 85 per cent are caused by a virus.

The first antibiotics were chemicals produced by fungi which inhibited the growth of bacteria under laboratory conditions. Sir Alexander Fleming's discovery of penicillin in 1928 stemmed from the discovery that bacteria would not grow on a culture medium on which the mould, *Penicillium notatum*, had accidentally grown. It was more than 10 years before the substance responsible for this effect on bacteria—penicillin—was isolated. Many antibiotics are laboratory-made descendants of these naturally occurring compounds.

Antibiotics have produced a dramatic improvement in the treatment of previously lethal diseases such as tuberculosis, meningitis and pneumonia. Unfortunately, some bacteria develop resistance to some antibiotics, such as the bacterium responsible for gonorrhoea and certain types of staphylococcal infection (e.g. boils, abscesses, carbuncles) previously destroyed by penicillin alone.

Antibodies

Chemical proteins produced by the body in response to ingested or inhaled substances and in an attempt to neutralize any potentially toxic effect. The formation of antibodies is a major defence mechanism, and is used therapeutically in immunization when a potentially toxic but neutralized substance—the antigen (e.g. polio virus, typhoid)—is injected. This produces antibodies which combat infection with the fully virulent organism.

Antibodies against the blood cells of babies with Rhesus incompatibility can cause their death but this can be prevented by careful ante-natal care (*see* Rhesus disease in the newborn).

Anticoagulants

Drugs used to decrease the clotting effect of blood. They are commonly used to treat patients with clots in the deep veins of the calf, and also to prevent clots forming on the damaged valves after cardiac surgery for the insertion of artificial valves. The most commonly used anticoagulant is warfarin, which can be taken by mouth. Heparin may be used initially but is only effective by injection and is rarely given for more than a few days.

Anticoagulants differ from most drugs because the dose must be carefully tailored to each patient as individual sensitivity varies widely. Frequent blood tests are required to prevent excess anticoagulation, which might cause spontaneous bruising and bleeding. Once a control dose is established, less frequent testing is required. However, other medicines may alter the effects of the anticoagulant, so aspirin and many of the drugs for arthritis or epilepsy must be prescribed with special care. The safest course is to take no other drugs at all (even Anadin and Alka-Seltzer contain aspirin) without consulting your doctor.

If, while taking warfarin, bleeding from the rectum, in the urine, from the nose or any spontaneous bruising occurs, medical advice must be sought immediately.

Antidepressants

Drugs given to alleviate depression (page 75) and should always be taken under medical supervision. Unfortunately, they are not always effective and other forms of treatment may be required. The most commonly prescribed antidepressant is amitriptyline (Lentizol, Triptafen, Tryptizol). Other frequently used antidepressants include nortriptyline (Allegron, Aventyl), doxepin (Sinequan), protriptyline (Concordin) and imipramine (Tofranil). Some of these preparations have sedative properties, which are helpful if insomnia or anxiety is also a problem. Those with sedative effects should be avoided in the daytime, particularly in drivers and those working with machinery. Lithium (Priadel), may be used in

manic depression.

Different patients respond to different antidepressants and it may be necessary to try more than one before any improvement occurs. Side-effects include drowsiness, dryness of the mouth, blurring of the vision, constipation, sweating and even dizziness. Very often these pass off in a few days as tolerance to the drug develops. Many antidepressants do not begin to work for 2–3 weeks and it is wise to persist for at least that time even if there has been no obvious improvement.

Antihistamines

A group of drugs which reduce some of the effects of histamine, a chemical released within the body as a result of allergy (page 16) and hypersensitivity, and responsible for many of their symptoms. Antihistamines are also sedative and many relieve nausea (*see* Travel sickness). Common examples are promethazine (Avomine, Phenergan), mepyramine (Anthisan) and cyclizine (Marzine).

Antiseptics

Chemicals which destroy bacteria. The stronger antiseptics—usually termed disinfectants—destroy living cells as well, which makes it impractical to use them in the mouth or on the skin.

Phenol was the first antiseptic, and many of the synthetic antiseptics are derived from it. Iodine is still used to cleanse the skin prior to surgical operations. The commonly used antiseptics for the skin are cetrimide, hexachlorophane and chlorhexidine. Most of the proprietary antiseptic ointments contain one of these compounds, and are used to treat simple cuts and abrasions.

It must be emphasized that poisonous quantities of some of these drugs may be absorbed if applied to the skin of newborn babies or if put in their baths.

Anxiety

Anxiety is experienced by everyone from time to time and is a normal response to adverse circumstances, such as an illness in a loved one, difficulties at work and financial problems. A few people become so anxious even about trivial matters that their normal life style and that of their immediate families is seriously affected. Typical features include faintness, dizziness, headache, tremor, sweating, poor concentration and memory, difficulty in sleeping, palpitation, diarrhoea, breathlessness and sexual difficulties. If the anxiety is a response to a

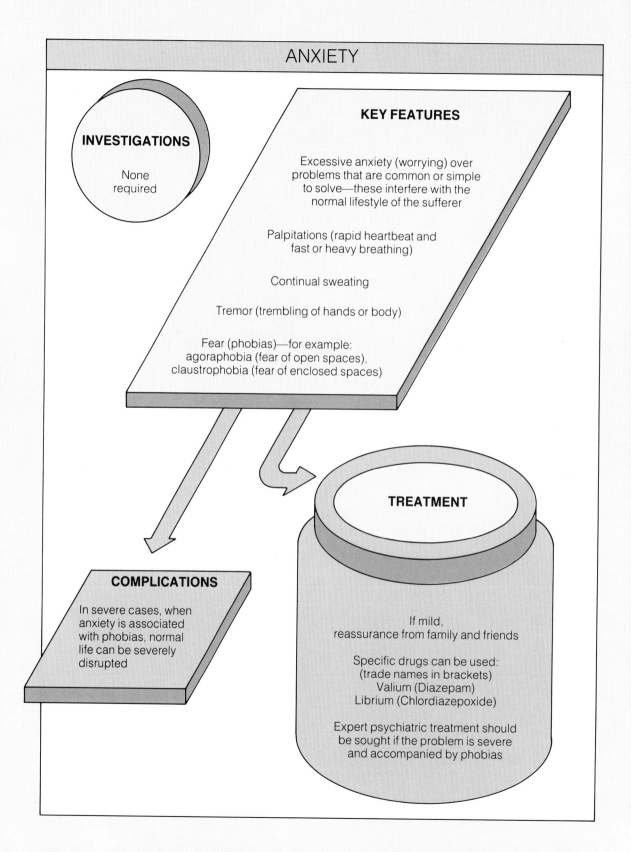

ANXIETY

INVESTIGATIONS

None
required

KEY FEATURES

Excessive anxiety (worrying) over
problems that are common or simple
to solve—these interfere with the
normal lifestyle of the sufferer

Palpitations (rapid heartbeat and
fast or heavy breathing)

Continual sweating

Tremor (trembling of hands or body)

Fear (phobias)—for example:
agoraphobia (fear of open spaces),
claustrophobia (fear of enclosed spaces)

TREATMENT

If mild,
reassurance from family and friends

Specific drugs can be used:
(trade names in brackets)
Valium (Diazepam)
Librium (Chlordiazepoxide)

Expert psychiatric treatment should
be sought if the problem is severe
and accompanied by phobias

COMPLICATIONS

In severe cases, when
anxiety is associated
with phobias, normal
life can be severely
disrupted

specific problem in a previously well-balanced individual it usually improves within a short time (e.g. 1–4 weeks), or when the problem resolves. If the symptoms persist or become sufficiently severe to disrupt a normal existence, medical advice should be obtained. (*See* Psychiatric treatment.)

Aorta

The major artery of the body (*see* diagram, page 253). It arises from the left ventricle of the heart and carries oxygenated blood to the entire body via its major divisions: the subclavian arteries to the arms; carotid and vertebral arteries to the brain; renal and mesenteric arteries to the kidneys and intestines; and iliac arteries to the legs.

Appendicitis

The pain usually begins in the middle of the abdomen, around the navel. Slight fever is common. The patient may vomit, and nausea is almost universal. Constipation is commoner than diarrhoea and this helps to distinguish it from gastro-enteritis. There is usually loss of appetite, so anyone who can tackle a meal is unlikely to have appendicitis. In 12–24 hours the pain moves to the right side of the lower abdomen, and there may be an area of tenderness here if gentle pressure is applied with the flat of the hand.

Many people worry unnecessarily that they have appendicitis, and this is reasonable because acute appendicitis is the commonest surgical emergency. If there is any doubt, it is important to seek medical advice.

The operation to remove the infected appendix is a simple one, taking about twenty minutes. A small incision is made low down on the right side of the abdomen over the spot where the appendix is usually found. The stay in hospital is normally only a few days, and the stitches are removed after 5–9 days. In fit young people, full activity can be resumed after about 4–6 weeks. (*See* chart, page 26.)

Appendix
(LATIN: *APPENDERE*, TO HANG UPON)

A small blunt-ended tube about the size of the little finger, attached to the caecum of the large intestine (*see* diagram, page 265). When it becomes obstructed, the subsequent infection produces the symptoms of appendicitis *(see above)*.

Appetite

Excess appetite is common in the overweight and their children. It is also a feature of an over-active thyroid gland (page 224).

Diminished appetite is usually caused by acute gastritis or food poisoning, and returns to normal as the acute infection settles.

Persistence of a decreased appetite, particularly if there is loss of weight, is a feature of nearly all serious illnesses—including depression and anxiety—and requires expert medical assessment.

Arterial disease
(ATHEROSCLEROSIS, ARTERIOSCLEROSIS)

The arteries are strong thick-walled vessels which carry the blood away from the heart. About 70 times a minute as the heart contracts and empties they are subjected to a sudden surge of blood under pressure. The blood is ejected into the largest artery—the aorta—and then flows into distributing arteries to the rest of the body. The repeated stress on the inner wall of the artery can damage it, and plaques or patches of cholesterol may form on the roughened area. Once in the wall of the artery, the cholesterol plaque slowly enlarges, to produce slow and progressive narrowing of the blood vessel, decreasing the flow through it. This commonly affects the coronary arteries, to cause heart attacks, and the cerebral vessels, resulting in strokes.

Roughening of the normally smooth inner lining of the artery may allow a blood clot to form. The clot then enlarges and suddenly occludes the artery, resulting again in a sudden diminution of blood flow.

Causative factors
Arterial disease is common in rich countries and is the commonest cause of death in the Western world. There are a number of factors which influence its development.

Smoking Moderate smokers have twice the chance of dying from a heart attack than non-smokers. Heavy smokers are even more at risk. They may also develop narrowing of the arteries to the leg, causing pain in the calf on exercise (intermittent claudication) and sometimes gangrene.

Obesity The overweight tend to have a high fat and cholesterol level in their blood and take little exercise.

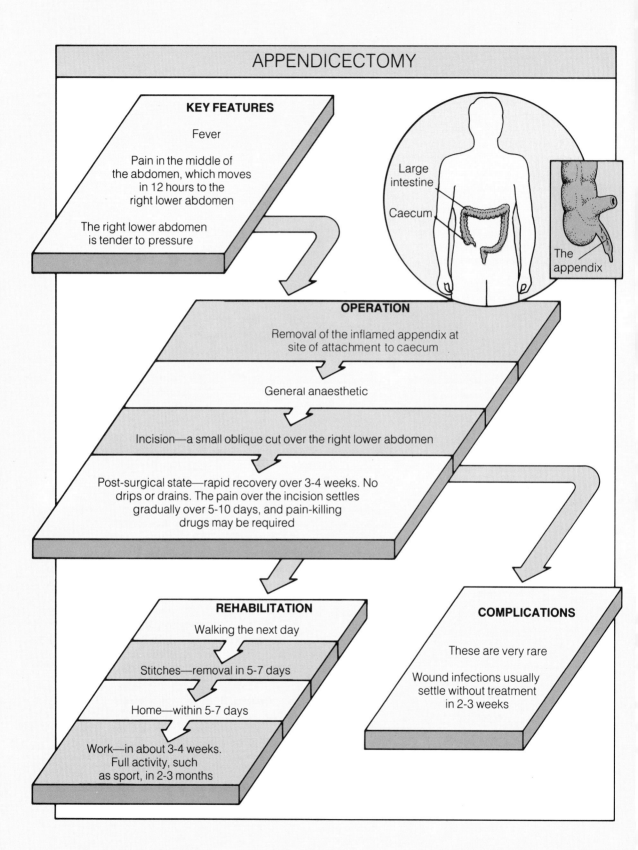

APPENDICECTOMY

KEY FEATURES

Fever

Pain in the middle of
the abdomen, which moves
in 12 hours to the
right lower abdomen

The right lower abdomen
is tender to pressure

Large
intestine

Caecum

The
appendix

OPERATION

Removal of the inflamed appendix at
site of attachment to caecum

General anaesthetic

Incision—a small oblique cut over the right lower abdomen

Post-surgical state—rapid recovery over 3-4 weeks. No
drips or drains. The pain over the incision settles
gradually over 5-10 days, and pain-killing
drugs may be required

REHABILITATION

Walking the next day

Stitches—removal in 5-7 days

Home—within 5-7 days

Work—in about 3-4 weeks.
Full activity, such
as sport, in 2-3 months

COMPLICATIONS

These are very rare

Wound infections usually
settle without treatment
in 2-3 weeks

Stress Long-term stress is thought by many experts to make coronary artery disease more likely, though this is difficult to prove. In the USA there has been a recent interest in the 'Type A' personality, who is a highly competitive, aggressive individual, driving himself hard at work and often obsessed with time-watching and keeping to deadlines. This type of personality seems more likely to have a heart attack or a stroke because of progressive arterial disease. An episode of acute stress may precipitate such an event in a susceptible person.

Untreated high blood pressure This increases the risk of coronary artery disease and strokes.

Diabetes Diabetics are more prone to coronary artery disease, strokes and arterial disease of the legs.

Prevention
There is a great deal which can be done to reduce the personal risk of developing arterial disease and its associated problems.
1 *Stop smoking.*
2 *Lose excess weight.* (*See* charts of ideal weights, page 292.)
3 *Take regular exercise.* Exercise is not dangerous provided it is taken slowly at first and the amount of activity increased gradually day by day (*see* Exercise).
4 *Diet.* A reduction in the consumption of saturated animal fats and their substitution with the poly-unsaturated variety may also reduce the risk, although there is no definite evidence about this.
5 *Stress.* Try to discipline recurrent stress at work or at home. Working hard at a job you basically enjoy is fine, but otherwise allow yourself periods of adequate relaxation and holidays.

Arteriosclerosis
SEE ARTERIAL DISEASE

Arthritis

Inflammation of a joint. The two common types of arthritis are osteoarthritis and rheumatoid arthritis. Gout is a less common cause of joint inflammation. Arthritis is rarely severe and most can be helped by modern medical and surgical treatment.

Osteoarthritis
This affects the large weight-bearing joints, such as the hip, knee and the spine. Clearly the greater the weight (in the obese), the earlier the arthritis tends to appear. In some women the joints of the hand may be the main target. Pain and stiffness in the arthritic joints are the first signs and do not usually develop until later in life, often in the over-50s. Almost all people over the age of 70 have some osteoarthritis, but it is usually mild.

The joints subjected to the greatest strain are the most likely to be affected. If the knee is involved, there may be local pain, stiffness and swelling of the joint. With the hip, the pain may make walking impossible. If present in the lower spine, there may be backache, and, in the upper spine, pain and stiffness in the neck. Osteoarthritis is more common in joints which have been injured in the past and often affects several joints.

Treatment
The initial treatment is rest for the affected joint and reduction of pain by means of pain killers (analgesics). Aspirin or paracetamol are usually very effective but, if not, drugs such as ibuprofen (Brufen), indomethacin (Indocid) or naproxen (Naprosyn) may help. It may be necessary to relieve the stresses and strains on worn joints by transferring to lighter work. Energetic hobbies may unfortunately have to be curtailed but this degree of severe arthritis is very rare.

An exciting development has been the use of artificial joints. In those severely disabled by painful arthritis of the hip, new ones may dramatically improve their range of activity and life style.

Rheumatoid arthritis
Differs from osteoarthritis in several respects. It affects younger people, often starting before the age of 40. Women are three times more likely to develop it, and the smaller joints, such as the fingers, toes and wrists, are usually affected first. Later the elbows, shoulders, ankles and knees may become involved. The other main difference is that patients with active rheumatoid disease often feel generally ill, with exhaustion, weight loss and often a slight fever. This does not happen in osteoarthritis, where pain and stiffness are confined to the joints. Unless pain is severe, general health is not affected. The stiffness in the joints in rheumatoid arthritis is worst first thing in the morning and improves later after moving around. The disease follows an unpredictable 'up and down' course with weeks or months when the joints improve, only to be followed by a period of pain and stiffness. This is why it is difficult to evaluate the different treatments, as it is not always possible to know whether improvement has been a result of treatment or would have happened anyway.

The cause of rheumatoid arthritis remains uncertain. Some experts consider that the antibodies which usually attack organisms from outside to combat infection 'mistake' parts of the joint for damaging organisms foreign to the body and attack them in the same way as they would bacteria. This induces a response from the patient's blood cells which then 'reject' the joint tissues in error.

Treatment

Only patients with severe rheumatoid arthritis can tell what it is like to suffer gnawing pain and stiffness in the joints and muscles year after year, at the same time seeing their physical capabilities steadily diminishing. Not surprisingly, many people become depressed, and treatment of this depression is one of the most important parts of therapy. However, a great deal can now be done to relieve the worst symptoms, using drugs, physiotherapy and surgery.

In the initial, acute phase of the disease the affected joints should be rested. Occasionally the joint has to be immobilized in a plaster of Paris splint. When the acute phase has passed, gentle exercises, under the supervision of a physiotherapist, will relieve the inevitable joint stiffness and strengthen muscles which have not been used. Local treatment in the form of wax baths or radiant heat may speed recovery. Drugs to relieve pain are extremely effective. Many of the drugs used in rheumatoid arthritis, as well as relieving pain, have an anti-inflammatory action (local inflammation within the joint is the cause of the symptoms). Aspirin and paracetamol are effective in mild disease; other commonly used preparations are ibuprofen (Brufen), indomethacin (Indocid) and naproxen (Naproysn). They all act in the same way, and should be taken with food as they sometimes cause gastritis if taken on an empty stomach. Rarely, these drugs are insufficient; gold injections or a course of oral penicillamine (Distamine) may be used, but require skilled supervision and regular blood tests to make sure the dose and length of course are properly tailored to the individual patient.

Steroids such as hydrocortisone can be injected directly into inflamed and painful joints.

Occasionally oral steroids, such as prednisolone, may be used to reduce inflammation if many joints are involved and unresponsive to conventional therapy. The dose must be reduced to a minumum because steroids have serious side-effects, especially if given over-generously. They should be taken only under medical supervision, and if someone is on a regular steroid he should carry a card stating it. Steroids should not be stopped suddenly.

The fear of rheumatoid arthritis is based on seeing a small number of severely and sometimes tragically disabled sufferers. However, the outlook is not always bad. With careful management 65 per cent of patients suffer only minimal disability and are able to maintain a fully active life style; 30 per cent of people with rheumatoid arthritis suffer some disability which means that they must curtail some activities. Only 5 per cent are severely disabled by the disease.

Other causes of arthritis include gout, tuberculosis, gonorrhoea, and acute bacterial infection which rapidly produces an acutely red, hot, swollen and painful joint. Acute rheumatic fever is now very rare. Mild transient arthritis with temporary pain and stiffness is not uncommon in many viral infections, such as mumps, measles, German measles and glandular fever.

Arthroscopy

The technique whereby the inside of the joint can be examined through a flexible telescope. Before it was available, the only way to see inside a joint was to open it surgically. Arthroscopy is much simpler and quicker, and may avoid the need for further surgery. It is particularly useful for examining the knee joint, to decide whether or not to operate on a suspected torn cartilage. Some surgeons have also perfected a technique of removing a torn cartilage through the arthroscope.

Artificial insemination

One method of treating infertility where the male partner is infertile. Sperm from a donor is placed in the upper vagina near the cervix of the female partner to fertilize her egg (ovum). (*See also* Infertility.) For some couples the advantage over adoption is that the wife produces a child, but considerable emotional stresses can be set up within the marriage.

Artificial kidneys

Better known as kidney machines, these are used for patients with severe renal failure. The patient's blood is circulated on one side of a semi-permeable membrane which has a pure clear solution on the other side. This removes toxic chemicals normally filtered by the healthy kidneys, whilst leaving the blood cells and protein to return to the patient. (*See also* Kidney failure *and* Kidney dialysis.)

Asbestosis

Inhalation of asbestos fibres sets up a reaction within

the lung tissue which becomes progressively damaged. This reaction eventually destroys the fine inner lining cells of the lung across which body gases move. The patient may suffer severe breathlessness on effort. There is unfortunately no known cure. It is now known that the disease can be prevented by damping asbestos before cutting it, and by wearing special masks which filter the inspired air to exclude asbestos fibres.

Ascorbic acid
(VITAMIN C)

An essential ingredient of a healthy diet, which maintains the integrity of body tissues (particularly small blood vessels) and prevents leakage of blood from their walls. Vitamin C is present in potatoes and in fresh fruit, particularly citrus fruit such as oranges.

Severe lack of vitamin C causes scurvy (page 204). This is exceedingly rare in the UK except in the elderly on a 'bread, butter and jam' diet. (*See also* Vitamins.)

Aspirin
(ACETYLSALICYLIC ACID)

Aspirin is the most widely used analgesic and anti-inflammatory drug. It is used to control pain caused by minor injury or infection, and is particularly effective for joint and bone pain and the pain of muscle tears and strain. It is often prescribed for arthritis, not only because it relieves pain but also because of its anti-inflammatory properties. It is also effective in lowering high temperatures, especially in children.

Many preparations contain aspirin as the active ingredient; e.g. Disprin, Solprin, Aspro, Aspro

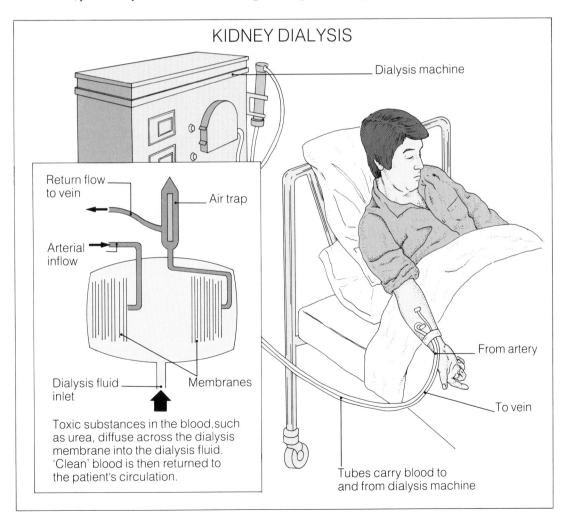

KIDNEY DIALYSIS

Dialysis machine

Return flow to vein

Air trap

Arterial inflow

Dialysis fluid inlet

Membranes

Toxic substances in the blood, such as urea, diffuse across the dialysis membrane into the dialysis fluid. 'Clean' blood is then returned to the patient's circulation.

From artery

To vein

Tubes carry blood to and from dialysis machine

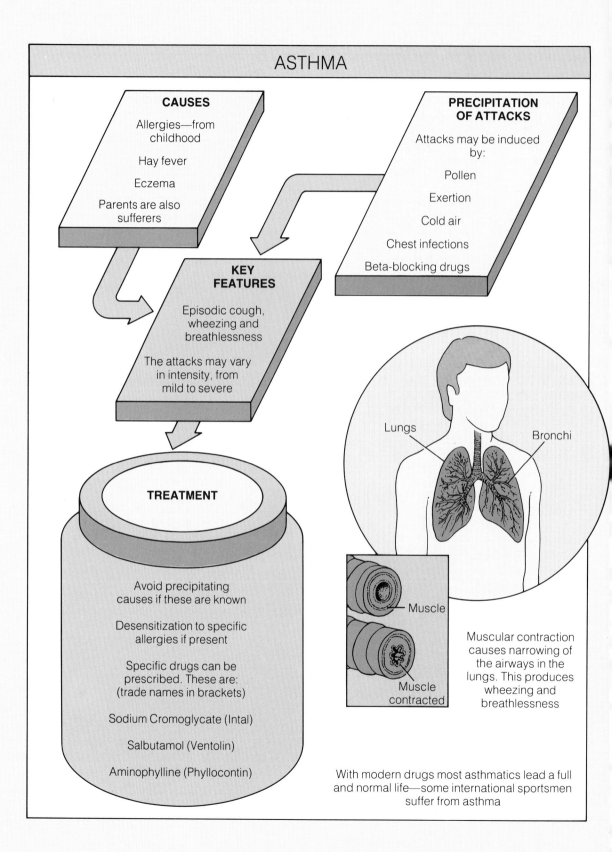

ASTHMA

CAUSES

Allergies—from childhood

Hay fever

Eczema

Parents are also sufferers

PRECIPITATION OF ATTACKS

Attacks may be induced by:

Pollen

Exertion

Cold air

Chest infections

Beta-blocking drugs

KEY FEATURES

Episodic cough, wheezing and breathlessness

The attacks may vary in intensity, from mild to severe

TREATMENT

Avoid precipitating causes if these are known

Desensitization to specific allergies if present

Specific drugs can be prescribed. These are: (trade names in brackets)

Sodium Cromoglycate (Intal)

Salbutamol (Ventolin)

Aminophylline (Phyllocontin)

Lungs

Bronchi

Muscle

Muscle contracted

Muscular contraction causes narrowing of the airways in the lungs. This produces wheezing and breathlessness

With modern drugs most asthmatics lead a full and normal life—some international sportsmen suffer from asthma

Clear, Anadin, Alka-Seltzer and Lem-Sip, and special low-dose preparations available for children.

Side-effects of aspirin
Aspirin may irritate the stomach lining and cause pain and even small ulcers which can bleed. It is best taken with food and avoided if there has been previous gastritis (page 108) or stomach ulcers (page 216). Some people are allergic to aspirin and develop a rash or even asthma. It is dangerous when taken in overdosage.

Aspirin is safe if used sensibly and with care, and effective if used for the right reasons. If not, the side-effects can be serious. It should not be used to promote sleep or mental relaxation, because aspirin has no direct effect on either unless the insomnia is due to persistent pain.

Asthma

An attack is recognized from the characteristic wheezing on breathing out. Asthmatics become very short of breath and often prefer to sit up in a chair, with the arms folded in front on a table, in order to assist breathing. Milder forms of asthma in children may begin with recurrent coughing at night or wheezing on exercise. The cause of the wheezing is temporary narrowing of the airways (bronchi), caused primarily by contraction of the muscles round and within their walls, which go into spasm. In addition, inflammation within the bronchial wall causes the cells to swell and to increase production of sputum, both of which further narrow the airways. The lungs themselves are not primarily affected by asthma, but if it persists they may become secondarily damaged.

Precipitating factors
Allergy Spasm of the muscles in the walls of the bronchi may be precipitated by an allergy to the house dust mite, which is a common offender. Other allergies include pollens (*see also* Hay fever), animal hair belonging to cats, dogs or horses, moulds and certain foods. Asthmatics may also suffer from other allergic disorders such as eczema and hay fever.

Infection Virus infections in the nose or throat, or bacterial infections of the lung (e.g. bronchitis), may trigger an attack.

Exercise Exercise-induced asthma is recognized from the wheeze or cough which only comes after exercise. This is relatively common in children, who tend to grow out of it.

Irritants in the air Examples include cigarette smoke and petrol fumes. Sometimes, cold air alone may precipitate an attack.

Emotion The degree to which emotional factors trigger asthma remains uncertain. Asthma is a most unpleasant and sometimes horrifying condition, and it would be surprising were asthmatics calm at the onset of an attack. Also, many minor attacks settle rapidly as soon as medical aid has arrived, which suggests an emotional overlay if not necessarily a trigger.

Even the most severe episodes can be controlled if treatment is started quickly and it is extremely important to reassure the patient and to call for medical support if an attack does not settle rapidly with the usual treatment.

Treatment
The treatment of asthma has improved dramatically in the last few years. Asthmatics who are allergic to cats, dogs or horses should avoid them. Children who wheeze are often allergic to house dust and the bedroom may be the room where this collects most readily. For this reason, these children often develop their worst wheezing at night and in the early morning. If dust is the allergen, this is more difficult to eradicate even in the cleanest home, but the advice given in the list below should be tried.

Desensitization to one or two specific allergies is sometimes effective, but most asthmatics are sensitive to many and so it is impracticable.

Anti-dust measures in the bedroom
1   Avoid unnecessary clutter and furniture which may collect dust.
2   Dust with a damp cloth (when the child is not there) at least twice a week.
3   Do not make the bed with the child in the room.
4   Keep the room will ventilated during the day.
5   Avoid feather mattresses and pillows. Foam rubber mattresses are better, and synthetic sheets (e.g. nylon) preferable.

Acute attacks
The most commonly used drug is salbutamol (Ventolin), which is available as tablets or in an inhaler. Inhalers are more effective because they deliver the drug straight to where it is needed (i.e. the bronchi). Once the inhalation technique has been correctly learnt, it is usually sufficiently effective to relieve sudden wheezing. If two puffs of Ventolin fail to improve the wheezing, it is usually because either it has not been taken correctly or the aerosol is

running out. Sometimes the airways may be too narrow for the Ventolin to be inhaled into the smaller airways. There is no value in taking more than two puffs of Ventolin every 4 hours, and more may produce shaking.

Oral steroids such as prednisolone, initially in a high dose and rapidly reducing over 1–2 weeks, can abort an acute attack; if so, it is worth while keeping a supply of prednisolone to be taken in the event of an acute attack. Oral prednisolone is extremely effective but does have side-effects if taken for any length of time, and it should be used only to prevent attacks becoming severe or in persistent asthma.

Medical advice should be obtained if an acute attack is not improved after using an inhaler, particularly in children.

Prevention of attacks

Sodium cromoglycate (Intal) by inhalation (one or two capsules twice daily) prevents asthma by blocking the release of histamine from the cells of the bronchi and preventing its muscle-constricting effect. Intal inhalations are of no value in acute attacks. If the combination of Ventolin and Intal is not sufficient, beclomethasone (Becotide) by inhalation may be added. This steroid preparation is given by inhaler and delivers the drug to the bronchi. It can therefore be given in a minute dose and does not produce the side-effects of oral steroids.

Inhalers and tablets available for treating asthma

Inhalers	Tablets
Atrovent	Alupent
Becotide	Bricanyl
Berotec	Nuelin
Bextasol	Phyllocontin
Bricanyl	Theocontin
Intal	Ventolin
Pulmadil	
Ventolin	

The treatment of asthma is now a very exact science. The combination of drugs such as Ventolin, Intal and Becotide should keep nearly every asthmatic almost completely symptom-free.

★ Medical advice must be obtained if an attack is severe or does not respond rapidly to inhalation therapy (or oral steroids in those patients experienced in their use). This applies especially to asthmatic children.

Astigmatism

Alteration of the angle of the visual image on the back of the eye. It is caused by variable curvature of the cornea, in front of the lens of the eye. It is rarely significant but, if severe, can be corrected with spectacles.

Atherosclerosis
SEE ARTERIAL DISEASE

Athlete's foot
(TINEA PEDIS)

An infection caused by a fungus (see Ringworm). The skin between the toes tends to become soggy and white and to peel easily. It may become inflamed, red and painful. The feet must be kept clean and dry, and anti-fungal powders and creams (e.g. Mycota, Tineafax, Tinaderm) applied regularly. Separate towels and bath mats must be used to prevent spread to other members of the household. (See illustration, page 235.)

Audiometry

The method of testing for deafness (page 72). Audiometry requires perfect quiet and is performed in a sound-proof room. Sounds of differing intensity are played into the ears, and the range of hearing detected is compared with normal.

Autistic children

Autism is a rare but very disturbing disorder for both the child and the parents. Parents first notice that their child never runs to them for comfort or reassurance. He is usually very difficult to 'get through to' and ignores his parents' questions, though he may listen intently to other noises, such as a car going by. The basic problem is that to the children the world is an incomprehensible muddle without any order. They are unable to arrange in their minds all the information arriving from the outside world. Whereas the normal child recognizes that the noises his mother makes when she speaks to him have some meaning, to an autistic child her words are a meaningless jumble of sound. He may be unable to grasp fairly simple concepts. If, for instance, his father's car is blue, he may be unable to grasp the fact that even if the neighbour's car is brown, it is still a car.

Very often parents seek medical advice when their child is about 2 years old because they think he may be deaf or retarded, or because of screaming attacks and difficulty controlling severe temper tantrums. Many of these children are highly intelligent, though their ability is 'locked away'. It is usually fairly easy to distinguish between autism and deafness—the deaf child will study the face intently

Asthma

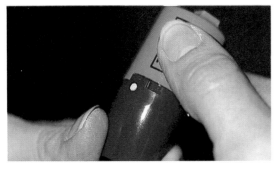

Hold inhaler upright by the mouthpiece.

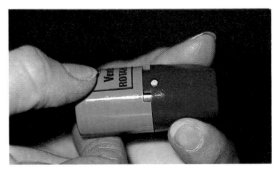

Rotate inhaler so dot is at end of channel.

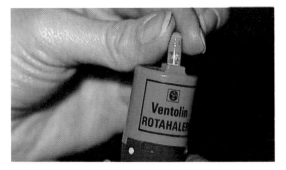

Insert the capsule.

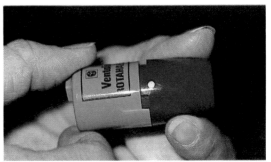

Rotate the inhaler in the opposite direction until it stops, to pierce the capsule.

Inhale through the mouth-piece in slow, deep even breaths.

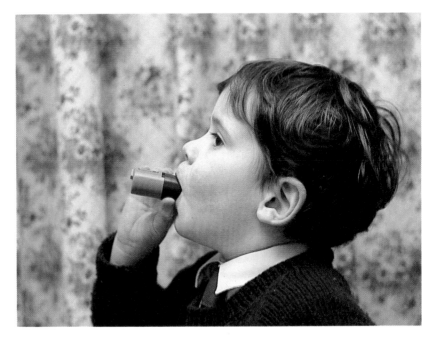

Defective Colour Vision

The four illustrations below are taken from a series of defective colour vision test charts developed by the Institute of Ophthalmology in London. They should not be used for self-diagnosis as they must be used together with the rest of the series in carefully controlled lighting conditions.

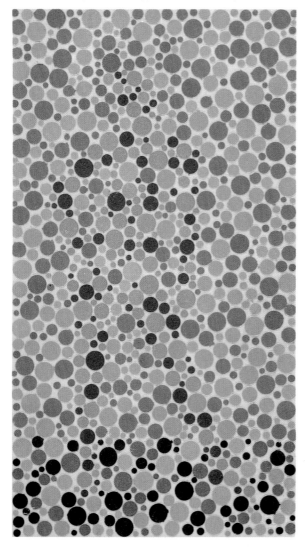

To a person with normal colour vision, the illustration above shows a woman with a purple hat and an olive-green bikini against a green background. Those with defective colour vision tend to see the bikini and the flesh as the same colour.

The umbrella in this plate may not be wholly visible to people with certain types of colour vision defect. They may be able to see only the handle, which they describe as a hockey stick.

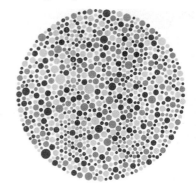

A red fork and a purple spade on a grey background. Some people with colour defective vision can see only the spade, others only the fork. A third group can see neither.

People with defective colour vision may be unable to identify the object, a teapot, in this plate since they will be able to see only the spout.

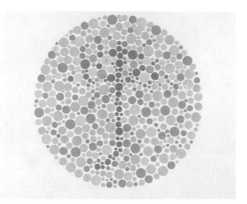

when someone is speaking to him and the autistic child will look away.

The causes of autism are unknown. It may be a form of psychiatric illness, like schizophrenia (page 200), but it is more likely to be due to a failure of normal brain development. The National Society for Autistic Children has parent groups which offer help and support to the families involved. They also produce a number of practical books on the subject.

Now that the special problems of autistic children have been recognized, it is becoming much easier to help them and their families.

Backache

Commonly caused by tearing or over-stretching of either the muscles of the back or the ligaments and intervertebral discs of the spine. The spine consists of 24 vertebrae, separated from each other by a cushion of cartilage with a soft centre, called the intervertebral disc. (*See also* Disc; *and* Spinal cord.)

The vertebrae are bound firmly together by tough ligaments, so that only little movement is possible between any one vertebra and the next. Over-stretching by excessive movement between two vertebrae exerts enormous strain on the ligaments and discs. Usually the ligament is stretched but if the back is stressed by sudden movement, the soft centre of the intervertebral disc may be squeezed out through the tougher outer coating. This 'slipped disc' causes severe backache; it may press on the sciatic nerve and lead to pain radiating down the back of the leg from the base of the spine (*see* Sciatica).

The pressure within the discs is least when lying flat but increases on standing up and on sitting. Bending over increases the pressure, and lifting at the same time puts the greatest stress on the discs.

Backache is very common, and 50 per cent of adults suffer from it at some time. As a result, 11½ million working days a year are lost in the United Kingdom, at a cost to industry of £220 million. Of this, £40 million are paid out in the form of sickness and invalid benefits and £60 million in general practice and hospital services.

Prevention of backache
The following should help prevent backache and

slipped discs. It applies particularly to the over-40s.
1   Avoid all sudden movements when the back is bent; e.g. leaping out of bed in the morning, or jumping up from sitting in a low chair.
2   Avoid any heavy lifting if possible, particularly if any twisting is involved. Postpone such movements until help is available. Those in physically demanding jobs where a lot of lifting is essential are more prone to back trouble. When lifting, try to bend at the knees and not at the back. Lift steadily without sudden jerky movements.
3   Avoid obesity. The greater the body weight, the greater the strain on the back.
4   Ensure that the bed is comfortable and that the mattress does not have a hollow in it. People with back problems often find a hard mattress or a board under the mattress of great benefit.

Treatment of backache
The majority of acute backaches are caused by sprains of the muscles or ligaments around the spine and clear up very quickly provided the back is rested. Rest alone resolves 50 per cent of backaches in 1 week, and 85 per cent after 2 weeks. Less often, slipped discs or arthritis are responsible and the pain persists for longer.
1   All lifting is banned.
2   If the pain is at all severe, go to bed. If necessary, have boards put underneath the mattress to ensure the bed is firm. Some find that the only comfortable place is lying flat on a firm bed or on the floor. Lie flat on the back with one pillow, and avoid sitting propped up because the back will then be bent as much as if you were sitting on a chair. It may be necessary to stay in bed for a week or two, before slowly getting up and about.
3   Avoid bending movements of the back, especially sudden and rotatory ones. It may be almost impossible to move the back at all because of the pain due to muscle spasm.
4   Local heat may afford great relief of the painful spasm in surrounding muscles.
5   Aspirin is one of the best drugs available to relieve the pain.

If the backache has not improved in 24–48 hours, seek medical advice. You should do this at the outset if the pain is associated with any weakness, numbness, tingling or pain in the legs, or if there is difficulty passing urine. When first getting up again, special care must be taken to avoid bending or lifting. Sitting for long periods in easy chairs is best avoided and it is safer to sit in a firm chair with a back support.

Treatment of severe backache

Requires expert guidance.

1 Stronger pain killers are available only on prescription, as are muscle relaxants which are given to relieve painful muscle spasm.
2 Expert physiotherapy will help relieve spasm. Different forms of treatment are available combined with muscle-strengthening exercises for the back to prevent further damage.
3 Manipulation must be performed with care and in expert hands can be rapidly, dramatically successful. Traction depends on a steady pull (rather than the sudden tug of manipulation) to gently separate the vertebrae and is of special use when the pain is due to a slipped disc.
4 Surgical belts and corsets provide support and also remind the sufferer not to bend or move suddenly. They are used for treatment of recurrent back problems. The back muscles must not be allowed to become flabby and weak while wearing a corset, and muscle-strengthening exercises should be performed. If the back is placed under strain by an unavoidable car journey or lifting, a corset may prevent serious pain or damage.
5 Surgery to remove the herniated part of the damaged disc is performed if other methods fail.

Bacteria

Small organisms which can be seen only with a microscope. They differ from viruses in that they can be grown in an artificial environment in which there are no living cells. Bacteria are responsible for many acute infections, including streptococcal sore throat, and some forms of pneumonia, meningitis and peritonitis.

Bad breath
(HALITOSIS)

Bad breath is a cause of great embarrassment and anxiety, but it rarely indicates serious disease. It is usually caused by eating foods rich in spices or garlic and settles after 2–3 days. It is common and persistent in smokers, whose breath may smell disgusting to all but themselves. Infections of the teeth and gums can be the source of the smell. Regular and scrupulous cleaning of the teeth and gums may be curative; if not, an early visit to a dental surgeon should trace the cause. Peppermints may help to disguise the smell—expensive preparations designed to sweeten the breath are rarely of more benefit. Chronic ulcers in the mouth are rarely the cause.

Baldness
SEE HAIR LOSS

Barber's rash
(SYCOSIS)

Due to bacterial infection occurring in the roots of the hair follicles in the beard area. The condition is made worse by shaving with an open razor and may be improved by changing to an electric razor or giving up shaving. Antibiotics are required only if the infection spreads from the hair follicles.

Barbiturates

A group of drugs which produce sedation, and are used to treat epilepsy. For many years they were the only drugs available for the treatment of insomnia, tension and raised blood pressure.

Short-acting barbiturates such as thiopentone are used as general anaesthetics, where they have an important place.

The main disadvantage of barbiturates such as phenobarbitone (Luminal), pentobarbitone (Nembutal), quinalbarbitone (Seconal), amylobarbitone (Sodium Amytal) and butobarbitone (Soneryl) is the occurrence of both psychological and physical dependence. It is easy for barbiturate taking to become a habit, so that true dependence or even addiction may follow. When this occurs, expert treatment in a specialized hospital unit may be needed to wean the addict from his drugs. It is dangerous suddenly to stop taking barbiturates after a long time. If given to an anxious patient, who may also be depressed, they may accentuate the depression. The elderly are particularly at risk from drowsiness and confusion. Finally, barbiturates are dangerous if taken in overdosage. Mild overdosage may happen when an older person forgets that he has taken his sleeping tablets and takes another. Barbiturates taken in overdose suppress respiration, which slows down or even stops.

Conclusion
Those taking barbiturates should be guided by their physician whether they should continue or stop them. Barbiturates are still safe when used under medical supervision, in particular for epilepsy and as general anaesthetics. If you have been on barbiturates regularly for any reason it is unwise to stop them suddenly.

The serious side-effects of barbiturates make

them unsuitable for routine use now that safer drugs are available.

Barium x-rays

Barium is opaque to x-rays (page 250) and is used in radiology to outline the intestinal tract.

A *barium meal* is performed to detect peptic ulcers and oesophageal acid reflux. The barium is drunk as a tasteless and rather unpalatable mixture, and the oesophagus, stomach, duodenum and small bowel are observed through an x-ray screen as they slowly fill and empty.

Barium enemas are used to examine the large bowel. Barium is passed through a narrow catheter into the rectum and pushed gently upwards by a combination of gravity and air to outline the bowel.

Both examinations are slightly uncomfortable but in no way painful. The information gained from them is often of great value in diagnosis and in planning treatment.

Battered babies

In Britain about 4,000 children are injured every year by their parents. Of these, about 400 die, and another 400 suffer permanent, often mental, disability. There is a big difference between the occasional hard smack delivered in a moment of exasperation and the continuing bullying suffered by some children.

Despite the horrifying figures and all the recent publicity, the significance of injuries to children is often overlooked and glib explanations from parents are accepted at face value. Sometimes, the parents of these children were themselves battered when they were young; they feel that their child is very demanding and screams a lot—and this may be true. Often the child is neglected as well as assaulted.

When physical violence towards a child becomes a frequent event and severe enough to give serious injuries then that child needs help. There are many agencies which can advise, including the local NSPCC inspector, the family doctor, and the Social Services Department. With expert advice and supervision, many families can be helped and the child's safety ensured.

BCG

Immunization against tuberculosis; it is discussed in the section on Tuberculosis.

Bed wetting
(ENURESIS)

Bed wetting at night (nocturnal enuresis) is very common. In children up to the age of 5 years it is not usually considered sufficiently abnormal to require treatment. Only very rarely is it a symptom of an underlying disease.

An understanding and patient approach by the parents will be of major help to the enuretic child. Wetting the bed at night is unpleasant for the parent who has to get up and change the sheets, but it is humiliating for the young child who may be made fun of by brothers and sisters, or even school friends.

Many older children who wet the bed at night despair of ever being able to stay dry (as do their parents). The parents may become more and more punitive in their attitude even though the child has no control over what he is doing at night. Bed wetting can be a sign of underlying emotional stress, particularly if the child has previously been dry at night. He will not be consciously aware of these stresses and it is very important to try to resolve any underlying conflicts within the family. A punitive attitude towards the bed wetting will only serve to make these conflicts worse.

Bed wetting results from failure to develop the skill of bladder control. A baby exerts no conscious control over his bladder and passes urine as soon as it is full. The older child soon learns to wait even if only for a few minutes.

There are several practical steps which may help.
1   If the child is to reach the toilet in time at night it should not be too far away and there must be adequate lighting so that he is not dissuaded from getting out of bed. A pot under the bed may be the best compromise.
2   Restriction of fluid intake for 1 or 2 hours before going to bed, and lifting the child when the parents go to bed is often curative.
3   Bladder training during the day, by encouraging the child to wait even for only a minute or two, will allow better night-time control.

If these measures are unsuccessful, medical advice should be sought. Imipramine (Tofranil Syrup) or amitriptyline (Tryptizol Syrup) taken at night are drugs often used in conjunction with a 'star chart'. Every morning the child is allowed to stick a star on the chart if he has had a dry night. This ritual, and the praise accompanying it, is often enough to encourage him. Another form of treatment involves waking devices, most commonly the 'bell and pad'. When the child passes urine, the pad becomes wet and a low-voltage electrical circuit is completed which rings a bell. He then has to get up, go to the toilet and finish passing urine, change the sheets, reset the alarm and go back to sleep. These alarms are safe in children over about 8 and must comply with government safety regulations. Although they appear to be a brutal way to tackle enuresis, these devices can be remarkably effective.

Bee and wasp stings
SEE STINGS

For emergency treatment of bee and wasp stings, *see* First Aid (page 276).

Bends
(DECOMPRESSION SICKNESS; CAISSON DISEASE)

Occurs in deep-sea divers who surface too rapidly. The nitrogen normally dissolved in the blood, comes out of solution and forms air bubbles which obstruct the arteries and blood supply to various body organs, usually the muscles and joints and sometimes the brain. Emergency treatment is to put the diver into a decompression chamber.

Benign growth

A swelling or tumour which is not malignant (*see* Tumour).

Beri-beri

A tropical disease caused by lack of vitamin B_1 (thiamine), usually associated with generalized vitamin deficiency and malnutrition. Thiamine deficiency results in failure of the heart to pump efficiently; it also causes damage to nerves, with numbness in the hands and feet and occasionally paralysis of the limbs.

Berries
POISONOUS

Deadly nightshade is very dangerous if eaten, as are laburnum seeds. For signs and emergency treatment, *see* Deadly nightshade. (*See also* Poisoning.)

Beta-blockers

A group of drugs used to treat high blood pressure (hypertension) (page 41), angina (page 19) and irregularities of heart rhythm.

The heart rate and blood pressure are controlled by special fibres of the sympathetic nervous system. Impulses are constantly relayed to the heart and blood vessels via these nerves to adjust the heart's output. In animals this system is vital for survival because the heart output can be rapidly increased in preparation for sudden physical activity if threatened by predators. This 'fight or flight' response is less vital to our survival but is responsible for the thumping in the chest indicating an increase in heart rate and blood pressure following a sudden shock, annoyance, excitement or love.

Beta-blockers partially block the action of the sympathetic nervous system and prevent stress to the heart and blood vessels. As a result they are very effective in decreasing blood pressure and in controlling angina. They slow the heart rate and reduce the amount of work performed by the heart both on exercise and at rest.

The commonly used beta-blockers are propranolol (Inderal), oxprenolol (Trasicor), atenolol (Tenormin), sotalol (Beta-Cardone) and timolol (Blocadren). The advantage of atenolol is that it needs to be taken only once a day. Practolol (Eraldin) has been withdrawn from use since it produced serious side-effects. These have not occurred with the others, which are very safe drugs. If taken in excess they can seriously slow the heart and may induce acute breathlessness in otherwise well-controlled asthmatics. Cold hands and feet are a rare and not serious complication. Beta-blockers are available only on prescription. Their official name usually ends in 'olol'.

Bilharzia
SEE SCHISTOSOMIASIS

Biopsy

A small piece of tissue removed at operation. This minor operation is usually performed under local anaesthetic and used to make a diagnosis or to follow the effects of treatment. It is not usually necessary to stay overnight in hospital. The tissues commonly biopsied are skin, lumps in the breast and enlarged lymph nodes; occasionally a needle is used to obtain a sample of liver or kidney tissue. After removal, the specimen can be examined microscopically or cultured for infecting organisms.

Birthmark
(NAEVUS)

Usually small and of no significance (*see* illustration, page 238), but may be unsightly on the face. Although they cause parents great anxiety, they can be safely left because most will disappear with time. There are four common birthmarks.

'Strawberry' naevus is a bright red lump which slowly enlarges and becomes raised above the level of the surrounding skin. It may occur in prominent places, such as the face or over the scalp. It may not be obvious until a few days after birth and then increases in size rapidly for up to 8 months. A static phase is usually reached which lasts for months until slow regression begins. The vast majority disappear and become almost indistinguishable from the surrounding skin, though some do not do so until the child is 7 years of age. If they are surgically removed, a small scar is inevitable. Nevertheless, this may be advisable if the naevus is in a prominent place and shows no signs of regression by the time the child is 6 or 7.

The 'stork mark' is so called because it looks as if the baby has been pecked on the face. It appears as a flat, pink lesion which becomes livid when the baby cries. Usually it occurs on the forehead, upper eyelids or the nape of the neck. Generally it regresses and disappears by the age of 2 years.

The 'port wine' naevus looks as if red wine has been spilt on the skin. It is often seen on the face, and does not fade with time.

Mongolian blue spots are large dark areas tinged with blue, often found over the buttocks in Negro or Oriental children. They disappear slowly after birth and are gone by the time the child is 5 years. They can be mistaken for extensive bruising and the parents even accused of assaulting the child.

Conclusion

Although birthmarks are a cause of great anxiety to parents, they are not dangerous and disappear spontaneously. If required, expert plastic surgery or laser therapy usually allows complete removal with a minimum of scarring.

Bites

SEE FIRST AID: DOG AND SNAKE BITES (PAGE 275)

Blackouts

Causes

There are many causes of transient loss of consciousness ('blackout').

Fainting

This is commoner in women than men and in people of a thin rather than a stocky build. The precipitating factor may be a sudden shock or pain, the sight of blood, or prolonged standing in warm, stuffy surroundings. The highly strung and emotional are more prone to faints. Recovery follows rapidly within a minute or two provided the head is kept low.

Acute anxiety

Acute anxiety may produce an overpowering desire to breathe rapidly and heavily. As a result, biochemical changes take place in the blood, to cause a marked reduction in carbon dioxide. This produces pins and needles in the fingers, cramps in the hands and feet, a sensation of light-headedness, discomfort in the chest and upper abdomen, and sometimes unconsciousness. Recovery follows rapidly within a few minutes.

Coughing (cough syncope)

A severe prolonged attack of coughing in someone who is overweight and bronchitic may result in loss of consciousness. Once consciousness is lost and the person is laid on the floor, the coughing stops, breathing restarts and consciousness rapidly returns.

Passing urine (micturition syncope)

This occurs in the elderly when they get up in the middle of the night to pass urine. The blood pressure tends to fall upon standing after leaving a warm bed and it falls further as the bladder empties. The brief period of unconsciousness which follows may be mistaken for a stroke, but the only danger is if the head is struck during the fall.

Postural changes

Many people feel slightly faint if they jump out of bed too quickly in the morning or leap up out of a chair. This is because the blood pressure falls with the sudden change of posture, particularly if moving from a warm to a cold environment, and it takes a moment or two for the body to restore the blood pressure and supply blood to the brain. In the elderly, fainting due to a fall in blood pressure on rising (postural hypotension) is common and due to the gradual deterioration with age in the reaction speed of the sympathetic nervous system to changes of posture. As a result they may lose consciousness, and elderly people who are prone to this should rise slowly from a sitting or lying position. Some drugs potentiate this and should be used only with careful medical supervision. These include: sedatives and sleeping tablets such as diazepam (Valium), nitrazepam (Mogadon) or chlorpromazine (Largactil); barbiturates such as butobarbitone (Soneryl), amylobarbitone (Sodium Amytal) or phenobarbitone; drugs used to treat blood pressure, such as guanethidine (Ismelin) or methyldopa (Aldomet); diuretics such as cyclopenthiazide (Navidrex-K), amiloride (Moduretic); and some antidepressants such as amitriptyline (Lentizol, Tryptizol).

Arterial disease (atherosclerosis, arteriosclerosis)
Some elderly people become dizzy or lose consciousness if they look up quickly or move their heads from side to side. Two of the four blood vessels running up the back of the vertebral column to the brain may become narrowed as the result of such movements and the supply of oxygen to the brain temporarily reduced. The problem can be avoided if care is taken not to turn or lift the head suddenly. Consciousness returns after a few moments, whereas strokes produce symptoms which last at least several hours.

Epilepsy   see page 93

Hypoglycaemia (low blood sugar) in diabetes

Slow heart rate
Rarely, in the middle aged and elderly, the heart rate may drop abruptly (30–40 beats per minute) and this is followed by sudden loss of consciousness. The attacks are brief but may recur. Repeated attacks can be dangerous, and medical advice should be obtained. If a slow pulse rate has been observed, associated with blackouts, a pacemaker can be inserted into the heart to maintain a normal pulse rate.

Emergency management of blackouts
The patient should be laid on his side on the floor, tight clothing loosened and dentures or broken teeth removed from the mouth. If 'fitting', he is probably an epileptic and should be left in this position until the fit stops.

If consciousness does not return within 1–2 minutes or if the pulse is absent (though this may be ★ difficult for the inexperienced to assess), an ambulance should be called immediately.

If breathing stops and there is no pulse, external cardiac massage (page 270) and mouth-to-mouth resuscitation (page 274) should be started immediately whilst awaiting the ambulance or medical assistance.

Everyone who loses consciousness unexpectedly other than in an obvious faint, or who is unconscious for more than 2 or 3 minutes, or who has a fit should seek medical advice urgently.

Brain tumours virtually never cause blackouts.

Bladder

The part of the urinary tract which stores the urine (*see* diagram, page 261). Urine, made by the kidneys, passes down the ureters into the bladder, which expands until its size stimulates the need to urinate (micturate). This act is conveniently controlled by the brain.

Bladder infection
SEE CYSTITIS

Bleeding

Frequently dramatic, it produces great anxiety—partly because small quantities of blood may look impressively large. Except following road accidents, bleeding is rarely sufficient to cause immediate danger to life but must always be acted upon urgently. The first-aid management of bleeding is discussed under First aid (page 269).

Bleeding in urine
(HAEMATURIA)

Bleeding from the kidney or bladder is usually caused by infection, stones or cancer. All are curable if treated quickly, so medical advice must be obtained.

Blindness

The commonest causes of blindness are trachoma (page 228) and, in the developed world, diabetes (page 78).

Other important causes of visual disturbance are short sight (myopia), long sight (presbyopia), cataract (page 53) and glaucoma (page 113). *See also* Glasses.

Colour blindness is discussed on page 63.
Sudden blindness—seek urgent advice.

Blood

The body contains about 7 litres of blood composed of 50 per cent plasma and 50 per cent cells.

The plasma contains clotting factors which prevent excess bleeding after injury—the best known are thrombin and prothrombin—and antibodies produced by the lymph nodes as a response to

BLOOD

Red cells

Platelets

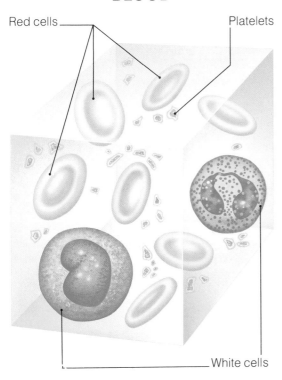

White cells

previous infection and immunization.

In every 1 cubic millimetre of blood are about 5 million red blood cells which contain the chemical haemoglobin, which carries oxygen from the lungs via the circulation to the tissues of the body. There are also 5,000–10,000 white blood cells, which are the first defence mechanism against infecting organisms, particularly bacteria.

See also Blood groups.

Blood groups

The 'ABO' system is used for grouping blood. It was discovered by Karl Landsteiner in Vienna in 1900 and he named the four blood groups A, B, AB and O.

Every individual has a specific blood group, which remains constant throughout life. The blood group depends upon the presence or absence of certain proteins in the red blood cells. The two proteins in ABO blood grouping are named A and B. The cells

of blood group A have the A protein on their surface; group B, the B protein; group AB, both; and group O neither.

Proportion of the UK population

Group A	42 per cent
Group B	8 per cent
Group AB	3 per cent
Group O	47 per cent

Only blood of the same group is used for transfusion. In an emergency, group O blood may be used because the O cells have neither protein on their surface and the recipient, even if he has antibodies to these proteins, will not destroy the transfused cells.

Another protein of importance is the Rhesus protein, discovered in Rhesus monkeys. About 85 per cent of Caucasians have this protein in their red cells and are 'Rhesus positive'. The remaining 15 per cent lack it and are 'Rhesus negative'. If a Rhesus-negative mother has a Rhesus-positive husband, their baby—if he is Rhesus positive—may develop Rhesus disease of the newborn (page 195). This can be avoided by good obstetric care.

The percentage of people with each blood group varies from nation to nation and from race to race. Blood groups have been used to trace likely patterns of human migration. Blood grouping is important medico-legally because blood found at the scene of a crime can be grouped and may be shown definitely not to have come from someone under suspicion. The opposite is not the case, because the person under suspicion and the true criminal could have the same blood group. This is also true in cases of disputed paternity: because blood groups are inherited in a predictable way it can only be proved that someone is definitely not a child's father.

Blood pressure
(HIGH BLOOD PRESSURE; HYPERTENSION)

The heart pumps blood into the circulation in sharp bursts at every beat. The blood pressure rises and falls in time with this, being greatest just after the heart contracts and least at the end of its relaxation phase. Both the high (systolic) and low (diastolic) levels are important, and the blood pressure is measured in millimetres of mercury (mmHg) and expressed as two numbers, one 'over' the other (e.g. 120/80).

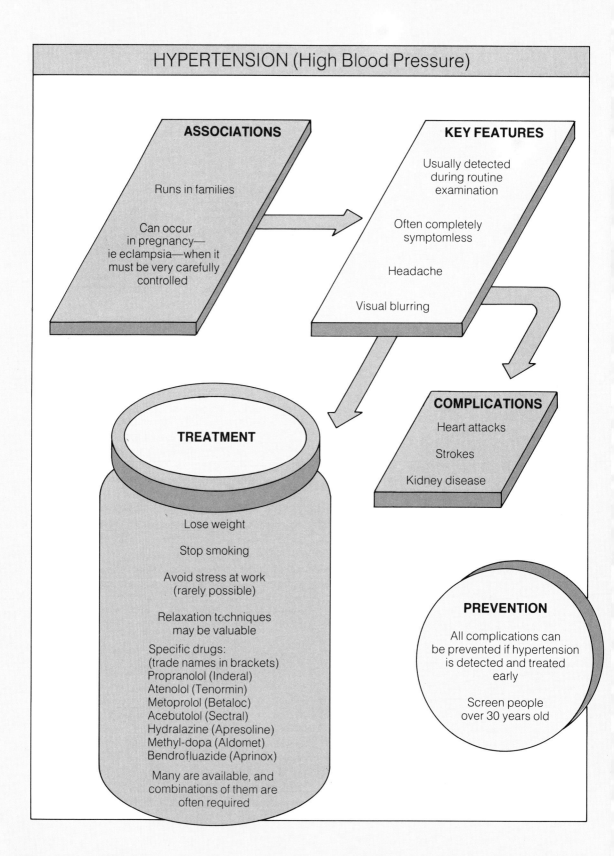

HYPERTENSION (High Blood Pressure)

ASSOCIATIONS

Runs in families

Can occur
in pregnancy—
ie eclampsia—when it
must be very carefully
controlled

KEY FEATURES

Usually detected
during routine
examination

Often completely
symptomless

Headache

Visual blurring

COMPLICATIONS

Heart attacks

Strokes

Kidney disease

TREATMENT

Lose weight

Stop smoking

Avoid stress at work
(rarely possible)

Relaxation techniques
may be valuable

Specific drugs:
(trade names in brackets)
Propranolol (Inderal)
Atenolol (Tenormin)
Metoprolol (Betaloc)
Acebutolol (Sectral)
Hydralazine (Apresoline)
Methyl-dopa (Aldomet)
Bendrofluazide (Aprinox)

Many are available, and
combinations of them are
often required

PREVENTION

All complications can
be prevented if hypertension
is detected and treated
early

Screen people
over 30 years old

It is difficult to define what a 'normal' blood pressure is because it changes from minute to minute and varies considerably depending on age, sex, weight and build. A level of around 120/80 mmHg is normal in a man of 40, but values in excess of this would be quite acceptable in someone of 65 because the pressure tends to increase with increasing years, without obvious complications.

It is well established that people with high blood pressure run a greater risk of suffering from strokes, heart disease and kidney disease. This risk is reduced if the elevated blood pressure is discovered early and reduced to normal levels with treatment. The only way of knowing whether high blood pressure is present is to measure it, because in the absence of complications there are usually no specific symptoms. It is for this reason that many doctors screen all their patients—particularly young men, in whom complications are more common.

In the majority of those who have high blood pressure no specific cause is ever found, though some experts believe that chronic stress may be an important factor. Short-term stress raises the pressure temporarily; for this reason, recurrent stress—whether at home or at work—is probably best avoided if possible. There is no evidence that hard work is harmful in any way. High blood pressure runs in families and may be inherited in the same way as eye colour, height and build. In a few, kidney disease and an excess of adrenal hormones cause high blood pressure. Specific treatment can then be recommended. The contraceptive pill may produce a rise in blood pressure, and all women on 'the pill' should have their blood pressure checked at least every year. Women known to have a high blood pressure should not take the pill.

Treatment

The drugs commonly used to treat blood pressure are:
1 Diuretics—which make the kidney eliminate salt and water; e.g. cyclopenthiazide (Navidrex) and bendrofluazide (Neo-NaClex, Aprinox). Food should have no added salt.
2 Beta-blockers (see Beta-blockers)—which reduce the work and output of the heart.
3 Drugs which reduce the resistance to the flow of blood through the circulation by relaxing the muscles in the vessel walls; e.g. methyldopa (Aldomet), guanethidine (Ismelin), hydrallazine (Apresoline).

If your family has a history of heart disease, heart attacks or strokes at a young age or high blood pressure, it is wise to get your own checked. Many family practices are attempting to screen all of their young and middle-aged patients for high blood pressure so that treatment may be started before any complications have occurred.

The drugs now available are both safe and effective, and if the blood pressure is kept under good control, life expectancy is normal and there is no greater risk of a heart attack or stroke. Despite the absence of symptoms it is vital to keep taking the drugs if the blood pressure rises without them. Some people like to maintain a check on their own blood pressures, and suitable machines are now available. They are most unsuitable for obsessive, worrying personalities, and may do more harm from the anxiety produced on finding a minimal rise of pressure.

Blood transfusion

The first attempts at blood transfusion took place in the fifteenth century. Until the discovery of blood groups in 1900 it was a procedure fraught with danger; many people were given blood incompatible with their own and died when their own antibodies attacked the transfused blood cells (see Blood groups).

Blood transfusion is now a routine and safe procedure. Precautions are taken to ensure that the patient receives only blood compatible with his own. In practice, this means giving him blood of his own group, although in a dire emergency group O Rhesus-negative can be used.

Transfusion can be life-saving following severe haemorrhage. Although the body compensates initially, a stage is reached when so much blood has been lost that there is insufficient for the heart to pump and maintain the circulation. The blood pressure falls and consciousness is lost. Blood must be given urgently to restore the volume of circulating fluid to enable the heart to pump efficiently and also to provide enough red blood cells to carry oxygen to the tissues.

Blood transfusion may be vital, and there is always an inadequate number of blood donors. Giving blood is not as uncomfortable as many believe. Provided you are in good health and not anaemic, it is in no way dangerous and the discomfort of a needle inserted into the vein of an arm by an expert is minimal.

Blood can be stored for 3 weeks at 4°C (39.2°F)—the temperature of a domestic refrigerator. After this it is not transfused but various vital fractions of the blood are taken to be used, for example, in treating haemophilia. A small amount of citrate is usually added to prevent the blood from clotting either during storage or when being transfused.

Blood vessels
ARTERIES AND VEINS

An artery is a blood vessel which takes blood away from the heart towards the tissues. The main artery from the left side of the heart is the aorta and contains oxygenated blood; that from the right side is the pulmonary artery and carries de-oxygenated blood returned from the tissues. An artery has thick walls which can be felt, and the pulsing of the heart beat can be felt. The pressure in the arteries is higher than in the veins—it is the 'blood pressure' usually measured by a doctor.

A vein returns the blood to the heart under low pressure and without pulsation. When cut, they ooze (sometimes fast) but do not spurt as a cut artery does. The blood is bluer in a vein because much of the oxygen has been removed by the tissues.

Blue babies

Many babies are blue immediately after they are born, but soon turn pink once they start breathing. A few babies remain blue or become blue in the first few months of life. When this happens it means that the blood is deficient in oxygen. This blue colour (cyanosis) is most obvious in the lips and tongue. The most common cause is a heart defect which has been present from birth.

The heart is not one but two pumps. The right side pumps blood round the lungs and the left round the body (*see* diagram, page 253).

Normally the two sides are separated by a partition but if there is a defect in it—a 'hole in the heart' (page 128)—or if the blood vessels leading out of the heart develop abnormally, blood leaks from one side to the other. If blue blood leaks from the right side to the left, it passes into the circulation round the body which is then supplied with low-oxygen blood. At some stage the heart defect must be repaired surgically if the child is to grow and develop normally, and to have a normal life expectancy. Often major surgery is deferred for some years until the child and the heart are larger, stronger and more easily operated upon. Unfortunately, in a very few cases the defect may be so serious that it cannot be rectified by even the best surgery.

Blurred vision

The commonest causes of blurred vision are short sight and long sight, neither of which is serious; both are easily corrected by wearing spectacles. Other causes include infection of the conjunctiva (*see* Conjunctivitis), cataract and, most important, ★glaucoma (page 113).

Boil

A small abscess or pocket of infection which forms around the base of a hair follicle, or in a sweat gland, just under the skin. Initially there is an ill-defined area of redness around the follicle, which becomes localized, red, hard and painful. The small amount of pus (consisting of dead bacteria and white blood cells which have destroyed them) eventually discharges, with relief of pain.

Antibiotics are not required for small boils. Warm dressings may give pain relief. It is unwise to prod or squeeze boils, especially if they are on the face, where scarring may follow. Larger boils on the face or around the eyes are always best seen by a doctor because antibiotics may be needed to ensure rapid healing and prevent the infection spreading.

Diabetics tend to get recurrent boils, but only a small number of those who get recurrent boils have diabetes.

★Bone fracture

The commonest fractures are of the radius at the wrist, caused by falls on the outstretched hand (Colles' fracture); the lower tibia and fibula in the ankle (Pott's fracture); the neck of the femur following falls in the elderly; the collar bone (or clavicle) from falls onto the shoulder, usually during sport. A march fracture is a fracture of one of the metatarsal bones of the foot.

If the bones remain in alignment, surgery may be unnecessary although they must be held immobile in plaster until the fractured ends unite. In displaced fractures, manipulation may be necessary to realign the bones before immobilization but, if not, surgery may be required. In these cases, internal fixation with metal plates or rods can be employed. If the skin above the fracture is open (compound fracture) there is an increased risk of infection in the bones, and surgery is necessary to close the wound. (For emergency treatment of fractures, *see* page 274.)

Bones

The skeleton (page 258; *and see* diagram, right) is composed mainly of calcium phosphate held together in a protein binding which acts in the same way as cement. Apart from its major function in the body structure, bone is a calcium store and calcium is essential for the health of all tissues—especially the action of muscles, including the heart muscle.

Bottle feeding
SEE UNDER INFANT FEEDING

Botulism

An exceedingly rare form of food poisoning (page 105).

Bowel

The intestinal tract from the duodenum to the rectum, and including both small and large intestines. (*See also* Digestive tract; Intestines; *and* the diagram, page 265.)

Brain

The part of the central nervous system contained within the skull, and in which all emotions and sensations are perceived and from which muscular activity is initiated. Motor impulses from the brain pass down the nerves in the spinal cord (the other part of the central nervous system) and from there through peripheral nerves to the muscles. Sensations pass from the skin and joints along the peripheral nerves to the spinal cord and up to the brain.

The brain has four major parts (lobes); these and their functions are shown in the diagram (page 257).

Brain tumours

There are two distinct types of brain tumour: a *primary* tumour arises from the tissues of the brain itself; *secondary* tumours arise as the result of spread from a cancer elsewhere in the body.

Primary brain tumours tend to occur at the extremes of life—in children or the elderly—and, with modern surgical techniques, are often removable. Many people have a disproportionate fear of

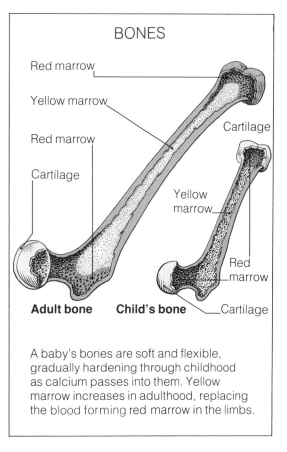

BONES

Red marrow
Yellow marrow
Red marrow
Cartilage
Cartilage
Yellow marrow
Red marrow

Adult bone   **Child's bone**   Cartilage

A baby's bones are soft and flexible, gradually hardening through childhood as calcium passes into them. Yellow marrow increases in adulthood, replacing the blood forming red marrow in the limbs.

developing one of these most uncommon tumours. Headaches are only very rarely caused by a tumour. Other features caused by them include epileptic fits in an adult who has never had them before, slowly developing strokes or persistent double vision.

Bran

A major constituent of unrefined foods and contains a high content of fibre. Foods with high and low contents of dietary fibre are described in the section on constipation (page 64).

Break-bone fever
SEE DENGUE

Breast disorders

Breast lumps are very common, and always raise the fear of cancer. They are usually simple cysts, but it is impossible to be certain until they have been carefully examined and investigated (*see* Mammogram). Cysts can often be emptied using a local anaesthetic and a syringe and needle. It is not necessary to remain in hospital, and once fluid is found the chance of a cancer can be refuted.

Breast cancer is a common disorder and, if detected early, can now usually be cured by a combination of surgery and, if required, radiotherapy.

Breast abscesses are common, particularly whilst breast feeding, and are hot and tender. They respond rapidly to antibiotics but may prevent further breast feeding.

Disorders of the nipple are discussed on page 159.

Breast feeding
SEE UNDER INFANT FEEDING

Breath, bad
(HALITOSIS) SEE BAD BREATH

Breath-holding attacks

Common in small children who wish to attract attention. The child may use the attack in situations of emotional stress when he has been hurt or has been disciplined. Breath-holding is often preceded by screaming. When the breath is held the child may go slightly blue around the lips and even lose consciousness for a few seconds. Once he becomes unconscious, normal breathing is re-established immediately.

These attacks are not dangerous though obviously very upsetting for the parents. It is unnecessary to try to wake the child since he will come round in a few seconds. Calmness about the whole problem, however difficult this may be, probably helps most in

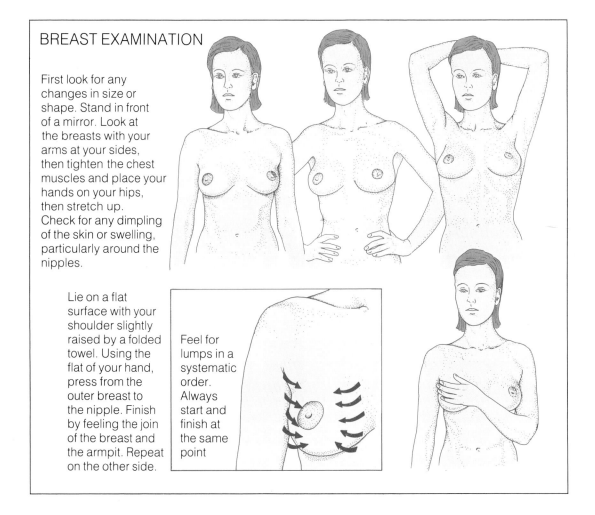

BREAST EXAMINATION

First look for any changes in size or shape. Stand in front of a mirror. Look at the breasts with your arms at your sides, then tighten the chest muscles and place your hands on your hips, then stretch up.
Check for any dimpling of the skin or swelling, particularly around the nipples.

Lie on a flat surface with your shoulder slightly raised by a folded towel. Using the flat of your hand, press from the outer breast to the nipple. Finish by feeling the join of the breast and the armpit. Repeat on the other side.

Feel for lumps in a systematic order. Always start and finish at the same point

BREAST LUMPS

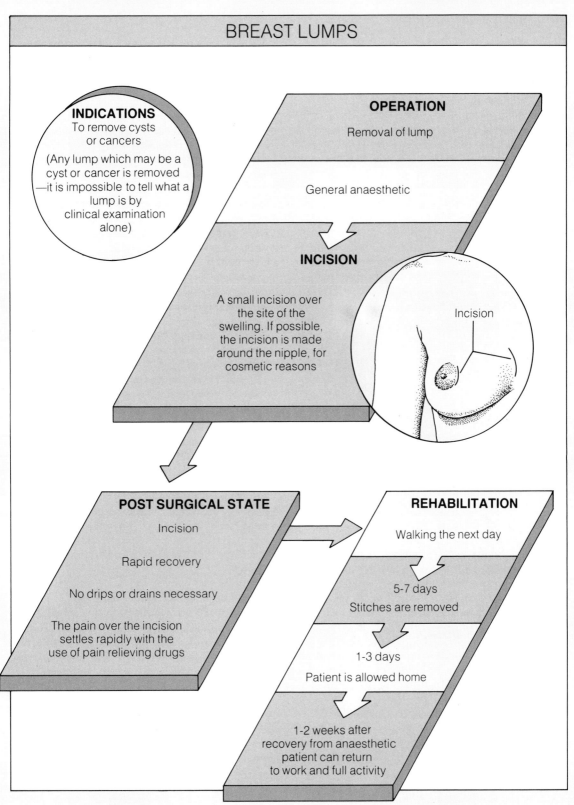

INDICATIONS

To remove cysts or cancers

(Any lump which may be a cyst or cancer is removed —it is impossible to tell what a lump is by clinical examination alone)

OPERATION

Removal of lump

General anaesthetic

INCISION

A small incision over the site of the swelling. If possible, the incision is made around the nipple, for cosmetic reasons

Incision

POST SURGICAL STATE

Incision

Rapid recovery

No drips or drains necessary

The pain over the incision settles rapidly with the use of pain relieving drugs

REHABILITATION

Walking the next day

5-7 days
Stitches are removed

1-3 days
Patient is allowed home

1-2 weeks after recovery from anaesthetic patient can return to work and full activity

47

the long run. All children grow out of the habit. (*See also* Tantrum.)

Breathlessness

This is common after unaccustomed exercise.

Breathlessness on mild exertion or at rest suggests disease of the heart or lungs (*see* Shortness of breath).

Breech delivery

The baby is born upside down, with buttocks appearing first. This mode of delivery results in slightly increased difficulty during labour, and it is therefore usual to attempt to turn the baby head-first (*see also under* Pregnancy).

Hospital delivery is recommended in view of the slightly increased complication rate during delivery.

★ Bronchiolitis

This infectious illness attacks children usually in the first few months of life. It is caused by one of the viruses (respiratory syncytial virus; RSV) which, in adults, causes the common cold. In young children, as well as the usual symptoms of a blocked, runny nose, wheezing may develop. Occasionally this becomes sufficiently severe to cause breathlessness, especially during feeding. Usually the infection resolves completely in a few days without any treatment.

An infant may find it tiring to suck, and becomes hungry and irritable when he fails to take his full feed. Very occasionally, in severe cases, admission to hospital may be necessary. A tube can then be passed into the stomach so that feeding can continue without the child having to suck. Humidification of the air in an incubator or 'oxygen tent' also helps respiration until the acute illness begins to subside.

Severe bronchiolitis is a very serious disease in infants, but with good nursing, modern incubators and careful monitoring of respiration and blood oxygen the outlook is invariably excellent, and there is no long-term damage.

Bronchitis

Infection of the bronchi, the airways which carry air from the atmosphere to the alveolar tissue of the lungs. It is common in industrialized countries where air pollution is widespread. It is so common in the United Kingdom that it has long been known as the 'English disease'. More working days are lost in the UK as a result than from any other disease; 20,000 people a year die from it. Smoking—the most intense atmospheric pollution—is the major cause.

The disease begins as a winter cough with sputum, which recurs year after year until it eventually persists throughout the year.

Normally the cells lining the bronchi are very efficient at removing the minute particles of dust present in the air. These particles become stuck in the normal mucus produced by the cells lining the bronchi and are then expelled by the action of fine hairs known as cilia which propel any debris up to the throat where it is swallowed with the saliva. If the bronchi become damaged by smoking, the cilia fail to function and at the same time the amount of mucus produced by the lining cells increases. As a result, the phlegm or mucus which is no longer cleared automatically from the air passages has to be expelled by coughing.

If this process continues, the bronchi become permanently damaged and allow infections to spread into the lung tissue (i.e. pneumonia). Progressive breathlessness follows and finally the sufferer may be short of breath even at rest.

Acute bronchitis may follow a heavy cold and affect those with no past history of chest disease. This invariably settles completely without damage to the lungs. Smokers are at much greater risk of recurrent bronchitis with eventual destruction of the lungs (i.e. chronic bronchitis).

Treatment
Smoking
Cigarette smoke paralyses the cilia—the fine hairs which line the large airways and which remove mucus and debris—and finally kills them. Once lost, they are never replaced.

Smokers with chronic bronchitis must be persuaded to give up the habit. The alternative is increasing incapacity with progressive breathlessness.

Coughs and colds
Chronic bronchitics are often given a supply of antibiotics for use should they develop a heavy cold or influenza. This is because there is a tendency for these infections to go rapidly to the lungs, which may become permanently damaged.

Bronchitics are advised to have an anti-influenza injection every autumn.

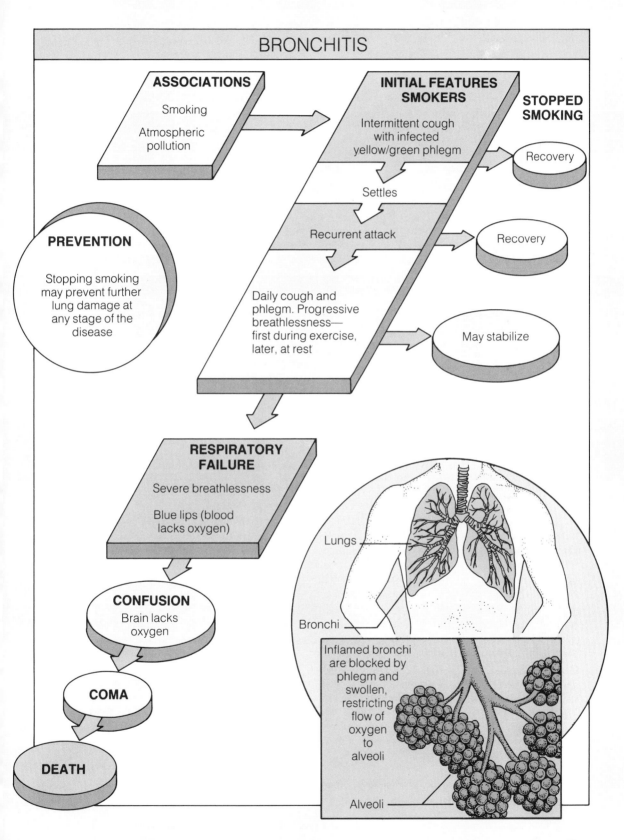

BRONCHITIS

ASSOCIATIONS

Smoking

Atmospheric pollution

INITIAL FEATURES SMOKERS

Intermittent cough with infected yellow/green phlegm

Settles

Recurrent attack

Daily cough and phlegm. Progressive breathlessness— first during exercise, later, at rest

STOPPED SMOKING

Recovery

Recovery

May stabilize

PREVENTION

Stopping smoking may prevent further lung damage at any stage of the disease

RESPIRATORY FAILURE

Severe breathlessness

Blue lips (blood lacks oxygen)

CONFUSION
Brain lacks oxygen

COMA

DEATH

Lungs

Bronchi

Inflamed bronchi are blocked by phlegm and swollen, restricting flow of oxygen to alveoli

Alveoli

Wheezing

Many people with chronic bronchitis wheeze. This may be due either to the bronchitis itself or to asthma. If there is an element of asthma (*see* Asthma), the temporary narrowing of the bronchi can be relieved by drugs, such as Ventolin in tablet or inhaler form, which act by relaxing the muscles within the walls of the large airways and allowing them to dilate.

Obesity

Overweight people are unable to expand their lungs properly and if they suffer from bronchitis should lose weight.

Bronchopneumonia

A pneumonia which affects any part of the lung tissue, and should be distinguished from lobar pneumonia in which a single anatomical lobe of the lung is involved. Bronchopneumonia is very much commoner (*see also* Chest infections; Pneumonia; *and* Lungs).

Treatment with physiotherapy and antibiotics is usually successful, except at the extremes of life, but it is also important to ensure a good fluid intake because large amounts of water vapour are lost due to the raised temperature and increased rate of respiration.

Bronchoscopy

A minor operation usually performed under an anaesthetic. It allows the surgeon to look down the throat into the windpipe (trachea) and to examine the large air passages (bronchi). Bronchoscopy has become much easier since the advent of the flexible bronchoscope. This is a thin telescopic instrument which can be passed gently down the trachea and bronchi without damaging their delicate linings. It has a light at one end and, looking through a magnifying eyepiece at the other, the bronchi can be seen clearly.

Bronchoscopy is valuable if someone is suspected of having inhaled small fragments of food or a button, for they can also be removed through the bronchoscope. The surgeon may be able to detect a cancer of the lung, and if necessary remove a small fragment of any suspicious tissue for examination under a microscope.

Bronchoscopy is a routine procedure in many hospitals, and lasts only a few minutes. The patient is usually asleep throughout and feels absolutely nothing. The throat may be sore afterwards but this clears in 3–4 days.

Bronchus

(GREEK: *BRONCHOS*, WINDPIPE)

The major airways to the lungs, starting from the lower end of the trachea (*see* diagram, page 255). At the level of the upper heart border, about one-third of the way down the breastbone (sternum), the trachea divides into right and left main bronchi; these, in turn, divide into smaller airways to the upper, middle and lower lobes of the right lung and the upper and lower lobes on the left.

Brucellosis

An infectious disease caused by bacteria and caught from cattle (*Brucella abortus* as it causes abortion in cattle) or goats (*Brucella melitensis*). It is an occupational disease of vets and cattlemen, who develop drenching sweats with fever, weight loss, muscle and joint pains, and depression sometimes with confusion and poor memory.

The disease is prevented by pasteurization of milk, and cured with antibiotics although a prolonged course may be required.

Bruise

Results from damage to small veins in the skin which leak blood into the surrounding tissues. The blue (low oxygen) blood gives the bruise its characteristic colour. An injury which leads to bruising is often followed by aching and stiffness in the affected muscle or joint.

There are many traditional remedies which are claimed to relieve bruises. Even the time-honoured treatment of a raw steak applied firmly to the injured area is not only expensive but makes little difference. There are creams available which are claimed to help but there is little evidence to suggest any benefit from them.

Provided the skin has not been broken, local warmth from a hot-water bottle or products such as Algipan, Ralgex or 'Deep Heat' may relieve the pain. Massage is often very soothing. Where there is bruising around a joint following a sprain, immersing the foot alternately in hot and cold water and an ankle support may give pain relief. Local warmth and the milder pain-killers (analgesics) such as aspirin remain the standby of treatment of bruising.

Bunion
SEE UNDER CHIROPODY

Burns
SEE UNDER FIRST AID (PAGE 270)

Burns—chemical

Most severe chemical burns occur in factories or at work and detailed treatments and the correct drugs are kept nearby.

In the home, all chemicals which fall onto the skin should be washed away under a running tap and not scrubbed. If a burn results and is very painful or ★extensive, medical advice should be sought immediately.

Chemicals in the eye are treated in a similar way, by washing the eye with copious quantities of tap water which can be applied either using a special eye cup, or by dipping the open eye into the water-filled ★palm of a hand or bowl of water. Medical advice should always be obtained after chemicals enter the eye.

Bursitis

Around many joints is a small fluid-filled cushion, or bursa, which protects the underlying bone. Inflammation of these bursae is common, and they become red, hot and tender. The commonest example is housemaid's knee (page 128).

Caesarean section

The name derives from the *lex cesari* law of early Rome, and describes the abdominal operation to deliver a baby which cannot be delivered normally through the vagina.

The operation is performed under general or spinal anaesthesia via an incision in the lower abdomen to expose the pregnant uterus from which the baby is delivered. Caesarean section is usually required if there is considerable delay during normal labour or if the baby shows signs of stress. (*See also* Pregnancy.)

Caisson disease
SEE BENDS

Calciferol
(VITAMIN D)

Present in milk, egg yolk and liver oils—especially fish (halibut and cod)—and is also manufactured in the skin on exposure to sunlight. Vitamin D is not present in breast milk, and breast-fed babies are usually given supplements until the age of 6 months.

Vitamin D is converted in the body to cholecalciferol, a chemical which is essential for the intestinal absorption of calcium, required for new bone formation. Dietary deficiency is rare in Britain, although it may occur in the children of Asian immigrants. The recommended daily intake of vitamin D is 400 international units. (*See also* Vitamins.)

Calorie

An international unit of energy. Scientifically it is properly a kilocalorie (1000 calories). Officially it has now been superseded by a new unit, the kilojoule, though this has not gained common acceptance; 1 kilocalorie approximately equals 4 kilojoules.

Cancer

From the Latin for crab, which describes the spreading nature of malignant tumours. Not all cancers are lethal, and some if detected early can now be cured (*see* Tumours).

Candida albicans

The biological name of the fungus which causes thrush (page 223).

Cannabis
(HEMP, POT, HASHISH, MARIHUANA)

Not an addictive drug, it does not produce tolerance

(i.e. an ever-larger amount is required to obtain the same euphoria), or dependence (physical and emotional need)—*see* Addiction. There is some evidence that fetal damage occurs if the mother smokes cannabis ('reefers' or 'joints').

The widespread use of cannabis throughout the Western world by stable members of society and of university staff has produced no serious complications and strongly suggests that it is not itself dangerous. However, not all users are responsible and there is a risk in the young of coming into contact with those who use and sell hard drugs such as heroin.

It is not certain why cannabis became so popular in the 1950s and '60s. Amongst the current younger generation it is viewed as passé and they have returned to alcohol, which may be more dangerous in the short and long term.

The law does not allow the possession or cultivation of cannabis.

Carbohydrates

Sugar, glucose and starch are pure carbohydrate and the major constituents of potatoes, bread, cakes and biscuits; they are part of a normal diet. Reduction of carbohydrate intake is frequently recommended to reduce weight (*see* Reducing diets, page 292).

Carbuncle

A large boil or coalescence of many boils (page 44). Before penicillin, people died from carbuncles, and still may become acutely ill.

Carcinoma

Derived from the Greek for crab (Latin = *cancer*), and used to describe malignant tumours. Not all are lethal, and if detected early, many cancers can now be cured. (*See* Tumour.)

Cardiac massage

The technique of pumping the heart when its own muscle has ceased to contract effectively. External cardiac massage is accomplished by regular and firm pressure on the lower breastbone (sternum). The technique is described on page 273.

Cardiogram
SEE ECG

Caries

Infection of the tooth pulp, and a common cause of toothache (page 228). The caries tends to spread, so it must be removed and the tooth cavity filled to prevent destruction and loss of the tooth.

Carpal tunnel syndrome

A disorder of the wrist, which causes pain, numbness and tingling in the hand. Discomfort may also be felt up the arm. The resulting pain is often worst during the night or early morning, becoming better if the arm is elevated. If allowed to continue, weakness of

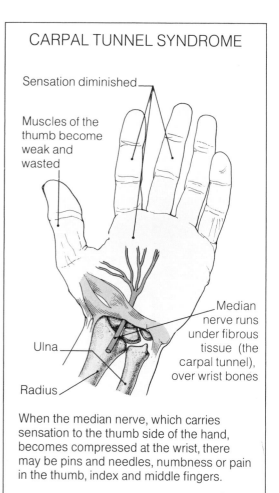

CARPAL TUNNEL SYNDROME

Sensation diminished

Muscles of the thumb become weak and wasted

Median nerve runs under fibrous tissue (the carpal tunnel), over wrist bones

Ulna

Radius

When the median nerve, which carries sensation to the thumb side of the hand, becomes compressed at the wrist, there may be pins and needles, numbness or pain in the thumb, index and middle fingers.

the thumb results. The pain is caused by compression of the median nerve as it passes in front of the wrist and through the carpal tunnel into the hand. There is just sufficient room for the nerve as it passes over the carpal (wrist) bones. If swelling occurs in this confined space, the nerve becomes compressed (*see* diagram, left).

The syndrome is common in rheumatoid arthritis, diabetes and in pregnancy. A previous fracture of the wrist may predispose to it.

Treatment with analgesics combined with a wrist splint worn at night is usually effective. Local injections of steroid at weekly intervals are relatively painless and often give dramatic relief.

If these measures are unsuccessful, the fibrous roof of the carpal tunnel can be split surgically to open the canal and decompress the nerve. The results of surgery are very successful.

Cartilages of the knee

Small pads of tough gristle which are half-moon-shaped and lie around the margins of the joint. Each knee has two cartilages: one on the outside and one on the inside. The top of the shin bone (tibia) is cup-shaped to take the rounded lower end of the thigh bone (femur). The cartilages deepen this shallow cup and allow greater joint stability. (*See* diagram, right).

The cartilages become damaged or split by a sudden twisting movement of the knee, particularly if it is slightly bent and taking weight at the same time. Soccer players may be tackled in just this situation, which explains why they suffer 'cartilage trouble' so commonly. A sudden severe pain is felt in the knee as the cartilage tears, and swelling follows. Continuing pain and intermittent 'locking' or 'giving way' of the knee frequently follow the acute injury.

The cartilage never heals once damaged, but it may cause little trouble. Aching may persist for some weeks after the original injury but slowly wears off if the joint is not again subjected to sudden twisting movements. This is impossible for athletes or sportsmen and the cartilage may have to be removed surgically. The cartilage is usually removed after opening the joint but recent developments suggest that they may in future be removed through an arthroscope inserted into the closed joint. Provided the muscles around the knee are exercised and strong, the stability of the joint does not suffer from removal of the cartilage.

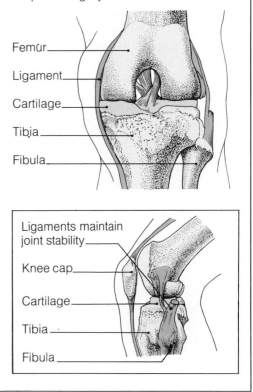

CARTILAGES OF THE KNEE

Injuries to the knee cartilages are 20 times more common in men, particularly in sportsmen. Sometimes damage will heal naturally or with the help of physiotherapy, but more often it requires surgery.

Femur

Ligament

Cartilage

Tibia

Fibula

Ligaments maintain joint stability

Knee cap

Cartilage

Tibia

Fibula

Cataract

Any opacity in the lens of the eye. Depending upon the density and site of the cataract, vision may be blurred or lost completely in the affected eye. Cataracts may follow trauma. They occur frequently in the elderly—earlier if they are diabetic.

Removal of a damaged lens from the eye restores sight but strong lenses must then be worn to compensate for the lost power of the removed lens.

(*See* chart, page 54; *also* Eye disorders, page 67.)

Catarrh

The excessive secretion of mucus from the lining of the nose and throat, usually the result of a common cold (page 63) or hay fever (page 119). This lining

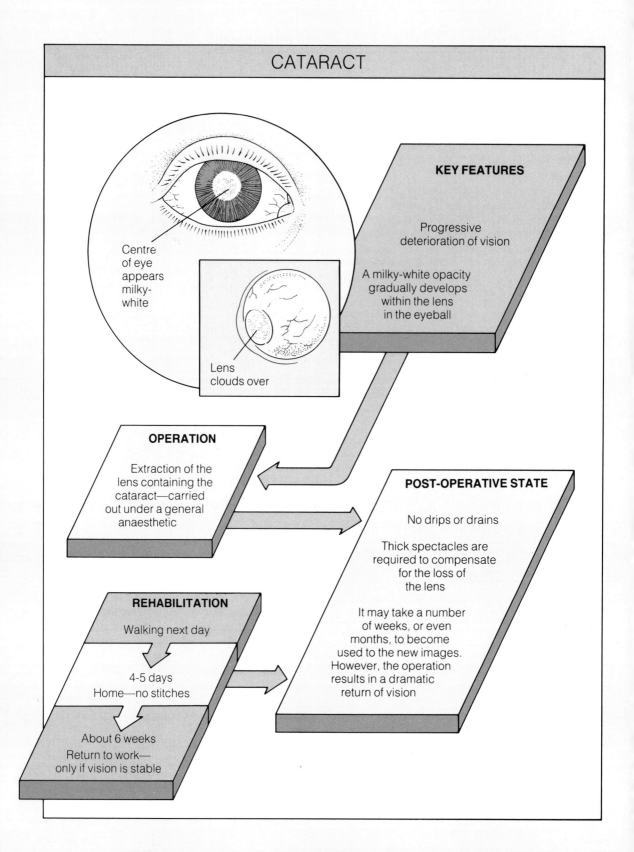

CATARACT

KEY FEATURES

Progressive deterioration of vision

A milky-white opacity gradually develops within the lens in the eyeball

Centre of eye appears milky-white

Lens clouds over

OPERATION

Extraction of the lens containing the cataract—carried out under a general anaesthetic

POST-OPERATIVE STATE

No drips or drains

Thick spectacles are required to compensate for the loss of the lens

It may take a number of weeks, or even months, to become used to the new images. However, the operation results in a dramatic return of vision

REHABILITATION

Walking next day

4-5 days
Home—no stitches

About 6 weeks
Return to work—only if vision is stable

normally secretes just enough fluid to keep moist, but it reacts to infection or irritation by secreting excess fluid in an attempt to clear the irritant. This results in nasal stuffiness or a running nose. There may be a blocked-up feeling at the back of the mouth and sneezing. Catarrh is not a serious symptom and settles in 2–4 days.

During the course of a heavy cold, it is common to become hoarse or to cough up white phlegm from the chest. If this becomes green, brown or yellow, this suggests that bronchitis has developed and medical advice should be sought, as a course of antibiotics may be required (*see* Bronchitis). Sufferers from previous attacks of bronchitis or asthma are more prone to this complication.

Persistent catarrh with blockage of the nose in children may be due to large adenoids. Steam or menthol inhalations (Vick) and decongestant nose drops or sprays—e.g. ephedrine preparations or xylometazoline (Otrivine) often help in the short term but should not be used for more than a few days. Ephedrine and ephedrine-like drugs are available in tablet or liquid form (e.g. Actifed) and act by constricting the local blood vessels and decreasing the blood supply which is the source of the secretions. Antibiotics have no place in the treatment of catarrh, which usually results from a virus infection.

Cauliflower ear

An occupational hazard of boxers and rugby football players. The flexible external ear (pinna) is squashed by a direct blow or while in the scrum and a blood clot (haematoma) then forms. The bruise disappears, but there may be permanent damage to the underlying cartilage and the normal corrugated shape of the ear never returns. The small, flattened puffy ear of a boxer or seasoned rugby player looks not unlike a cauliflower, albeit somewhat moth-eaten.

Cerebellum

Part of the brain and situated below the occipital cortex (*see* diagram, page 257). The cerebellum is connected to the brain stem and thence up to the rest of the brain and down to the spinal cord. It is partially responsible for the control of balance and the co-ordination of fine and coarse movements of the muscles controlling the limbs and speech. Disorders of the cerebellum may cause slurring of speech and a tremor which produces difficulties with fine movements as used in sewing and surgery.

Cerebral palsy

Paralysis of one or more limbs due to disease of the brain or cerebrum. This commonly occurs following strokes (page 217), and is a feature of a child who is spastic (*see* Spastic children).

Cerebrovascular accident
SEE STROKE

Cervical smear

The investigation performed to detect early pre-cancerous cells in the cervix of the womb (uterus). A small wooden spatula or spoon is inserted through a metal tube called a speculum, into the vagina and gently rubbed against the tissues of the cervix. In a similar procedure, the buccal smear, loose cells are removed from the inside of the cheeks for microscopical examination. The tissue removed is smeared onto a slide, stained and then examined under a microscope. If pre-cancerous cells are seen, the results of treatment are excellent and the development of a possible cancer avoided. Women of 35 years and over are advised to have a smear performed every year or two and there is growing evidence that this advice applies perhaps to even younger women if they have had a number of sexual partners or started sexual activity unusually young.

Cervix
(LATIN: NECK)

The neck of the womb (uterus) (*see also* Genital tract: female; *and* the diagram, page 263). It is a narrow part of the uterus, connecting its body to the top of the vagina. It is the part directly visible to the gynaecologist on examination.

Chapped hands

Occurs if they are not carefully dried. It is more common in those with the greatest exposure (e.g. housewives, fish merchants), but why some are more susceptible is unknown.

Prevention is by carefully drying the hands if wet, and by using gloves and, if necessary, barrier creams.

Chest

Contains the heart (page 120), the lungs (page 147), the oesophagus (gullet, page 116), the trachea (page 228) and numerous other internal structures. These are encased in the rib cage, enclosed at the back by the bones of the spine (i.e. the vertebrae) and in front by the breastbone (sternum). The relationships of these structures is shown in the section on Anatomy (page 251 onwards).

Chest infections

The common chest infections are acute bronchitis and pneumonia. Both produce fever, cough, infected sputum and variable degrees of breathlessness and wheezing.

The lungs (page 147) consist of many-branching tubes (the bronchi) which become progressively smaller and open into minute blind-ended sacs, or alveoli. The alveoli are richly supplied with blood and are the site of oxygen absorption. The bronchi serve only to deliver the air to the alveoli.

Infection in the bronchi is bronchitis (page 48) and infection within the alveoli is pneumonia (page 179). The distinction is important because when the alveoli are infected the exchange of oxygen is likely to be impaired. Bronchitis and pneumonia are caused by infection with bacteria and viruses, and worsened by irritants such as cigarette smoke.

Treatment
It is important to drink plenty of fluids to prevent dehydration as the result of the fever. Aspirin or paracetamol usually keep the temperature down. Steam or menthol inhalations help to remove the phlegm from the chest, but in severe chest infections physiotherapy may also be required.

The organisms which cause pneumonia are well known and respond rapidly to the correct antibiotics. In previously healthy individuals complete recovery can be confidently expected.

Bronchitis is caused by smoking or viruses, which do not respond to antibiotics—these are usually required only if bacterial pneumonia supervenes.

Chest pain

Caused by damage, infection or irritation of any of the structures within it (*see* Chest). By far the most common cause of pain is strain of the joints holding the ribs to the vertebrae and sternum, or of the slips of muscle between the individual ribs. This may result from lying in an uncomfortable position, or follow unfamiliar exercise or activity. Athletes commonly develop muscle and joint strains when beginning to train at the start of an athletic season.

Simple strains settle within 5–10 days and are partially relieved by local heat (e.g. a hot-water bottle) and aspirin. Occasionally a pulled intercostal muscle (between the ribs) may give painful symptoms for months because it is obviously impossible to rest it completely.

Certain types of pain indicate more serious disorders and are due to indigestion, oesophageal reflux (*see* Heartburn *and* Hiatus hernia), nerve irritation as in shingles (*Herpes zoster, see* Zoster), heart disease (*see* Angina), pulmonary blood clots (*see* Pulmonary embolus), and irritation of the pleura, the fine surface lining of the lungs (pleurisy, page 178). This last may be secondary to pneumonia (page 179).

Chickenpox

A common infectious disease, usually contracted in childhood. The illness is usually mild and the child is most infectious just before he develops the characteristic spots. He may feel slightly unwell but not sufficiently ill to go to bed and so remains up and about, passing on the virus to his friends and schoolmates.

The incubation period (i.e. the time between initial contact and the appearance of the clinical disease) is 15–18 days, but extremes of 7 and 26 days can occur. Although the illness may begin with spots, lethargy, headache and a sore throat often precede them for 1 or 2 days. Large numbers of small, round, white spots then appear which are slightly raised above the level of the surrounding skin. They look like blisters or small drops of water lying on the skin and are numerous on the head, face and body, with fewer over the shins and forearms. The spots become surrounded by small red areas of skin and then slowly dry and crust, leaving a faint scar. This scarring gradually fades provided there has not been too much scratching. The rash is very irritating and it is difficult to avoid scratching. (*See* illustration, page 235.)

Calamine lotion partially relieves the itching and is well worth using, because scratching can produce secondary infection as well as scarring. Antihistamines taken by mouth are sometimes useful at the height of the symptoms; they reduce skin irritation and produce sedation. Because the cause of the illness is a virus, antibiotics are useless except when secondary bacterial infection occurs.

Complications following chickenpox are rare.

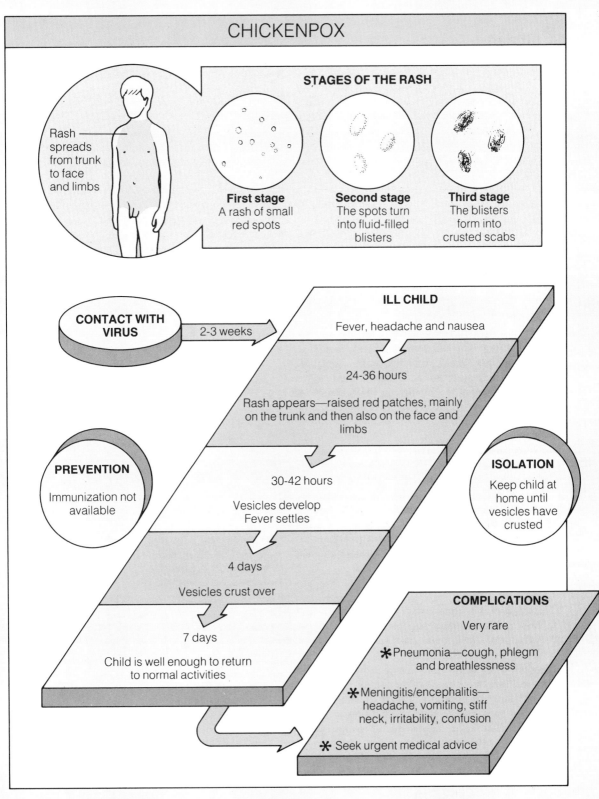

CHICKENPOX

STAGES OF THE RASH

Rash spreads from trunk to face and limbs

First stage
A rash of small red spots

Second stage
The spots turn into fluid-filled blisters

Third stage
The blisters form into crusted scabs

CONTACT WITH VIRUS

2-3 weeks

ILL CHILD

Fever, headache and nausea

24-36 hours

Rash appears—raised red patches, mainly on the trunk and then also on the face and limbs

30-42 hours

Vesicles develop
Fever settles

PREVENTION

Immunization not available

4 days

Vesicles crust over

7 days

Child is well enough to return to normal activities

ISOLATION

Keep child at home until vesicles have crusted

COMPLICATIONS

Very rare

* Pneumonia—cough, phlegm and breathlessness

* Meningitis/encephalitis— headache, vomiting, stiff neck, irritability, confusion

* Seek urgent medical advice

Chilblains
(PERNIOSIS)

Small painful red or purple patches which appear on the tips of the toes, the heels and the fingers. At first they itch but they may become painful. The cause is unknown but is believed to be the result of a combination of cold and damp. Chilblains are prevented by keeping the feet and body warm in the winter.

Treatment is disappointing and there is little evidence to support the use of large amounts of vitamin C, and ointments give only transient relief of pain. Corn pads take the pressure off the lesions and prevent them rubbing against footwear. Most chilblains disappear in the spring and prevention is the best remedy.

Chiropody

The art of foot care. Disorders commonly dealt with by chiropodists include bunions, corns, verrucas, hammer toes and ingrowing toe nails. Expert care of the feet is essential in diabetics, in whom the blood and nerve supply are defective.

Bunion
An uncomfortable and painful swelling at the side of the base of the big toe, caused by wearing poorly fitting shoes. Bunions are associated with hallux valgus, where the big toe is pushed against, and often over, the other toes. Initially the bunion is uncomfortable, and chiropody, local heat, rest and better-fitting shoes may be sufficient treatment. If not, the big toe may have to be straightened surgically.

Corns
Thick pads of skin which occur on any part of the foot in response to continual rubbing or pressure, and they consist of small, round, hard areas of callus with a central core containing skin cells packed tightly together. They result from poorly fitting shoes and abnormalities in the shape of the toes or feet. Corns are not dangerous but, if painful, can be removed.

'Corn pads' can be used to take pressure off a small, circular corn. Ointments or paints which dissolve away the excess layers of skin must be used with great care, as they may burn the skin around the corn. Paring down a corn with a scalpel blade should be performed only by a chiropodist because there is a danger of cutting into and infecting the normal surrounding skin.

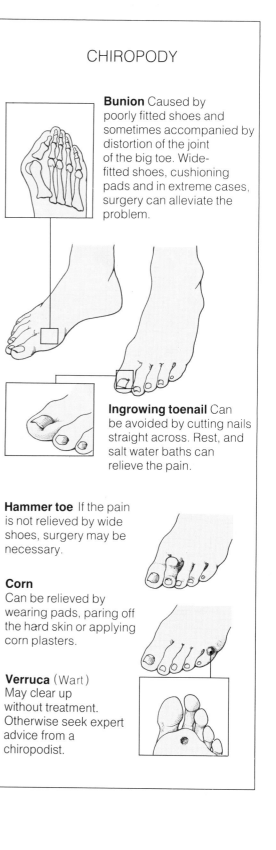

CHIROPODY

Bunion Caused by poorly fitted shoes and sometimes accompanied by distortion of the joint of the big toe. Wide-fitted shoes, cushioning pads and in extreme cases, surgery can alleviate the problem.

Ingrowing toenail Can be avoided by cutting nails straight across. Rest, and salt water baths can relieve the pain.

Hammer toe If the pain is not relieved by wide shoes, surgery may be necessary.

Corn Can be relieved by wearing pads, paring off the hard skin or applying corn plasters.

Verruca (Wart) May clear up without treatment. Otherwise seek expert advice from a chiropodist.

58

Hallux valgus (bent big toe)

The big toe may become bent over the other toes if tight or pointed shoes are worn. This crowds the other toes and predisposes to bunions, corns or hammer toes. Expert chiropody, with padding of the now prominent joint at the base of the toe, may relieve the symptoms, but if the toe becomes persistently uncomfortable and inconvenient, then it can be straightened surgically.

Hammer toe

A toe which has become excessively bent under by wearing shoes which are too tight. The prominent knuckle which forms may rub against the shoe, resulting in a painful corn. If the toe is not too stiff, it can be straightened with a small splint; otherwise surgery is required.

Ingrowing toe nails

Result from cutting the nails flush to the skin. This leaves the advancing edge of the nail below the level of the skin folds on each side, and, as the nail grows forward, the two edges penetrate the skin—which becomes infected. As a result, ingrowing toe nails are extremely painful.

They can be prevented by cutting the nails correctly, i.e. straight across to leave a small protruding corner of nail on each side. When the nail regrows it will then ride up over the skin instead of burrowing into it.

If the skin and tissues around the nail become infected, antibiotics may be required. If unsuccessful or if the infection recurs the entire nail may have to be removed surgically.

Verruca (plantar wart)

A wart growing on the sole of the foot. (Warts—page 247—are caused by a virus infection in the skin.) A verruca is often painful because it is pressed into the foot by the patient's weight. They can be confused with corns, and for this reason and in order to obtain correct treatment, an expert chiropodist should be consulted.

Verrucas are not serious and not very infectious. They are self-limiting and disappear within a year or two—which probably accounts for the apparent success of bizarre traditional remedies. Various medical preparations are used to speed the spontaneous disappearance. One method is to soak the verruca in formaldehyde solution (available on prescription) every day while protecting the normal surrounding skin with petroleum jelly (Vaseline).

School staff may over-react to the presence of a verruca and this can be resolved by wearing special protective socks (available from sports shops) whilst swimming or playing sports.

Chiropractice

A system of treatment based on the theory that disease is caused by an interference with nerve function and that this can be restored to normal by manipulation, particularly of the spinal column.

Chiropractice is not formally recognized by the medical profession.

Cholecystitis

Inflammation of the gall bladder, which produces pain in the upper abdomen (usually on the right side) with fever, nausea and vomiting. Gall stones (page 106) may be present, and if so can be removed with the inflamed gall bladder—the operation is termed cholecystectomy (page 60). The pain can be confused with indigestion and stomach ulcers (*see also* Abdominal pain).

Cholera

An acute infection of the bowel, caused by the organism *Vibrio cholerae*. This is ingested and produces a severe enteritis (*see* Gastro-enteritis) with profuse diarrhoea. The loss of fluid and salts from the bowel may be enormous (e.g. 10–20 litres, 17.5–35 pints) and, if left untreated, results in severe dehydration and even death. Cholera is transmitted in drinking water which has become contaminated by excreta from someone already suffering from the illness. Outbreaks occur where sanitation is poor.

Treatment consists of rapid replacement of the lost fluid and salts. Dacca Solution is widely used in the tropics and contains fluid and salts in exactly the same proportions as those lost in the diarrhoeal fluid. Prevention is much better than cure, and adequate sanitation by preventing faecal contamination of water supplies makes spread almost impossible. Vaccination is now available but it is effective for only a short time and must be repeated every 6 months to achieve adequate immunity. Travellers to the tropics or where sanitation standards may be poor should be vaccinated prior to departure if cholera is present in the area. It is, however, more important not to drink from sources which might be suspect, or to eat food washed in that water.

GALL BLADDER REMOVAL (Cholecystectomy)

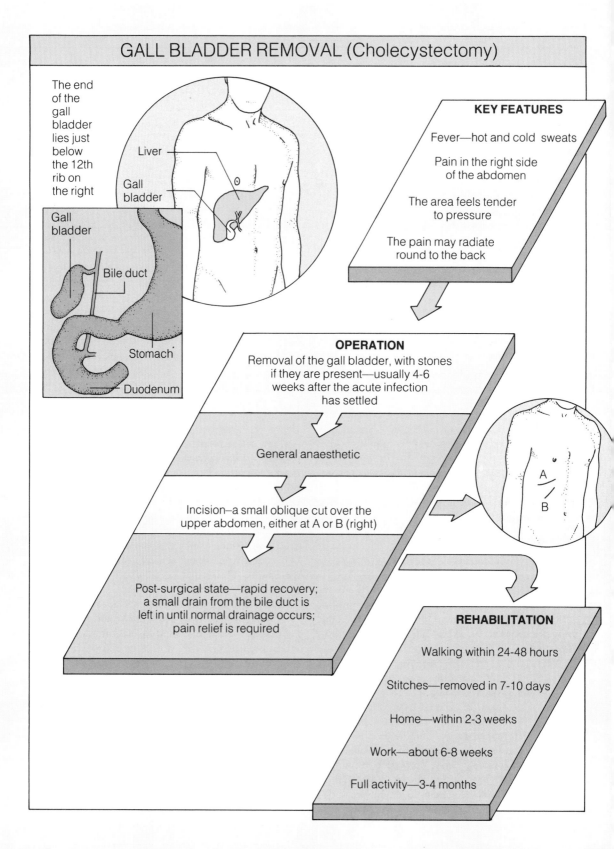

The end of the gall bladder lies just below the 12th rib on the right

Liver

Gall bladder

Gall bladder

Bile duct

Stomach

Duodenum

KEY FEATURES

Fever—hot and cold sweats

Pain in the right side of the abdomen

The area feels tender to pressure

The pain may radiate round to the back

OPERATION

Removal of the gall bladder, with stones if they are present—usually 4-6 weeks after the acute infection has settled

General anaesthetic

Incision—a small oblique cut over the upper abdomen, either at A or B (right)

Post-surgical state—rapid recovery; a small drain from the bile duct is left in until normal drainage occurs; pain relief is required

A
B

REHABILITATION

Walking within 24-48 hours

Stitches—removed in 7-10 days

Home—within 2-3 weeks

Work—about 6-8 weeks

Full activity—3-4 months

Cholesterol

A major constituent of fatty foods found in milk, butter, eggs and liver. Cholesterol may form stones in the gall bladder, and is laid down on the inner walls of blood vessels resulting in severe narrowing—a major cause of angina (page 19), heart attacks (page 120) and strokes (page 217). There is limited evidence that reduction of the dietary intake of cholesterol reduces the risk of heart attacks and strokes, but controlling the blood pressure (*see* Blood pressure) and stopping smoking (page 208) are more important.

Chorea
GREEK: *CHOREIA*, DANCE

Abnormal jerking movements of the limbs, which occurs in rheumatic fever (page 195) and Huntington's chorea (page 129). The commonest cause of abnormal movements is a tic or habit spasm in children, and they invariably grow out of them.

Chromosome abnormalities
SEE GENETIC DISORDERS

Chronic illness

An illness which persists for a considerable time, i.e. months or years. It is not necessarily severe and, indeed, may be quite mild. There may be acute episodes of worse illness during this period. Examples of chronic illness include rheumatoid arthritis, duodenal ulcer and chronic bronchitis.

Circulation
SEE HEART

Circulation disorders
SEE ARTERIAL DISEASE

Circumcision

The removal of the foreskin (prepuce) from the penis. Until recently it was common for male babies to be circumcised soon after birth, at the request of the parents, because it was believed to be more hygienic. Secretions can become trapped behind the foreskin, but in the adult regular washing with the foreskin pulled back is all that is required.

Forcible attempts to pull back the foreskin in babies and toddlers may cause infection because the foreskin is not designed to retract as in the adult.

Circumcision may be performed for religious reasons. The medical indication for circumcision is if the foreskin covering the end of the penis is so tight that the passage of urine is obstructed (phimosis). It is recognized from the foreskin ballooning out when urine is passed and a stream which is reduced to a trickle. Removal of the foreskin is curative. Circumcision may also be necessary if there is chronic inflammation of the end of the penis. There is a very small risk that the wound will become infected, or that the tip of the penis may be damaged at operation but this is extremely rare in the hands of a good surgeon.

Cirrhosis

A disease of the liver, usually caused by excessive consumption of alcohol. In its mildest form it can be diagnosed only by removing a small piece of liver tissue and examining it under a microscope (liver biopsy, *see* Biopsy). A blood test may give the first clue by showing abnormalities in liver function. If alcoholic cirrhosis is detected at this stage and the excessive intake of alcohol curbed, the disease often resolves of its own accord. However, if it is allowed to progress then ill health, liver failure and even death may follow. In chronic alcoholism, not only is there an excessive intake of alcohol but also a diet poor in protein and vitamins, as alcohol is taken to the exclusion of food (*see* Alcoholism).

The complications of cirrhosis are generalized infection, retention of fluid in the abdomen (which becomes extremely swollen), and bleeding from the oesophagus and stomach. There is no satisfactory treatment other than stopping alcohol in the early stages. The complications are treated as they arise. Antibiotics are given for infection, diuretics to remove excess fluid if it collects in the abdomen, and blood to replace the loss during bleeding.

Claustrophobia
(LATIN: *CLAUSTRUM*, BARRIER. GREEK: *PHOBOS*, FEAR)

An irrational fear of being cooped up in confined spaces such as lifts, crowded shops and streets, and tunnels. Everyone possesses this fear to a limited extent, but in the claustrophobic it may become an overpowering and incapacitating obsession.

Severe claustrophobia is very rare, and treatment

should be guided by a psychiatrist with special expertise and experience. Psychotherapy is often used but improvement can be expected only after months or even years of treatment.

Cleft palate

Cleft palate and hare lip (page 119) are common birth deformities which are usually correctable using plastic surgery (*see also* Palate, page 165).

Club foot
(TALIPES)

Minor degrees of club foot are common in newly born babies, probably as a result of pressure on the foot while in the uterus. This usually corrects itself within a few days.

Occasionally the feet remain permanently turned downwards and inwards so that they look towards each other. Alternatively, the feet become drawn up at the ankle joint so that the upper surface of the foot meets the lower part of shin.

The first variety is more difficult to treat but may respond to regular physiotherapy and splinting to restore normal posture and muscle strength. If this fails, orthopaedic surgery is required to realign the bones. Club foot with the foot drawn up to meet the lower tibia usually improves with physiotherapy and exercises.

Club foot and spina bifida (page 213) may occur together. Medical attention should be sought for any baby with club feet.

Coal miner's lung
SEE PNEUMOCONIOSIS

Cocaine

A drug of addiction, which produces elation and excitement like that with amphetamines ('speed'). It is usually taken as snuff ('snow') and may give rise to nasal ulceration. Tolerance does not occur.

Coeliac disease

A rare disease, usually of children who are unable to digest fats. This is caused by a decrease in area of the absorptive surface on the inner wall of the small intestine due to a sensitivity to ingested wheat

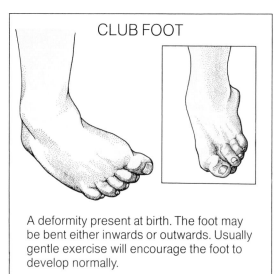

CLUB FOOT

A deformity present at birth. The foot may be bent either inwards or outwards. Usually gentle exercise will encourage the foot to develop normally.

gluten. As a result the child passes very large amounts of pale faeces.

Coeliac disease is cured completely by eating only foods from which gluten is totally excluded.

Coil
SEE UNDER FAMILY PLANNING

Coitus interruptus

A method of birth control (*see* Family planning).

Cold sores
(HERPES SIMPLEX)

Small superficial blisters which appear around the mouth and sometimes the nostrils during a cold, an attack of sinusitis or an acute chest infection. They are caused by the virus, *Herpes simplex,* which survives in the skin around the mouth in an inactive state until another infection lowers body resistance, allowing the virus to grow and form blisters. Cold sores are not serious and settle with the precipitating illness, which is usually not serious itself. The blisters should be kept dry and will heal completely after about 10 days. The exudate and crusts are potentially infective especially to small babies—handling and kissing should be kept to a minimum during the active phase of the disease. (*See* illustration, page 237.)

Colds

Recognized from the well known symptoms of running and stuffed-up nose, sneezing, sore throat and running eyes, with or without a fever. They are more common in the spring and autumn, but can occur at any time.

More than 150 viruses are known to cause colds, and each year different viruses spread through the community by coughing and sneezing, especially in large gatherings. Immunity to one virus gives no immunity to the others, and this, combined with the impossibility of predicting which virus or viruses will strike next, makes it impossible to develop an effective vaccine.

The frequent gathering of people indoors rather than out, particularly in schools, is an important means of spread. Research suggests that the cold viruses survive more easily at lower temperatures and a latent infection may be converted to an active form by a cooler environment.

What to do about a cold

Most colds get better on their own. Treatment is aimed at relieving the symptoms, although it will not shorten the illness. Sore throats are often relieved by aspirin gargles two or three times daily or sucking sweets or lozenges. If the cold causes streaming or a stuffy nose, steam or menthol inhalations and a decongestant spray or drops (such as Otrivine) often give relief.

Small babies who are unable to breathe through their noses while sucking may become breathless during feeds. Nose drops given just before each feed may help, and any marked shortness of breath must be reported to the doctor. Older children who find it difficult to sleep because of catarrh or a cough, may obtain relief from a night-time dose of a syrup (e.g. Actifed) which dries up the nasal secretions. Simple cough linctuses are ineffective and none of the proprietary products is better than codeine linctus.

Antibiotics are valueless in virus illness including colds unless secondary infection by bacteria supervenes. Sinusitis, laryngitis, bronchitis and asthma may follow a simple cold. People who suffer from severe chronic bronchitis or asthma may need a course of antibiotics if they frequently develop bacterial infections of the lung following colds.

Aspirin for sore throat and to reduce the fever, with a tot of whisky or hot lemon, are still as effective as any treatment for colds. Vitamin C taken for prevention or for treatment has no proven effect.

★ Colic

A sharp griping pain, coming in waves, which makes the sufferer roll about in agony. Colic is caused by severe contraction in a muscular tube attempting to remove an obstruction. It is a characteristic feature of intestinal obstruction (page 136), kidney stones (page 141) which have passed into the ureter, and gall stones (page 106) in the bile ducts.

Collapse
SEE BLACKOUTS

Colon
(GREEK: *KOLON*, LARGE INTESTINE)

The major part of the large intestine, stretching from the caecum to the rectum (*see also* Intestines). Its prime function is to reabsorb water which has passed through the small intestine.

Colour blindness

The retina, the light-sensitive back layer of the eye contains two types of cell: rods and cones (*see* Eye). The cones contain pigments which determine colour vision, and deficiency or absence of these pigments results in colour blindness. The defect is genetically determined and present from birth. About 8 per cent of men and 0.4 per cent of women are colour blind to some degree, and the most common variety produces confusion between red and green. Very often the sufferer from colour blindness is unaware of his disability unless he has a job where colour differentiation is important.

The presence of defective colour vision can be determined by the use of special charts (page 34).

★ Coma

A state of unconsciousness but excluding normal sleep. Loss of consciousness is considered with blackouts (page 39).

Compound fracture

A fracture which has broken the skin. There is an increased risk of bone infection, and the fractured bones must be realigned, the wound cleaned and the skin closed surgically under full anaesthesia to prevent further damage.

★Concussion

Loss of consciousness from a head injury. If mild (e.g. head injury during a boxing contest), consciousness may return rapidly—even within seconds; but severe damage (e.g. following a traffic accident) may result in days or months of unconsciousness. It may follow a small bleed into the brain, and even if consciousness is regained rapidly a careful medical assessment is essential.

Condom

The alternative name for sheath (see Family planning).

Confusion
SEE DELIRIUM; AND DEMENTIA

Congenital dislocation of the hip
SEE UNDER DISLOCATION

Conjunctivitis

The conjunctiva is a thin membrane which covers the front of the eyeball. Because the eye is exposed infection, irritation and damage are common. The symptoms of conjunctivitis are redness, grittiness and watering (page 67). When the inflammation is due to a virus or to allergy (as in hay fever), the discharge from the eye is watery. When the infection is bacterial the fluid is sticky and may be yellow or green. The discharge is most noticeable in the morning when the eyelids may be stuck together.

Babies and children under a year old sometimes have a persistently watering or sticky eye due to blockage of the duct (the naso-lacrimal duct) which drains the tears from the eye into the nose. This is not a serious condition and usually resolves spontaneously by the child's first birthday as the facial bones grow. Occasionally a minor operation is needed to unblock the duct.

Treatment
Antibiotic eye drops are required for bacterial conjunctivitis. When caused by viruses and hay fever, decongestant eye drops relieve the symptoms but not the cause. Conjunctivitis is not normally dangerous, being sufficiently uncomfortable for most patients to seek treatment early. Metal workers and welders are at special risk and should always wear protective goggles when working to prevent damage from hot metal splinters. Medical advice should always be obtained for a baby with a sticky eye.

Constipation

Normal people may have between three bowel actions per day and three per week. Normally the bowel wall is stretched by the presence of a stool, and this induces a desire to defecate. If this is ignored or consciously over-ridden, the stool becomes dry, hard and difficult to pass and the bowel becomes chronically stretched. The reflex may be lost and constipation is the inevitable result. When the rock-hard motion is finally passed it may produce a small tear of the anus, a fissure, with a slight amount of bleeding. (Note Any bleeding from the rectum should be reported to your doctor.)

Treatment
The best treatment for constipation is to eat a diet rich in roughage. Examples of such foods and of fibre-free foods are given below.

High-fibre foods
  Bran
  'All Bran', 'Bran Buds', 'Bran Flakes', 'Sultana Bran'
  Root crops, such as potatoes and carrots, with their skins

Medium-fibre foods
  Peas, beans, lentils, groundnuts
  Whole cereals, whole wheat meal, wholemeal bread, oatmeal, brown rice, whole rye crispbread, whole grain breakfast cereals, maize meal, millet meal, root crops such as potatoes, cassava and yams (without their skins), plantains, figs, dates, bananas

Low-fibre foods
  'Bran Flakes', 'Sultana Bran'
  Brown bread
  Leaf and root vegetables, most soft fruits (except those mentioned above)
  White bread, white rice, maize cornflour, most breakfast cereals

Fibre-free foods
  All fats, vegetable and animal; milk, cheese, sugar, meat, fish, eggs
  Beverages, beer, wine, tea, coffee, alcohol and most fruit juice drinks.

Many of the drugs used in the treatment of constipation (e.g. Isogel, Normacol or Fybogel) are bulk laxatives and add roughage to the diet. Senna (Senokot) works by irritating the muscles of the bowel, which respond by forcibly pushing the stool out. The danger with Senokot and similar laxatives is that the bowel may eventually not act without them. They should be used only for a few days at a time.

Note In the middle aged and elderly, constipation developing over a few weeks or months for no obvious reason (such as a change of diet or immobility) can result from partial blockage of the bowel and medical advice should be sought. This applies also to babies who are constipated from birth.

Contact lenses
SEE GLASSES

Contraception
SEE FAMILY PLANNING

★Convulsions
IN CHILDREN: *SEE* FEVER
IN ADULTS: *SEE* EPILEPSY

Corn
SEE UNDER CHIROPODY

Cornea

A transparent covering in front of the iris and pupil (*see under* Eye). Transplants of cornea can often restore sight when blindness is due to opacity of the cornea (page 68). Corneal ulcer is described on page 69.

Coronary arteries

The arteries which supply blood to the muscle of the heart. Narrowing or obstruction may cause a heart attack (page 120) or angina (page 19).

★Coronary thrombosis

A thrombus or clot in one of the coronary arteries which supply blood to the heart muscle is a common cause of heart attacks (or 'coronaries'). The features are described on page 120.

Corticosteroids
SEE STEROIDS

Cot death
(SUDDEN INFANT DEATH SYNDROME)

The sudden, unexpected and unexplained death of an infant usually between the age of 4 weeks and 6 months is called a cot death. Typically the baby appears well when put to bed, only to be found dead the next morning.

The cause of cot deaths is unknown although a number of theories have been suggested. They are more common in the late winter or early spring months when respiratory infections are at their height, and some authorities believe that a sudden overwhelming respiratory infection is responsible. Another theory is that these babies fail to clear their tracheas whilst asleep and the secretions obstruct air flow—if the baby is deeply asleep it cannot overcome the obstruction. Cot death is very unusual in breast-fed babies and cow's milk allergy has been suggested as a possible cause.

Cot deaths are tragic events with, at present, no known means of prevention. There is no evidence to suggest that cot deaths are more likely to happen to subsequent children of the same family.

The psychological effects of this tragedy on both parents cannot be over-emphasized. If required, expert advice can be obtained to enable them to recover from their loss and to discuss future pregnancies.

Cough

This common symptom is caused by irritation of any part of the respiratory tract. It may involve the upper part (i.e. the nose, mouth, throat, pharynx and larynx) or the lower part (i.e. the trachea, the main breathing tubes (bronchi) and lungs).

By far the commonest cause of cough is infection of the upper tract by viruses, particularly the common cold viruses. They infect and irritate the throat or pharynx (*see* Pharyngitis), and can inflame the tonsils at the back of the throat (*see* Tonsillitis). Inflammation of the nasal sinuses (*see* Sinusitis) may spread to involve the pharynx and cause cough. Infection of the larynx (*see* Laryngitis) is less common and so is infection of the trachea (*see* Tracheitis), the bronchi (*see* Bronchitis) or the lung (*see* Pneumonia). The cough is a nervous reflex in response to irritation of the delicate surface lining of the airways, clearly developed in an attempt to remove the irritation.

Usually the cough disappears within 2–4 weeks as the infection clears, although it may persist for a few more weeks, often more noticeably at night. Even coughs which persist for more than 5 or 6 weeks usually disappear on their own, but it is important to seek medical advice because in some rare cases more serious lung disease may be present. This is particularly so in smokers, in whom lung cancer and bronchitis are relatively common (page 208). Tuberculosis of the lung (page 230) is no longer a common cause of coughing.

Treatment of simple coughs is necessary if they are severe or prevent sleep. Cough linctus can be obtained from a chemist or doctor and commonly contains small amounts of codeine, a cough suppressant.

Most coughs are not serious and disappear on their own, but if the cough persists after 5 or 6 weeks, it is important to seek medical advice.

Cramp

Painful spasm of a muscle or group of muscles which undergo powerful sustained contraction. The cause is unknown. Though painful, cramp is not serious and usually settles in a few minutes; if it is recurrent, treatment with quinine may relieve it. Cramp is relieved by gently stretching the muscle—e.g. bending the foot up at the ankle if the calf muscle is affected.

Cramp after heavy work or exercise in a hot climate is prevented by taking salt tablets.

Recurrent cramp in the calves is due to narrowing of the arteries to the legs, so that insufficient blood and oxygen reach the calf muscles during exercise. The pain disappears after 1 or 2 minutes, only to recur on further exertion. This is known as intermittent claudication (limping) and can be corrected surgically by inserting an artery graft to bypass the obstructed blood vessel.

Cretinism

Thyroid under-activity during fetal life or in early infancy causes poor development and slow growth with mental retardation. If detected early, the process can be completely corrected by replacing the absent hormone with thyroxine—which must be taken regularly for the remainder of life.

Crohn's disease
(REGIONAL ILEITIS; REGIONAL ENTERITIS)

A disease of the bowel which usually affects young adults. Segments of the small intestine and, less commonly, the large intestine become inflamed and this may lead to colicky abdominal pain. The patients often feel generally unwell, with loss of appetite and weight, and fever.

Crohn's disease varies from very mild, with few if any attacks of abdominal pain and diarrhoea, to severe with chronic ill health and frequent acute attacks. Although the cause remains unknown, treatment is becoming more effective. It must be very carefully supervised, and this is best achieved in specialist departments.

Prednisolone is used to suppress the intestinal inflammation. Rarely, the intestine becomes obstructed and this must be relieved surgically.

★ Croup

A barking seal-like cough caused by laryngitis which occurs in young children up to the age of 4. Severe croup is rare, but can be both alarming and dangerous.

It is important to distinguish between croup and 'wheezing' because the treatment of the two conditions is different. Both follow catarrhal colds and both tend to produce noisy breathing, but the noise of croup is barking and harsh, and occurs when the child breathes *in*, while wheezing is higher pitched and almost musical in quality and loudest on breathing *out*.

Croup is a serious complication of acute laryngitis in small children (*see* Laryngitis). In adults the larynx is a rigid tube made of rings of hard cartilage. In the young child the walls are softer and the larynx is more 'plastic'. When it becomes seriously inflamed it may collapse if a deep breath in is taken. The turbulence produced by the air passing through a narrowed larynx produces the characteristic 'honking' noise of croup.

Treatment
Croup usually occurs at night and the child may have been noted to have a hoarse voice and a cold. Any difficulty in breathing or any attack of noisy breathing lasting more than a few minutes should always be reported to your doctor immediately. If the child is drowsy or blue or so out of breath that he is unable to talk or walk, notify your doctor immediately or take him direct to hospital.

Eye Disorders

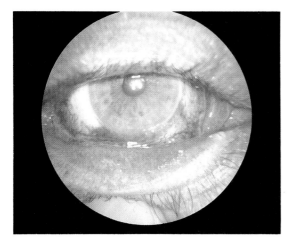

Conjunctivitis *The eye is red, painful and feels 'gritty'. It is usually caused by a virus but the infection may be bacterial and require antibiotics.*

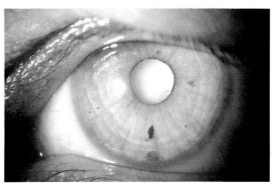

Cataract *The lens of the eye becomes opaque and obscures vision. It may follow injury and is common in diabetes. The lens is removed to restore vision.*

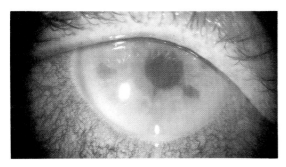

Iritis *Inflammation of the iris causes pain in the eye which is red, particularly around the iris. Visual acuity is reduced.*

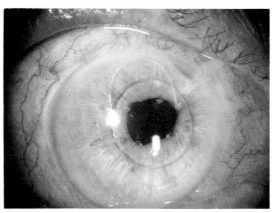

Acrylic lens *This may be inserted into the eye to replace the lens removed for cataracts, and further improve vision.*

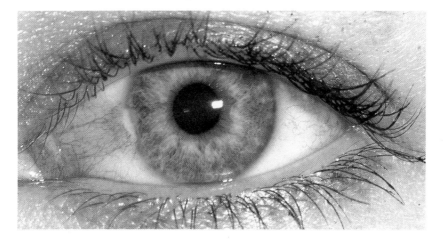

Pterygium *A small leash of blood vessels on the surface of the inner side of the eye. The conjunctiva overlying the pupil is not affected and vision is normal.*

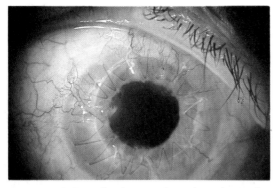

Corneal graft *Corneal grafts are used to replace a damaged or scarred cornea which is obscuring vision. The operation is very successful.*

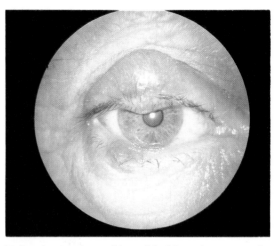

Meibomian cyst *A cyst of the eyelids. It is not dangerous and rarely causes symptoms but if it becomes infected or is unsightly it can be removed.*

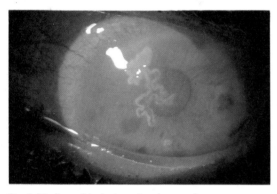

Dendritic (branching) ulcer *An ulcer on the cornea caused by Herpes simplex virus. It is stained brilliant green by the dye fluorescein.*

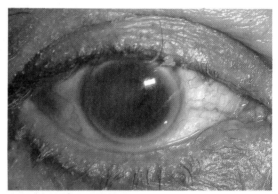

Arcus senilis *A white circle around the cornea, common in the elderly. Occasionally it is associated with an excess of fats in the blood. There is no danger to vision.*

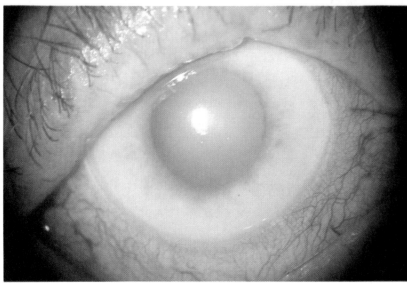

Glaucoma *Increased pressure within the eyeball causes progressive loss of vision in the elderly. There may be no pain initially, unless the rise of pressure is sudden. Seek urgent medical advice.*

Corneal ulcer and corneal scarring *Ulcers follow injury e.g. metal splinters in welders or infection–usually Herpes simplex virus. Ulcers are demonstrated by fluorescein dye dropped into the eye. Corneal ulcers may leave a scar and vision is affected if the scar lies over the pupil.*
Seek urgent medical advice.

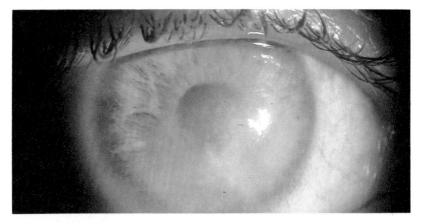

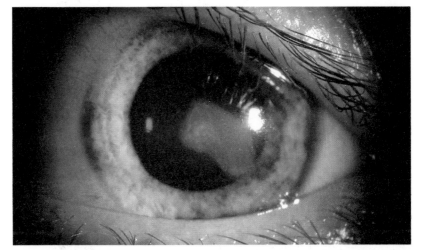

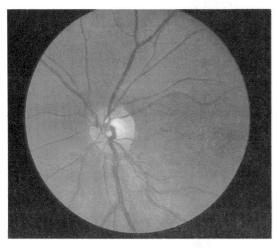

Normal fundus *The appearance through an ophthalmoscope. The optic nerve is seen as a pale central disc from which the blood vessels spread across the retina.*

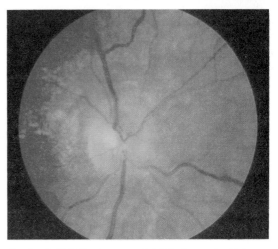

Fundus–in high blood pressure *Initially the arteries thicken. If the blood pressure is not controlled blood and serum seep out to form red haemorrhages and yellow exudates on the retina, with diminished vision.*

69

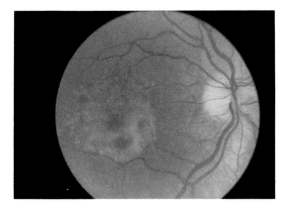

Macular degeneration *The macula is the area of greatest visual acuity. Degeneration causes marked visual deterioration.*

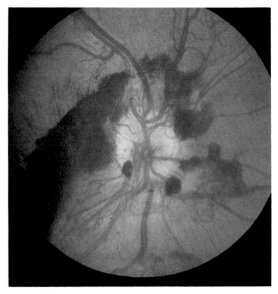

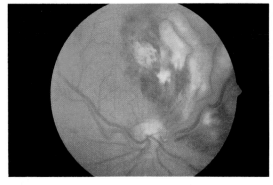

Branch vein occlusion *Blockage of a retinal vein prevents blood flow to a segment of the retina which loses its visual acuity. The remaining retina remains normal.*

Diabetic retinopathy *In severe uncontrolled diabetes vision can deteriorate as the result of infection, cataracts, and retinal damage from leaking retinal arteries.*

Jaundice *The conjunctiva appears yellow due to the high levels of bile in the blood. The commonest causes are virus hepatitis and alcoholic liver disease.*

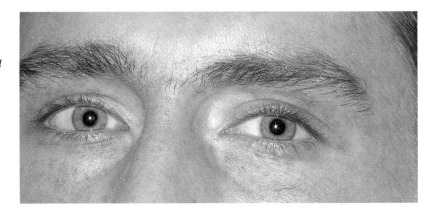

The most effective first aid for croup is to put the child in a warm room and to fill a sheet tented over the child with steam from a boiling kettle. The episode usually settles within a few minutes if steam is inhaled, and by the time the doctor arrives may be well under control. If not, the child may require admission to hospital for observation during the period of acute infection.

Cushing's disease

A rare disorder resulting from over-activity of the adrenal gland (page 13) or the pituitary gland (page 177). There is over-secretion of steroid hormones into the blood and this in turn may cause high blood pressure, diabetes and rapid gain of weight.

Cyanocobalamin
(VITAMIN B$_{12}$) *SEE UNDER* VITAMINS

Cyst

A round fluid-filled lump usually found in the breast, ovary or skin. Sometimes cysts contain fluid under high pressure and feel solid.

Breast cysts
A lump in the breast should always be reported to your doctor. Often they are cysts and this is confirmed by removing the contained fluid through a fine needle. They are benign and in no way cancerous.

Ovarian cysts
The ovaries are the female reproductive organs which produce eggs (ova) monthly at the time of ovulation. One of the commonest disorders of the ovaries is cyst formation. The majority are benign and of no consequence, but they may bleed or twist and cause severe abdominal pain. Sometimes their sheer size causes problems and they may grow to the size of a football. Large cysts have even led to a mistaken diagnosis of pregnancy.

If one ovary is removed because of a cyst, the other takes over the production of female hormones and egg production each month (normally they take it in turns).

Sebaceous cysts ('wens')
These occur in the skin and can appear almost anywhere, although the majority are found on the forehead, scalp, neck and back. The cyst contains greasy secretions originally produced by a sweat gland which has become blocked. They are very common, benign and in no way dangerous. If they are large, unsightly or rub on clothing, they can be removed easily. A local anaesthetic is used for the operation which takes 20–30 minutes, and there is no need to stay in hospital.

Cystic fibrosis

A serious disease of childhood which affects the lungs and pancreas, causing recurrent chest infections and poor absorption of food. The diseased lungs produce a sticky, tenacious secretion which is so difficult to cough up that recurrent chest infections occur. Each bout of infection leaves the lungs slightly more damaged than before and the child's general health suffers from the repeated infections. Modern treatment with antibiotics and vigorous chest physiotherapy cannot prevent these episodes but helps to resolve them.

The normal pancreas provides digestive juices which break down ingested food and allow its absorption. In cystic fibrosis the pancreas becomes blocked by sticky secretions and fails to produce digestive juices in adequate amounts. This leads to chronic diarrhoea, poor weight gain and ill health.

The diagnosis of cystic fibrosis should be suspected in a young child with recurrent chest infections, diarrhoea, general ill health and failure to gain weight. Each chest infection should be treated vigorously with antibiotics and physiotherapy but the long-term outlook for these children is unfortunately poor because the lungs become progressively damaged. The disease is transmitted genetically.

Cystitis
(GREEK: *KYSTIS*, BLADDER; *ITIS*, INFLAMMATION)

Acute infection of the bladder, causing lower abdominal pain, pain on urination (dysuria) and frequency of micturition, sometimes with blood in the urine and fever. Drinking large quantities of water may relieve symptoms. Medical advice should be obtained so that the urine may be cultured for bacteria and the correct antibiotics prescribed.

If cystitis persists or recurs, further detailed investigation—including x-ray of the kidneys and possibly cystoscopy—is necessary to exclude the presence of stones or abnormal renal anatomy.

Cystoscope

A narrow telescope which is inserted into the urethra and used to look into the bladder.

Cystoscopy is usually required to investigate the passing of blood in the urine (haematuria)—usually due to stones or cancer in kidneys or bladder—and for recurrent bladder infection (cystitis).

Modern cystoscopes possess a burning tip (diathermy) which both cuts and coagulates severed blood vessels. They may be used to remove enlarged prostatic tissue obstructing the outflow of urine from the bladder. This operation (transurethral resection) prevents the need for the major operation of prostatectomy through the abdominal wall.

Cytology

The art of staining and studying cells to detect infection or cancer. This is commonly performed on cells taken from the cervix (page 55) of the uterus to detect very early cancer cells (cervical smear, page 55).

D and C
(DILATATION AND CURETTAGE)

The most commonly performed gynaecological operation, being carried out to investigate the cause of irregular, painful or heavy periods (page 171), infertility (page 134) and bleeding from the vagina after the menopause.

In this operation the neck of the womb (cervix) is gently dilated so that a small curette can be passed carefully through it and specimens of lining tissue obtained by gentle scraping. The lining tissue from the inner wall of the uterus (the endometrium) is examined under a microscope and gives information about the uterus and ovarian hormone production, and may detect cancer cells.

Dandruff

The shedding of flakes from the scalp. It is caused by excessive drying of the scalp, usually due to washing with strong shampoos.

The best treatment is to wash the hair less often. It is important to choose the mildest type of shampoo, and when shampooing to use only one application and not massage the scalp for too long. There are many shampoos available for treating dandruff and different ones suit different people. Those based on zinc or selenium are probably the most effective. For some patients none is effective.

Dandruff which is very severe is uncommon although it does occur. A small number of skin diseases may mimic dandruff and if the scalp does not clear easily, medical advice should be sought.

Deadly nightshade
(*ATROPA BELLADONNA*)

The berry in particular is poisonous and is very dangerous if eaten, usually by children. The skin becomes dry and hot and the heart slows. If ingested, nausea and vomiting should be induced by putting the fingers in the back of the throat, or swallowing salt water, and the child taken immediately to the Accident and Emergency Department of a hospital.

Deafness
IN ADULTS

Deafness is an increasing problem because the number of elderly is growing and also more people are suffering the result of long-term exposure to noise.

Between 1½ and 2 million adults in the UK have significant hearing loss, and in about a third of these the loss is serious. About 100,000 people suffer from hearing loss produced by noise. Excessive noise damages normal ears and accelerates the normal deterioration in hearing that takes place with increasing age.

As well as noise-induced deafness and the deafness that comes on unavoidably in old age, there are other less common causes. Ear infections, though commoner in children, may cause deafness if left untreated. Ménière's disease produces a slowly progressive deafness and is usually accompanied by attacks of ringing in the ears, nausea, vomiting and vertigo. Otosclerosis is a disease in which the bones of the middle ear become fixed and are no longer able to vibrate and transmit sounds from the outside (*see* Ear). This produces deafness in the 15–30 age group but, if detected early, surgical repair is dramatically successful in about 90 per cent of sufferers. Alternatively, a hearing aid can be used. Deafness

D & C (Dilatation and curettage)

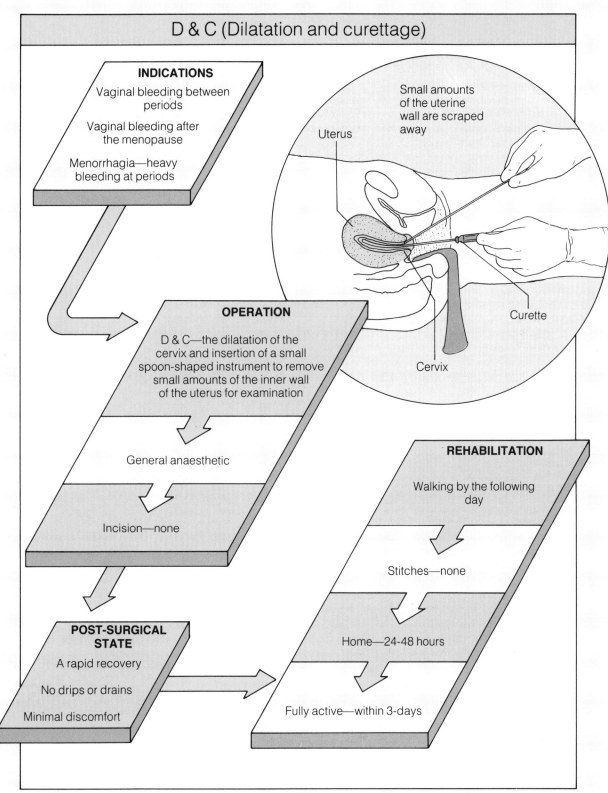

INDICATIONS

Vaginal bleeding between periods

Vaginal bleeding after the menopause

Menorrhagia—heavy bleeding at periods

Small amounts of the uterine wall are scraped away

Uterus

Curette

Cervix

OPERATION

D & C—the dilatation of the cervix and insertion of a small spoon-shaped instrument to remove small amounts of the inner wall of the uterus for examination

General anaesthetic

Incision—none

REHABILITATION

Walking by the following day

Stitches—none

Home—24-48 hours

Fully active—within 3-days

POST-SURGICAL STATE

A rapid recovery

No drips or drains

Minimal discomfort

also occurs if there is a deficiency of thyroxine (*see* Thyroid disease).

Noise and deafness

Sound is measured in decibels (dB). A loud sound of 120 decibels causes discomfort, but exposure to 140 decibels gives pain and the ear may be permanently damaged. Even much lower noise levels may produce damage if the ear is exposed to them for long periods. The International Standards Organization has determined the noise levels which can be tolerated at work. The upper limits are 91 decibels at the lowest frequency noise that the human ear can pick up (250 hertz (cycles per second), a low rumble) and 70 decibels for the highest frequencies (8,000 hertz (cycles per second), a high-pitched whistle). Deep, low-frequency noises are much less damaging than high-frequency ones—it is common experience how much more unpleasant and piercing a shrill whistle is compared with the low rumble of a lorry.

Loud noises are also less dangerous if exposure is brief. In industry, the worker who rotates his job to prevent exposure to constant high noise levels is not so likely to damage his hearing. Also the younger worker is less at risk.

Industrial noise can be reduced by improving the design of machinery and by wearing protective ear plugs and ear muffs. These can reduce the amount of noise by 20 and 25 decibels respectively (i.e. 45 decibels if they are both worn).

The avoidance of unnecessary noise in our everyday lives may also be important. Traffic noise inside cars may reach 115 decibels. Pop music is usually played at a level around 110 decibels with peaks reaching over 120 (higher nearer the loudspeakers). This is equivalent to continuous exposure at 95 decibels, a level at which the International Standards Organization have advised no more than 1½ hours' exposure. Habitual exposure to these noise levels may result in permanent damage.

In a recent study, 20 per cent of school leavers had significant noise-induced hearing loss. This may go unnoticed in the young but it becomes a major disability in the old.

Treatment

The avoidance of excessive noise is the best insurance against premature deafness. Apart from a few exceptions—e.g. wax (page 247), hypothyroidism (page 224) and otosclerosis (*see above*)—there is usually no dramatic treatment that can be offered once deafness has occurred.

Hearing aids are often a great help but it may be difficult for very old people to get used to them and an ear trumpet may be more valuable. Lip reading is a skill which most people can master but again the elderly find it difficult. The speaker's face should be in a good light and not camouflaged by a beard or moustache. The 'dead pan' speaker or the person who talks with a pipe or cigarette in his mouth may defeat the best lip reader.

The problems encountered by the deaf are formidable and the older the age at which it appears, the more difficult it is to adjust either at work or socially. They may be considered rude or even stupid, and their embarrassment and loneliness can result in severe psychological ill health.

Deafness
IN CHILDREN

About 20 children in every 1,000 have significant deafness, usually resulting from partially treated ear infections (*see* Ear infection: glue ear). Early detection is extremely important because deafness creates difficulty in the child's learning to speak. This leads to serious problems when starting school.

The signs of normal hearing development in children are:

2–3 months	Reacts to a sudden noise by frowning or blushing
5 months	Turns his eyes towards the source of a sound
6 months	Turns his head towards the source of a sound

After this, deafness is usually discovered either by formal testing in a baby clinic, when speech is noted to be delayed, or on starting school. The usual speech milestones, though there are considerable individual variations, are:

1 year	Says one or two words with meaning
18 months	Says about 20 words with meaning
21–24 months	Puts words together
2½ years	Uses about 250 words

Any child in whom deafness is suspected should be seen by a doctor and, if confirmed, by a specialist, to ensure that no reversible lesion is left too long and also for advice about the management of ear infections, including 'glue ear' (*see* Ear infection).

Decompression sickness
SEE BENDS

★Delirium

Acute confusion which is usually temporary and the result of a severe general illness, injury, or infection with high fever. The confusion passes when the illness subsides or when the temperature returns to normal. The elderly are especially prone to episodes of delirium when they are ill. Delirium and confusion in the elderly are commonly caused by drugs (e.g. phenobarbitone and sedatives).

During the period of confusion, violent behaviour may occur as the result of vivid hallucinations. When he recovers, the patient often has little or no memory of what has taken place. Treatment with sedatives is frequently required for a short time in the acute stage.

Delirium tremens

This form of delirium occurs in alcoholics during alcohol withdrawal and is a sign of severe alcoholism. Hallucinations are frequent and take the form of sinister insects or animals.

Alcoholics who develop delirium tremens on stopping alcohol also have severe liver disease with partial destruction of many or all of the liver cells. They must stop drinking entirely or premature death is inevitable. Special treatment units exist in many large psychiatric hospitals to help alcoholics stop drinking. (*See also* Alcoholism.)

Delivery

Delivery of a child at birth is straight-forward and uncomplicated in the hands of an experienced midwife or obstetrician. Very occasionally, delivery requires the use of obstetric forceps. These instruments are carefully designed to cradle the baby's head and help the mother to ease the baby out. If delivery is delayed or obstructed, the baby can be delivered by Caesarean section (page 51). (*See also* Pregnancy.)

Dementia

The slow progressive loss of intellect due to degeneration and death of brain cells. Normally throughout life there is gradual loss of brain cells which are not replaced. The number lost is only a small proportion of the total and is of no significance. However, if there is also injury or infection, or, in the elderly, diminution of blood supply, the rate of loss increases and dementia results.

The first signs of dementia are slight absent-mindedness, memory impairment, or a tendency to repeat oneself. In the early stages, depression and frustration may accompany dementia if some insight is retained. Severely demented patients may spend most of their time mentally confused.

Old people are especially prone to dementia which develops as the blood and oxygen supply to the brain gradually decreases with age; if it is severe, they become incapable of looking after themselves.

The modern tendency is for more and more of these old people to be admitted to institutions, either hospitals or old people's homes. Medicine has little to offer except that in hospital they can be supervised constantly and their general well-being safeguarded. Unfortunately, moving old people away from familiar surroundings and friends, when already a little confused, tends only to make things worse. Most demented elderly people are quietly and benevolently confused and are not violent, noisy or aggressive. Many elderly people need care and greatly appreciate the efforts made on their behalf. What they miss most of all is company, particularly from their children and grandchildren.

Dengue fever
(BREAK-BONE FEVER)

A mosquito-borne infection which causes fever and severe muscle cramps (hence 'break-bone fever') and joint pains. It invariably settles within 3–4 days. It is common only in the tropics.

Depression

An excessive down-swing of mood. Nearly everyone's mood varies from day to day and this is normal. It is not uncommon to feel on top of the world one day and a bit 'down in the dumps' the next. However, when such episodes last for longer than 1 or 2 weeks, or when the depression of mood is interfering with daily life, medical advice should be sought.

There are two types of depression. In the first, the trigger for the depression is obvious, such as a bereavement, a personal or family upset, or loneliness. This is called reactive depression. In the second type, endogenous depression, there is no obvious precipitating factor. Endogenous depression tends to occur in those who have always had downward swings of mood, but there is considerable overlap between the two forms.

It is usually obvious when someone is depressed,

but the signs are not always clearly defined. Insomnia or early morning waking is an early pointer; often there are daily mood swings and things seem blackest in the early morning, becoming less depressing as the day wears on. Other symptoms are poor appetite, loss of energy, inability to concentrate, and a feeling of worthlessness, inferiority and hopelessness, and dejection and uselessness often with guilt for the trouble being caused to friends and relatives. Suicidal feelings are common. Perpetual worrying over minor physical symptoms may be the first sign. Perhaps an unspoken fear of cancer may be a trigger.

Depression sometimes occurs as part of a manic-depressive psychosis when the patient undergoes wide-ranging mood swings alternating between wild elation and energy, and deep depression with withdrawal. Depression also occurs in schizophrenics (*see* Schizophrenia).

Treatment

Antidepressant drugs have an important role in treatment but are by no means the whole answer. In reactive depression it is far more important to tackle the situation which has triggered it. The help of close family and friends should be enlisted to provide support. If the person can be encouraged to discuss his worries and anxieties, and understand why he feels depressed, this often helps him surface from his depression.

Above all, sympathy is needed. It is of no help to advise the depressed to 'pull yourself together'—it may even be harmful because his inevitable failure to do so may depress him further.

If the depressed person finds it difficult to discuss things frankly with his immediate family, it may be valuable to enlist the aid of the local doctor, priest or a family friend.

Antidepressants should be used only under medical supervision, because they have serious side-effects if taken without due caution. They help to elevate the mood but take 2 or 3 weeks before starting to exert their effect. The most widely used antidepressants belong to the tricyclic group of drugs, e.g. amitriptyline (Tryptizol, Lentizol), imipramine (Tofranil), and trimipramine (Surmontil).

Psychotherapy aims to help the patient by talking to him in depth about his feelings and problems, in the hope that greater understanding will allow him to come to terms with them. Group psychotherapy is often helpful because it enables depressed people to meet and discuss similar problems with each other. This relieves the feeling of isolation.

Electro-convulsive therapy (ECT) is still considered by many psychiatrists to be a most valuable form of treatment for some types of depression. There has been controversy surrounding ECT over the past few years because it has been difficult to establish how valuable it is, and because of its side-effects; the critics of ECT point to evidence which suggests that it may impair memory. The patient is always given a general anaesthetic beforehand and is asleep at the time of the treatment and remembers nothing of it. While unconscious, electrodes are placed on each side of the skull and an electric current is passed across the brain. ECT sometimes dramatically lifts depression and is now reserved for people with very severe depression particularly if they have suicidal feelings, and in whom other forms of treatment have been unsuccessful.

Post-natal depression (puerperal depression)

Some 50 per cent of mothers experience depression about 3 days after childbirth, which lasts for 2 or 3 weeks. This results from a combination of exhaustion from labour and the 9 month pregnancy and an abrupt and large change in blood hormone levels on delivery. Fatigue, exhaustion, mild anxiety and crying are common, and although upsetting to both parents, particularly when they are meant to be overjoyed, is rarely serious and settles rapidly. The husband's role is vital, and the problem should be explained to him so that he will appreciate the need to remain understanding and not worry about transient personal rejection—the depression will almost certainly disappear within a few days. Severe depression is rare but more serious with marked irritability, temper and, in the extreme, rejection of both husband and baby.

The outlook for the mother with mild post-natal depression is excellent provided she receives adequate support. The depression usually lifts in a few weeks although it may recur with subsequent deliveries. If depression is severe, expert treatment is required from a psychiatrist.

Dermatitis
(ECZEMA)

Inflammation of the skin; the term is used interchangeably with eczema. It occurs most frequently in exposed areas of skin, usually of the hands and face. Initially there may be little to see despite considerable skin irritation. The skin becomes dry and cracked, or red, weeping and shiny. If it is scratched and the skin broken, secondary infection may follow. (*See* illustration, page 238.)

When allergy is the trigger, the degree of

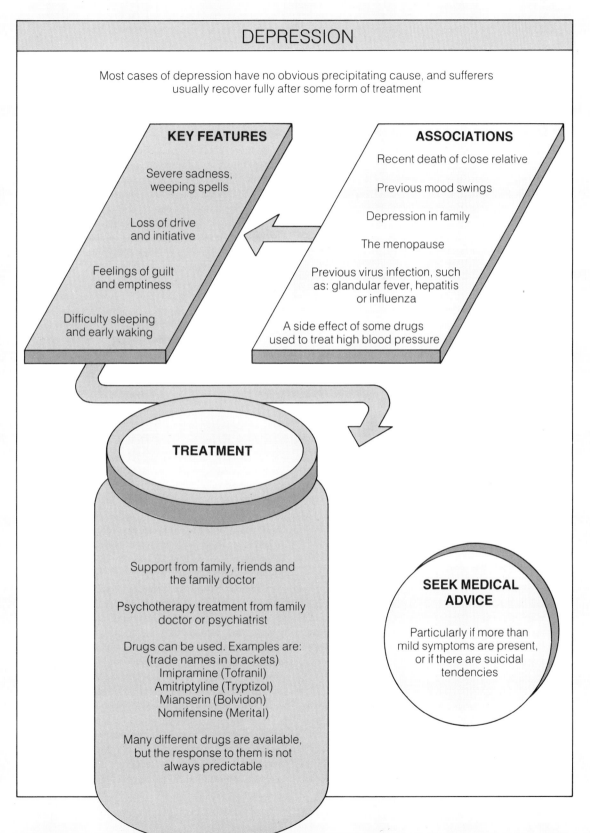

DEPRESSION

Most cases of depression have no obvious precipitating cause, and sufferers usually recover fully after some form of treatment

KEY FEATURES

Severe sadness, weeping spells

Loss of drive and initiative

Feelings of guilt and emptiness

Difficulty sleeping and early waking

ASSOCIATIONS

Recent death of close relative

Previous mood swings

Depression in family

The menopause

Previous virus infection, such as: glandular fever, hepatitis or influenza

A side effect of some drugs used to treat high blood pressure

TREATMENT

Support from family, friends and the family doctor

Psychotherapy treatment from family doctor or psychiatrist

Drugs can be used. Examples are: (trade names in brackets)
Imipramine (Tofranil)
Amitriptyline (Tryptizol)
Mianserin (Bolvidon)
Nomifensine (Merital)

Many different drugs are available, but the response to them is not always predictable

SEEK MEDICAL ADVICE

Particularly if more than mild symptoms are present, or if there are suicidal tendencies

inflammation varies from month to month in an unpredictable way. Allergic eczema may co-exist with asthma and hay fever. Mental stress or tension often make it worse but it is impossible to know which comes first, since eczema is an upsetting condition if inadequately treated.

Smallpox vaccination is no longer given routinely in childhood, but it is still requested by certain countries before entry. No one who has eczema should, on any account, be vaccinated, because a serious and even fatal spreading eczema may result.

If eczema is mild it can often be controlled by the regular use of a moisturizing cream. In more severe cases, creams containing zinc and castor oil are often effective; if not, steroid creams (e.g. hydrocortisone, Betnavite) are used. All steroids are potentially dangerous and should be used only with expert supervision.

Contact dermatitis

Occurs when and where the skin comes into contact with an agent to which it is sensitive (e.g. man-made fibre, metal in rings, or chemicals). The clue to the cause is the site on the body. Nickel clasps on underwear are a common cause of contact dermatitis. Patch testing by a specialist can help to identify the underlying causes which can be avoided.

Infantile eczema

Common in children who have a family history of allergy such as hay fever or asthma. The areas usually affected are the cheeks, scalp, body and in skin flexures (particularly behind the knees, in front of the elbows, around the wrists and ankles and on the neck). The dermatitis fluctuates in severity and in most children it gradually fades away over 5–10 years.

Napkin dermatitis *see* Nappy rash

Solar dermatitis

Results from over-exposure to sunlight. Some people are especially susceptible to sunlight (e.g. redheads) and they are well advised to sunbathe with great caution and to use creams which block ultraviolet light.

Varicose eczema

Occurs over the lower leg and ankles in people with severe varicose veins, and is caused by sluggish circulation of blood. There is often considerable irritation, and if the skin is broken by scratching there is a danger of ulcer formation. Creams may relieve the symptoms but the defective veins may have to be removed surgically.

Desensitization

A technique used to treat hay fever or asthma if there is sensitivity to one specific substance such as grass pollen, mould, cat fur or bee stings. It is rarely successful because sensitivity to a single substance is uncommon. Since desensitization is by no means 100 per cent successful even to one substance, multiple sensitivity makes success even less likely. The procedure involves injections at weekly intervals with quantities of the sensitizing substance which are so minute that no skin reaction occurs—nevertheless, antibodies to the sensitizing substance are formed within the blood stream. The dose is steadily increased, with the gradual development of greater amounts of 'blocking antibodies', and this results in tolerance to the larger doses met in everyday life. (*See also* Hay fever.)

Diabetes mellitus
(GREEK: *DIABAINEIN*, TO PASS THROUGH; LATIN: *MELLITUS*, HONEYED)

Diabetes mellitus means 'sweet flowing urine' and refers to the excess of glucose in the urine of uncontrolled diabetics. The normal pancreas (page 166) produces insulin, which lowers the level of glucose (sugar) in the blood. Small amounts of insulin are secreted all the time and this prevents the concentration of sugar in the blood rising too high. In diabetics, effective insulin is not present in sufficient quantities. As a result the sugar in the blood is not metabolized.

There are two main types of diabetes mellitus: one which arises early in life (sometimes in childhood), and the other which develops in middle or old age, in people who are usually overweight. They are often referred to as 'juvenile onset' and 'maturity onset', respectively. (*See* chart, page 80.)

The first symptoms of diabetes in the young are excessive thirst, frequent passing of urine, weight loss and general exhaustion. Female diabetics often get vaginal thrush (page 223).

In young diabetics treatment consists of a strict diet and regular injections of insulin. The diet is aimed at reducing the intake of refined carbohydrates (bread, cakes and sugar), excess of which raises the blood sugar above normal levels. A higher proportion of the diabetic's diet is made up of fibre and protein. A diet is also necessary to ensure that the number of calories taken in per day is correct and properly distributed throughout the day and that the weight is maintained at a reasonable level.

Regular injections of insulin, which is slowly

absorbed by the body over a period of hours, replace the insulin which is no longer made by the pancreas. Without insulin the sugar level would rise and coma would follow. If too much insulin is given, however, there is a danger that coma may be produced by a precipitous fall in the blood sugar. The experienced diabetic learns to keep himself in balance, and knows that more exercise than normal or less to eat means that less insulin will be required to maintain normal levels of blood sugar.

★ **Diabetic emergencies**
Coma due to excessive blood sugar levels (*hyper*glycaemic coma) develops slowly and often follows an infection such as a heavy cold. The diabetic becomes slowly more and more drowsy, his tongue becomes dry, respiration becomes rapid and the breath may smell aromatic and sweet from acetone. In *hypo*glycaemic coma (too little sugar in the blood) the patient becomes sweaty, shaky, disorientated and often unco-operative or aggressive, rapidly losing consciousness.

In any semi-conscious diabetic it is always worthwhile to give him some sugar by mouth. Sweet tea or a lump of sugar may be enough. If he is unwell because his blood sugar is too high this will not raise the level to any significant extent, but if it is low, it may be sufficient to prevent the blood sugar falling so far that consciousness is lost. If this does happen he should be taken to hospital or a doctor immediately.

Insulin is required for nearly all young diabetics. The purified forms of insulin now available are highly effective in controlling the blood sugar. In the future, diabetics can look forward to implants of insulin which will be injected only every few months. It is hoped that these implants will regulate the rate at which insulin is released according to the level of the blood sugar, simulating the normal pancreas.

Treating the high blood sugar in diabetics solves only part of the problem since there are other biochemical abnormalities which cannot be treated. These predispose to arterial disease (atherosclerosis) as well as kidney, eye (page 70) and sometimes neurological damage. The better the control of the sugar levels, the less frequent are these complications.

Diabetes which comes on in middle or old age is usually mild. A diet is needed to reduce weight but the blood sugar can be kept at a reasonable level with tablets. Insulin injections are rarely necessary.

All diabetics should be encouraged to take special care of their feet and to have chiropody if necessary. This is because the circulation to the feet is frequently diminished. As a result minor sores occur where the shoes rub and these may become infected.

Diabetics cannot accurately assess their blood sugar at all times but they can get a good idea by testing their urine. As a general rule, the higher the blood sugar level the more glucose leaks out into the urine through the kidneys. All diabetics are taught how to test their urine to determine how much glucose it contains, which gives an early warning of sugar levels outside the control range.

The main fear of the majority of young diabetics is the daily self-injection. However, virtually all of them become expert at injection techniques (shown on page 104) and all other aspects of diabetic control.

Dialysis

This is the basic principle upon which artificial kidneys work. Some thin membranes such as cellophane (and a large number of other natural and artificial membranes) allow water and simple small molecules such as salt and sugar to pass through them whilst big molecules and cells cannot. In this way toxic chemicals such as urea, which are normally filtered out of the body by the kidneys, are removed from the blood in a kidney dialysis machine. The blood cells and proteins are returned to the patient. (*See also* Kidney failure; *and* Kidney dialysis.)

Diaphragm

The dome-shaped muscle which divides the chest from the abdomen. It is attached to the inner margins of the lower ribs and moves up and down in response to stimulation by the phrenic nerves, themselves driven by the respiratory centre within the brain. As the diaphragm moves down, it lowers the pressure within the thorax and air flows in from the atmosphere to compensate for this change. When the diaphragm relaxes, it moves up and air is expelled.

Diarrhoea
IN BABIES AND YOUNG CHILDREN

Breast-fed babies usually have loose motions and this is normal. However, the consistency of the stool sometimes becomes even more watery than usual. The most common cause is viral gastro-enteritis which produces epidemics of diarrhoea and vomiting in the winter months. In adults, the loss of fluid is of little consequence. A small baby, however, which develops profuse diarrhoea, possibly accompanied by vomiting (the other hallmark of gastro-enteritis), may become dehydrated and very ill in a few hours.

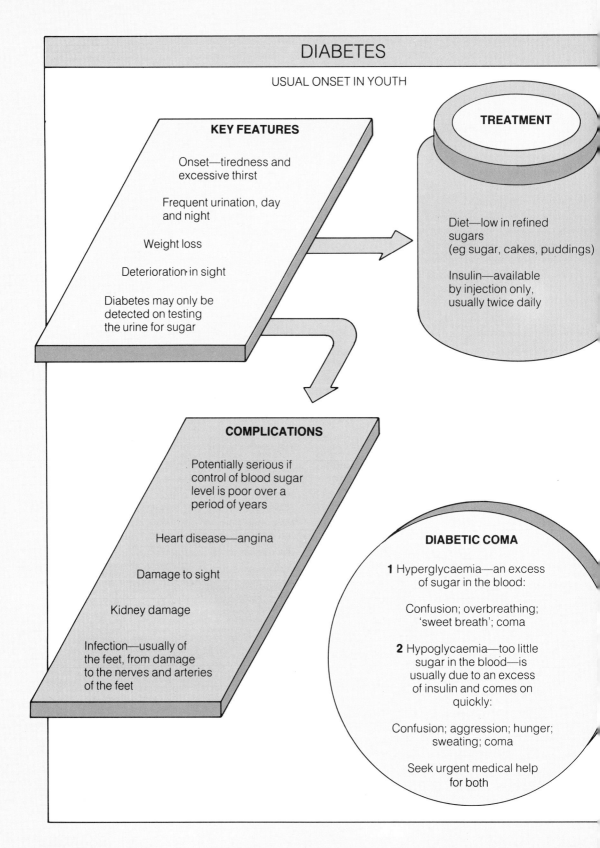

DIABETES

USUAL ONSET IN YOUTH

KEY FEATURES

Onset—tiredness and excessive thirst

Frequent urination, day and night

Weight loss

Deterioration in sight

Diabetes may only be detected on testing the urine for sugar

TREATMENT

Diet—low in refined sugars (eg sugar, cakes, puddings)

Insulin—available by injection only, usually twice daily

COMPLICATIONS

Potentially serious if control of blood sugar level is poor over a period of years

Heart disease—angina

Damage to sight

Kidney damage

Infection—usually of the feet, from damage to the nerves and arteries of the feet

DIABETIC COMA

1 Hyperglycaemia—an excess of sugar in the blood:

Confusion; overbreathing; 'sweet breath'; coma

2 Hypoglycaemia—too little sugar in the blood—is usually due to an excess of insulin and comes on quickly:

Confusion; aggression; hunger; sweating; coma

Seek urgent medical help for both

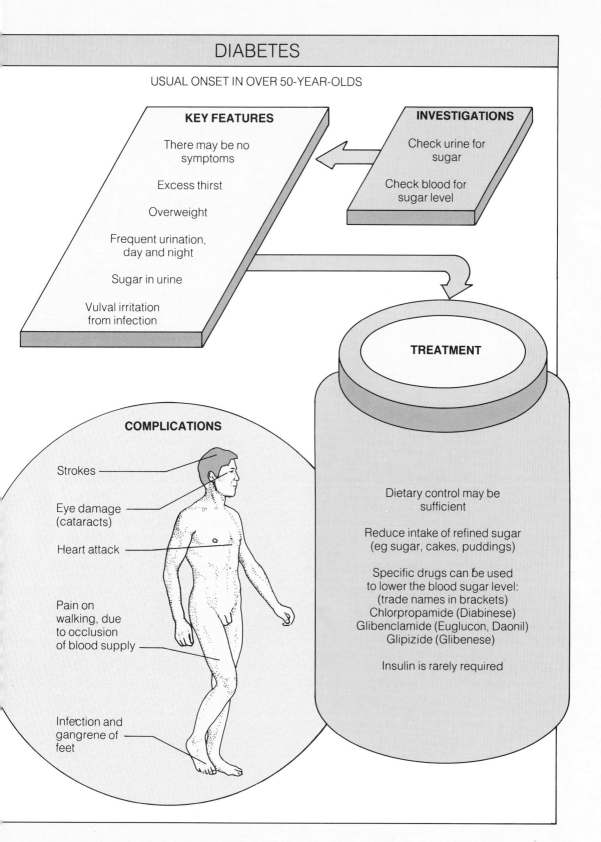

DIABETES

USUAL ONSET IN OVER 50-YEAR-OLDS

KEY FEATURES

There may be no
symptoms

Excess thirst

Overweight

Frequent urination,
day and night

Sugar in urine

Vulval irritation
from infection

INVESTIGATIONS

Check urine for
sugar

Check blood for
sugar level

TREATMENT

Dietary control may be
sufficient

Reduce intake of refined sugar
(eg sugar, cakes, puddings)

Specific drugs can be used
to lower the blood sugar level:
(trade names in brackets)
Chlorpropamide (Diabinese)
Glibenclamide (Euglucon, Daonil)
Glipizide (Glibenese)

Insulin is rarely required

COMPLICATIONS

Strokes

Eye damage
(cataracts)

Heart attack

Pain on
walking, due
to occlusion
of blood supply

Infection and
gangrene of
feet

Breast-fed babies develop gastro-enteritis much less commonly than bottle-fed babies. Profuse diarrhoea in a baby should be reported to your doctor. If bottle fed, the child should be given boiled water only until the symptoms subside, followed by the slow reintroduction of milk over 24–36 hours; i.e. start with quarter strength milk (one part milk and three parts water) followed by half, three-quarter and then full strength milk, provided the diarrhoea does not recur. The fact that the baby is not getting many calories for a short while does not matter. It is far more important to stop the diarrhoea and prevent excessive fluid loss and dehydration. Salt may be added to the water in a concentration of a 'pinch per pint' and no more but only under guidance.

If the baby screams excessively or becomes limp, drowsy or unresponsive after an episode of diarrhoea, it should be seen by a doctor as a matter of urgency, because it may be severely dehydrated. Other signs of severe dehydration might be a sunken fontanelle (the soft part of the top of the baby's head), a vacant and glazed expression, sunken eyes or a dry tongue and mouth. Dehydration to this degree is rare, even in small babies. If the doctor cannot be contacted, the baby should be taken, without delay, to the nearest hospital.

Diarrhoea also occurs in babies who are under-fed, the stools becoming loose and green. Some babies develop loose, smelly motions when they are weaned and started on cereal foods, but only if these symptoms persist is it necessary to consult the doctor (see Coeliac disease).

Some children who have an attack of gastro-enteritis during an epidemic, or who develop diarrhoea in the course of a 'heavy cold', may take a long time to recover fully. In these situations, the persistent diarrhoea may be due to intolerance to one of the sugars present in milk. This intolerance is ★ precipitated by the initial virus infection and usually settles within a few days. Until it does, it is best to exclude lactose from the diet by making up the feeds with special milk powder.

★ Medical advice should be obtained if diarrhoea affects very young infants, if there is blood in the motions, if features of dehydration occur (see above), if the child is ill, or if it persists for more than 48 hours.

Diarrhoea
IN ADULTS

As in children, the most common causes of diarrhoea in adults are viral gastro-enteritis and food poisoning. There may be a fever accompanied by nausea and vomiting. Colicky pain in the abdomen sometimes occurs and tends to be worse immediately before the bowels are opened.

The best treatment is to rest the stomach and bowel by drinking only clear fluids (e.g. water and squashes) and having nothing to eat. The major problem is dehydration but in adults this is rare and less dangerous. Drugs such as codeine or kaolin reduce the diarrhoea. Severe diarrhoea in these epidemics usually subsides after 24–48 hours and a light diet can then be taken. Even at this stage it is probably best to avoid dairy products such as milk, butter, eggs or cream for a few days.

If the diarrhoea persists for longer than a few days you should seek medical advice. Diarrhoea which persists after returning from an area of poor sanitation may require investigation to exclude rare tropical conditions, particularly if blood is passed with the diarrhoea. This may be due to inflammation of the bowel following bacillary or amoebic dysentery.

Occasionally a tendency to diarrhoea develops slowly over several months in a middle-aged or elderly person who previously had a regular or even slightly constipated bowel habit. Further investigation may be needed to ensure that a bowel tumour is not present.

Conclusion
Diarrhoea is usually caused by a virus infection. Reasonable precautions should be taken to prevent it spreading to other members of the family by ensuring that everyone washes their hands after defecation and before eating. No one with diarrhoea should be allowed to prepare or touch food for consumption by others whether in the home or outside. Medical advice should be sought if symptoms persist for more than 48 hours, if blood accompanies the diarrhoea or if the patient's condition deteriorates.

Diet
(GREEK: *DIAITA*, WAY OF LIFE)

A balanced diet contains all of the constituents required for growth in children and to maintain health in adults—i.e. carbohydrates, proteins, fats, vitamins and chemicals such as iron and calcium.

Special diets are required in diabetes (page 78) to reduce the intake of sugar and carbohydrate. In kidney failure (page 141) the protein and potassium intake must be decreased because protein waste products and potassium cannot be excreted by the diseased kidneys. In liver failure, protein reduction is often necessary.

Weight reduction is best achieved by reducing the total intake of calories (*see* Reducing diets, page 292).

Hypersensitivity of the gut wall to specific foods may result in diarrhoea; e.g. gluten can cause coeliac disease (page 62), abdominal pain and various other allergic symptoms and must occasionally be excluded from the diet.

High-fibre diets containing bran and wholemeal bread are strongly recommended for the treatment of constipation, diverticular disease (page 85) and spastic colon (page 212). For foods containing fibre, *see* Constipation.

Dietary fibre

Plant and vegetable matter is composed of cellulose and cannot be completely digested or absorbed. Dietary fibre consists of cellulose, which remains in the bowel and adds bulk to the faecal material. It also absorbs water, which further increases the weight and softness of the stool. The colon and rectum are better able to deal with this soft bulky material than the small hard stool which is the usual result of our highly refined diets.

African races such as the Bantu, who consume high-fibre diets, pass stools which average 200–400 grams (7–14 ounces) a day and values of over 1 kilogram (2.2 pounds) have been recorded, whereas Western man has a daily stool weight of only 100 grams (3.5 ounces). The reflex stimulus to defecate is produced only when the rectum is sufficiently full. Difficulty arises if the quantity of the stool produced is insufficient to stimulate the reflex or if the motion is so hard that it can only be pushed out by straining. Bantus suffer virtually no constipation, diverticular disease, appendicitis, piles or cancer of the colon (*see* Diverticular disease; Appendicitis; Piles).

For foods containing fibre (e.g. bran and wholemeal bread), *see* Constipation.

Difficulty in swallowing
SEE SWALLOWING DIFFICULTY

Digestive tract
(LATIN: *DIGERERE*, TO SEPARATE)

The body tissues involved in the absorption and excretion of food, from the lips to the anus. Food is first chewed and coarsely ground and mixed in the mouth with saliva from the salivary glands which also partially digest it. The food is passed down the gullet (oesophagus) to the stomach. Here it is further broken down and mixed with the digestive enzymes and hydrochloric acid secreted by the stomach, by the muscular contractions of the stomach wall.

The food is eased on by smooth, co-ordinated contractions of the stomach into the duodenum, where it meets the pancreatic enzymes (pancreozymin and secretin) which digest proteins and fats, and bile which digests and emulsifies fats. The mixture passes on to the jejunum and ileum of the small intestine, where the fat and protein components are absorbed and available to the body to build up and replace its own fats and protein-containing tissues—especially muscle. Water, essential chemicals (e.g. sodium, potassium, calcium) and vitamins are also absorbed in the small intestine. The remaining unwanted material passes on through the large intestine and out of the body. The large bowel, like the bladder for urine, acts as a reservoir so that defecation need only take place in safety (in animals) and at convenience (in man). In health, the muscular wall of the entire tract produces smooth ripples of contraction which pass along the wall and move the food. If the contractions become more active—particularly if the intestine is obstructed—abdominal colic results (page 63).

Digoxin

The digitalis group of drugs are used for the treatment of heart diseases. Originally the digitalis drugs were obtained by extraction from leaves of the foxglove plant (botanical name, *Digitalis purpurea*). They were impure and often of unknown potency and action. Digoxin has been the standard compound for 50 years.

In certain types of heart disease the heart muscle becomes weakened and unable to contract maximally. The output of the heart decreases and produces symptoms of heart failure such as shortness of breath on exercise or when lying flat. The ankles may swell.

Digoxin increases the force of contraction of the heart, and in heart failure produces a dramatic improvement in exercise tolerance. Digoxin is also used to treat an irregular heart beat. It is potentially dangerous with side-effects of nausea and loss of appetite, and for this reason it should be taken only under medical supervision.

Diphtheria

This is a serious infection which has been virtually eradicated in the developed world by routine childhood immunization. The illness is caused by a bacterium which infects the throat and occasionally the larynx at the upper end of the trachea. The bacterium releases a chemical toxin into the blood which causes fever, headache and vomiting and occasionally even damages the heart muscle.

Most people recover but up to 10 per cent may die if not previously immunized and if not correctly treated with anti-toxin and antibiotics. Diphtheria is totally preventable by immunization in childhood.

Disc
(INTERVERTEBRAL DISC)

Discs are fibrous rings of tissue surrounding a cushion of jelly. They separate the individual bones of the spine (vertebrae) and allow a degree of elasticity and mobility as well as functioning as shock absorbers.

Slipped disc
The cause of many types of backache. The disc may slip forward or sideways, to cause backache (page 35) or sciatica (page 203). The fibrous ring of a disc may slip or the central jelly may rupture through it—sideways or forwards—to cause backache. If a nerve is compressed as a result, shooting pain down the nerve and weakness of muscles supplied by that nerve may follow (e.g. sciatica from pressure on the sciatic nerve of the leg). The discs most often affected are those in the neck (causing cervical spondylosis) and those in the small of the back (the lumbar spine).

Pressure on the nerves in the neck causes numbness and pins and needles in the fingers, and occasionally shooting pains down the arm. The pressure is relieved by wearing a collar which partially fixes the vertebrae in the neck. Pressure on the nerves in the lower (lumbar) spine causes shooting pain down the back of the leg, along the route (distribution) of the sciatic nerve. The pain is usually relieved by lying flat on the back on a hard bed (or on the floor).

Medical advice should be obtained if there is any suspicion of nerve pressure or sciatica.

Discharge

Discharge of fluid commonly follows infection in the vagina (*see* Vaginal discharge), the nose (*see* Colds), the ear (*see* Ear infection) and the penis (*see* Venereal diseases). The discharge and pus contain the infecting organisms, and white blood cells which act to destroy the organisms. Discharges are thick and creamy if full of white pus cells, and thin if they consist mainly of serum (*see* Blood).

★ Dislocation

The displacement of the two articular surfaces of a joint from their normal position. The stability of a joint depends on the tone and strength of the muscles around it. The range of movement of a joint is limited by the 'staying' action of its surrounding ligaments. The close fit of the surfaces of the joint is also important.

Dislocation occurs most commonly with the shoulder joint because the socket formed by the shoulder blade (scapula) is very shallow. It often follows a sporting accident and there is no fracture. The joint is very painful and virtually no movement is possible. Sometimes the humerus slips back into place of its own accord but usually it has to be replaced under deep sedation or full anaesthesia. The hip joint rarely dislocates because the head of the thigh bone (femur) fits exactly into the deep cup (acetabulum) of the pelvis.

Other joints where dislocation occurs, but where there is usually an associated fracture, are the ankle, elbow and wrist.

First aid following dislocation
The first step is to get the patient to hospital. An x-ray can then be performed to exclude any associated fracture and the dislocation treated by an expert. On the way to hospital the joint should be immobilized in a position of comfort to diminish or prevent pain.

Congenital dislocation of the hip
This occurs in babies and is present from birth. Doctors in hospital or the Infant Welfare Clinic usually examine babies for this soon after birth. It is important to make the diagnosis early so that treatment can be started as soon as possible. Initially it may be sufficient to keep the legs splayed apart with an aluminium or plaster of Paris splint. This encourages the head of the thigh bone (femur) to adopt its correct position in the socket of the pelvis. In older children over 3 years, or where these measures fail, an operation may be necessary to realign the bones and fix them in position.

Disseminated sclerosis

Another name for multiple sclerosis (page 154).

Diuretics

Drugs which act on the kidney to increase the urinary excretion of salt and water. This is achieved by allowing more salt to leak out of the kidneys. Living organisms always excrete salt well diluted with water, and, the kidney being no exception, water follows the salt loss induced by diuretics. The potassium which also tends to leak out has to be replaced. The effect of diuretic treatment is undone if unlimited salt is eaten in the diet.

Diuretics are prescribed to treat heart disorders where there is retention of fluid in the body (*see under* Ankle swelling). The quick-acting drugs frusemide (Lasix) and bumetamide (Burinex) are the most commonly used at the start of treatment with the cheaper, gentler thiazides (*see below*) reserved for maintenance therapy.

The thiazide group of diuretics (page 284) is also used to reduce high blood pressure. Examples are cyclopenthiazide (Navidrex) and bendrofluazide (Neo-NaClex).

When diuretics are taken by mouth there may be no noticeable increase in the amount of urine passed during the day. If they are taken in the evening, however, the patient may have to get up during the night to pass urine. For this reason diuretics are usually taken in the morning and certainly no later than mid-afternoon.

Diuretics should only be taken under medical supervision because they have potentially serious side-effects. The major side-effect is to deplete the body of potassium, which is important for the satisfactory function of the heart and muscles. Potassium is replaced by an adequate potassium intake in the diet, usually with tablets. An alternative is to give potassium-retaining drugs with the diuretics.

Diverticular disease

Diverticula are small pouches which appear as 'blow-outs' along the side of the descending and sigmoid colon of the large intestine. This part of the bowel contracts to push faecal material downwards and then out of the body. The wall of this part of the colon is thin, and if high pressures develop as the result of constipation, it produces small areas of 'ballooning' of the bowel wall at points of weakness.

These small pouches, or diverticula, may become infected (diverticulitis), bleed, or perforate (when peritonitis may follow). They are almost universally present in the elderly. Usually diverticula produce no problems and are discovered as an incidental finding during an x-ray investigation or operation for an unrelated disorder.

Diverticular disease is more common in the developed world where a low-roughage diet is eaten, tending to produce small hard stools which are often difficult to pass without straining. Even severe diverticular disease can usually be treated very successfully by taking a high-roughage diet including regular bran and wholemeal bread.

Dizzy spell

The sensation of light-headedness or impending blackout. This feeling together with weakness is common during many illnesses, particularly if there is a fever, pain or emotional disturbance. It may also occur after exercise and when hungry. Many of the conditions which produce dizzy spells can also lead to blackouts (page 39).

In most people, from time to time the blood pressure may drop sufficiently for the brain to become temporarily short of oxygen; this is the commonest cause of dizziness. This occurs when standing quickly, particularly after sitting or lying relaxed for an hour or two in a warm room. This is because the blood has pooled in the veins of the legs and has to be returned to the heart by the leg muscle pump before the heart can pump it to the brain. Guardsmen, who stand still on parade on a hot day, may faint because the leg muscles cannot pump efficiently. This is why they 'work' their calf muscles whilst on parade.

Virus infections (e.g. colds, sinusitis, influenza or viral gastro-enteritis) are a common cause of dizziness because they cause a slight fall of blood pressure upon standing. This is not a sign of serious illness, and, as with the other situations mentioned, will respond quickly to lying down.

Viruses also produce dizziness if they infect the labyrinth—the balancing organ of the inner ear. This causes difficulty in balancing, and vertigo—an uncomfortable spinning sensation. Falls are subsequently very common. Posture makes little difference and the dizziness is equally bad whether lying or standing. Sudden movement of the head from side to side tends to make it worse. Ménière's disease (page 151) causes vertigo, often accompanied by hearing loss and nausea.

In the elderly, dizzy spells caused by irregularity of the heart rhythm may be accompanied by palpitations. Narrowing of the arteries to the brain may lead to faintness on looking up or after any sudden head movement. Sometimes high blood pressure may be responsible.

If dizziness or dizzy spells persist for more than 24 hours, or if there is a spinning sensation or vomiting, medical advice should be sought.

Dog bites
SEE UNDER FIRST AID (PAGE 275)

Double vision

Transient blurring of vision often occurs in association with feeling faint and usually goes away as soon as the dizziness subsides. Another frequent cause is alcohol intoxication, when the sufferer may see double for some hours. Double vision after a blow to the head must be taken seriously, although simple concussion may be the cause if the casualty was knocked out. Double vision after a head injury should always be reported to a doctor immediately, especially if it is accompanied by any drowsiness, headache or nausea.

Double vision which occurs for no obvious reason in someone previously well should also be reported. It is an unusual symptom and requires expert assessment.

Some adults who had squints as children may grow up with double vision. This is now rare because most children have squints corrected successfully early in life. Some who did not actually squint in childhood may have a 'lazy eye' and see double when tired.

Down's syndrome
SEE MONGOLISM

Drowning
SEE UNDER FIRST AID (PAGE 274)

Drug addiction
SEE ADDICTION

Drugs

Chemicals prescribed for the relief or investigation of diseases or symptoms. The majority of drugs are prescribed for the common disorders of pain, infections, anxiety and depression. About 50 per cent of patients do not take the drugs at all or fail to complete the course.

Addiction and dependence (page 13) are serious complications of drug therapy.

Duodenal ulcer

The duodenum is the first part of the small intestine immediately beyond the stomach. It is particularly prone to ulceration, though less so than 10 or more years ago. The features and treatment are described with stomach ulcers (page 216) and summarized opposite.

Duodenum
(LATIN: *DUODENI*, TWELVE AT A TIME)

The first part of the small intestine, connecting the stomach with the ileum (*see* diagram, page 265). It is about 12 fingers' breadth in length (hence *duodenum*). The pancreatic and bile ducts open into it, and pour their digestive secretions onto the food previously mixed and partly digested in the stomach.

Dysentery

An infection of the bowel which results in profuse diarrhoea, with or without bleeding. The infection is usually caused by eating food or drinking water contaminated by a specific group of bacteria called Shigella. Other organisms such as amoebae (amoebic dysentery) are less commonly found. Dysentery is more common in the tropics and in countries where the standards of hygiene and sanitation are poor.

Great care has to be taken after dysentery is confirmed, to prevent its transmission. Careful washing of the hands after defecation and before eating is always important but especially if dysentery has been reported. Those in the catering trade who could be infected with dysentery as judged by contacts or symptoms must be prevented from handling food until cleared.

Treatment with kaolin mixtures and codeine tablets often reduces the diarrhoea. Antibiotics are not normally required because the infection usually settles spontaneously after a period of 2–10 days. Dehydration may result from the diarrhoea, so an adequate intake of fluid is essential throughout the illness.

Dysentery should be reported to the local public health authorities, who will check the extent of its spread and, if possible, find the original source.

DUODENAL ULCER

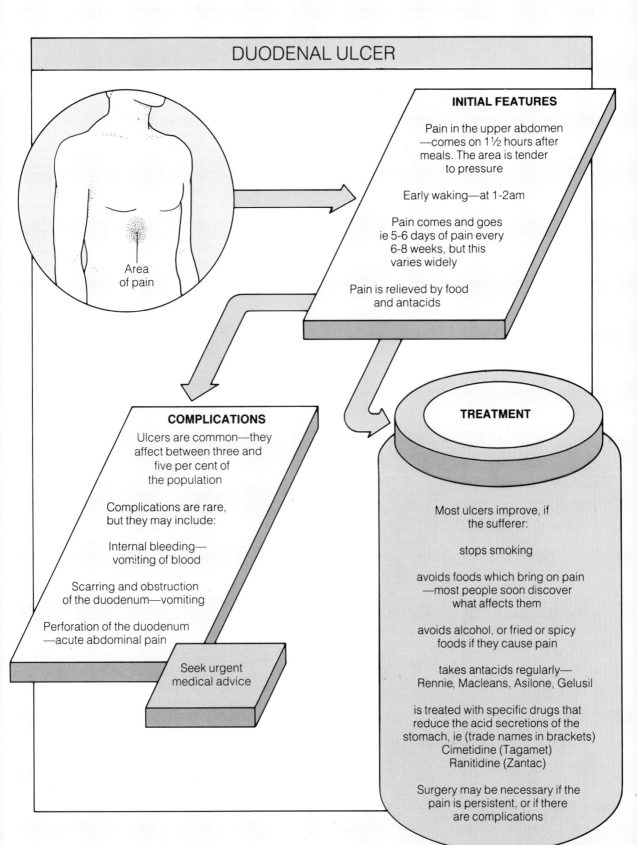

Area of pain

INITIAL FEATURES

Pain in the upper abdomen
—comes on 1½ hours after
meals. The area is tender
to pressure

Early waking—at 1-2am

Pain comes and goes
ie 5-6 days of pain every
6-8 weeks, but this
varies widely

Pain is relieved by food
and antacids

COMPLICATIONS

Ulcers are common—they
affect between three and
five per cent of
the population

Complications are rare,
but they may include:

Internal bleeding—
vomiting of blood

Scarring and obstruction
of the duodenum—vomiting

Perforation of the duodenum
—acute abdominal pain

Seek urgent
medical advice

TREATMENT

Most ulcers improve, if
the sufferer:

stops smoking

avoids foods which bring on pain
—most people soon discover
what affects them

avoids alcohol, or fried or spicy
foods if they cause pain

takes antacids regularly—
Rennie, Macleans, Asilone, Gelusil

is treated with specific drugs that
reduce the acid secretions of the
stomach, ie (trade names in brackets)
Cimetidine (Tagamet)
Ranitidine (Zantac)

Surgery may be necessary if the
pain is persistent, or if there
are complications

87

Dyslexia
(GREEK: *DYS*, DIFFICULT; *LEXIS*, WORD

There are some children of normal intelligence and ability who find it very difficult to learn to read. Their abilities in other directions are normal and they appear to have no emotional problems. Dyslexia is a poorly understood disorder, whose existence was not appreciated until a few years ago. The cause remains unknown.

The early recognition of children with reading and writing difficulties is very important. Assessment by an educational psychologist may be valuable. Some parents are reluctant to ask for this, for fear that they might appear to be criticizing the school. In this case, referral through the family doctor may be a better plan. Once the problem is recognized, intensive help in reading and writing can be given by teachers with a special skill in dyslexia. The children can be told that they are not stupid but will have to work particularly hard at these skills. Special allowance should always be made for them in public examinations to enable them to realize their full potential despite their difficulties.

Dysmenorrhoea
(GREEK: *DYS*, DIFFICULT; *MEN*, MONTH; *RHOIA*, TO FLOW)

Painful menstruation—a common and unpleasant sensation but rarely serious. For features and treatment, *see under* Periods.

Dyspepsia
(GREEK: *DYS*, DIFFICULT; *PEPTEIN*, TO DIGEST)

A common condition marked by heartburn and a burning and sore upper abdominal discomfort, often precipitated by some foods and relieved by others (especially milk).

Antacid drugs often give relief. The commonest cause is oesophageal reflux (page 194). (*See also* Hiatus hernia; Indigestion; *and* Stomach ulcer.)

Ear

The organ of hearing and balance, the ear has three parts (*see* diagram, opposite). The outer ear is like a funnel, which receives the sound and transmits it to the eardrum. The middle ear transmits and amplifies the vibration of the eardrum via three small bones (the malleus, incus and stapes) across a disc-shaped cavity from the eardrum to the inner ear. The inner ear receives the vibrations into a coiled shell-like structure known as the cochlea. From here nerves relay the sound impulses to the temporal lobe of the brain. The semicircular canals consist of three fluid-filled tubes and contain hair-like nerve endings which are stimulated by the movement of small calcium stones within the canals. These stones move as the head is tilted backwards, forwards or from side to side, and the nerves relay these impulses to the brain, a mechanism seen in some invertebrate animals such as crayfish. Damage to the labyrinth, as in acute infectious labyrinthitis, can cause sudden loss of balance (*see* Vertigo).

Ear infection

★ Otitis media
Infection of the middle ear, which commonly follows throat infection with swelling of the adenoids which blocks the Eustachian tube. Normally the small amount of fluid from the middle ear drains via this tube, and when it becomes blocked the secretions collect and become infected. Middle ear infection occurs chiefly in children because their smaller tubes are more likely to block and also because swelling of the adenoids is more common in childhood. Otitis media causes severe pain and deafness, often with a marked fever. In children, nausea and vomiting is frequent. The eardrum appears red and inflamed, and may be ballooned outwards into the external ear canal. Otitis media is a serious condition requiring antibiotic therapy to prevent perforation of the eardrum, and backward spread of infection into the air sinuses of the mastoid bone (mastoiditis).

Otitis externa
Inflammation of the external ear canal, caused by local damage; it is common in children who push sticks and dirty fingers into their ears. It is seen, rarely, in adults who have used the same technique to remove wax. The skin lining the canal becomes infected and discharges pus, sometimes with blood. Otitis externa is not serious and usually responds rapidly to regular cleaning plus antiseptic solutions. Occasionally, local antibiotics and even steroids are necessary. The ear canal *must* be kept dry, so bathing

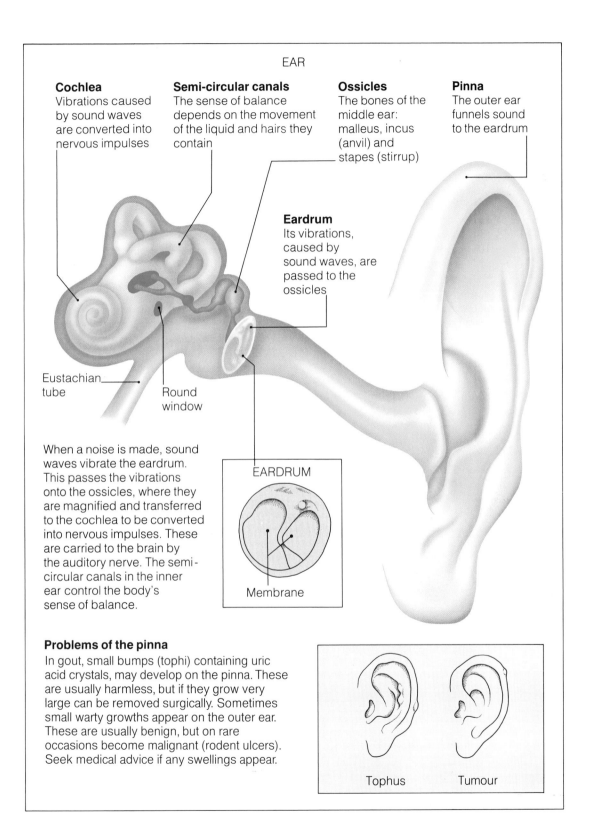

EAR

Cochlea
Vibrations caused by sound waves are converted into nervous impulses

Semi-circular canals
The sense of balance depends on the movement of the liquid and hairs they contain

Ossicles
The bones of the middle ear: malleus, incus (anvil) and stapes (stirrup)

Pinna
The outer ear funnels sound to the eardrum

Eardrum
Its vibrations, caused by sound waves, are passed to the ossicles

Eustachian tube

Round window

When a noise is made, sound waves vibrate the eardrum. This passes the vibrations onto the ossicles, where they are magnified and transferred to the cochlea to be converted into nervous impulses. These are carried to the brain by the auditory nerve. The semi-circular canals in the inner ear control the body's sense of balance.

EARDRUM

Membrane

Problems of the pinna
In gout, small bumps (tophi) containing uric acid crystals, may develop on the pinna. These are usually harmless, but if they grow very large can be removed surgically. Sometimes small warty growths appear on the outer ear. These are usually benign, but on rare occasions become malignant (rodent ulcers). Seek medical advice if any swellings appear.

Tophus

Tumour

is forbidden and ear plugs are worn when hair washing and bathing.

'Glue ear' (chronic serous otitis media)
Sticky fluid collects in the middle ear, sometimes following untreated otitis media, and prevents the transmission of sound across the middle ear to the receptor nerves of the inner ear. If not detected in early life, affected children may appear to be slow learners and subnormal purely because they cannot hear. Treatment by a specialist is simple and curative.

See also Earache.

Earache

The commonest cause is infection in either the external ear (otitis externa) or the middle ear (otitis media). (These are discussed under Ear infection.) The pain of a severe sore throat or a bad tooth may be felt in the ears in the absence of any ear infection. If the Eustachian tube becomes blocked, pain in the ears may result even though there is no infection present. While the blockage persists, the pressure on the two sides of the thin, flexible eardrum (tympanic membrane) cannot be equalized and the membrane is then drawn into the middle ear by the negative pressure from within which cannot be equalized with the outside atmosphere. As the drum becomes stretched, pain is produced. Deafness in one or both ears may also occur. Rapid changes of height (e.g. in an aeroplane) may cause pain in the ear. Here, on descent, as the air pressure decreases outside, the tympanic membrane may be pushed outwards by a stronger pressure from within unless the Eustachian tube is unblocked. Usually repeated swallowing is sufficient since the act of swallowing tends, automatically, to open the Eustachian tube and thus allow pressures within the ear to equalize with the pressure outside. Other causes of earache include boils or foreign bodies (e.g. beads in the outer ear).

If antibiotics are prescribed for an ear infection the full course must be taken. Failure to do this may mean that the bacteria are not completely eradicated even though the pain and temperature subside.

Decongestant nasal drops are sometimes useful because they help to unblock the Eustachian tube and aid drainage of infected material from the middle ear. During the acute stage of an ear infection, when there is severe earache and fever, regular doses of analgesics such as aspirin will help to relieve both. If deafness in the absence of other symptoms persists

for more than 24 hours, medical advice should be obtained. Anyone, particularly a child, who develops earache or deafness in association with fever, nausea or vomiting should be seen by a doctor as a matter of urgency.

Perforated eardrum
If middle ear infection is untreated, fluid builds up behind the eardrum and may burst through. The discharge emerges through a small tear in the eardrum, which usually closes spontaneously when the infection has subsided. Recurrent ear infections with a chronically discharging ear may produce a small hole in the drum which fails to close. This does not necessarily affect hearing, but people with these perforations must usually avoid getting water into the ear, or they become dizzy or develop middle ear infection because the perforation allows the entry of bacteria. When swimming they must avoid putting their heads under water or use ear plugs. Cold winds blowing into the ear may have a similar effect, and this can be prevented by wearing an ear plug on the affected side.

Discharge from an ear must not be allowed to continue without specialist assessment.

ECG
(ELECTROCARDIOGRAM)

When the heart beats there is a wave of electrical activity which passes through it from top to bottom. An electrocardiograph is a sensitive instrument which can detect these minute voltages from metal plates (electrodes) placed on the surface of the body.

ECGs are a useful aid in diagnosing or excluding heart attacks as a cause of chest pains. The ECG shows a number of characteristic features following a heart attack, but this is not invariably so and the tracing can sometimes be normal. In these circumstances a series of ECGs is of great value. The other chief use of the ECG is in the detailed understanding of dysrhythmias—where the heart is irregular or abnormally fast or slow. Extra beats can also result in unpleasant palpitation and the ECG can determine which part of the heart is giving rise to them. Having an electrocardiogram is totally painless. Recording electrodes (metal plates) are attached to the limbs by elastic bands and to the chest by a rubber sucker. The entire recording takes no more than 10 minutes. In '24-hour monitoring' of the ECG a small cassette recorder is attached to two standard leads and carried from a belt under the clothes. Expert analysis of the ECG over 24 hours

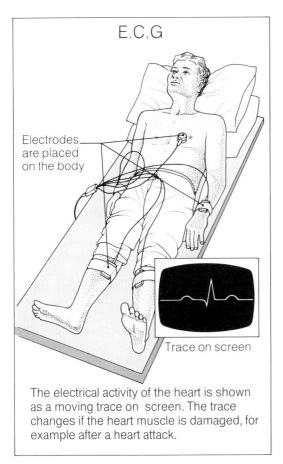

E.C.G

Electrodes are placed on the body

Trace on screen

The electrical activity of the heart is shown as a moving trace on screen. The trace changes if the heart muscle is damaged, for example after a heart attack.

will determine whether transient symptoms are related to alteration in heart rate or rhythm.

Eclampsia
(TOXAEMIA OF PREGNANCY)

A condition of pregnant women, characterized by raised blood pressure, ankle swelling, and loss of protein into the urine.

If severe and untreated there is an increased risk both to the developing child and to the mother. Admission to hospital for expert supervision and treatment may be necessary. The main object of therapy is to reduce the blood pressure to normal values and treatment is invariably successful. (For a more detailed account, *see under* Pregnancy.)

ECT
(ELECTRO-CONVULSIVE THERAPY)

Used in the treatment of very severe depression when other forms of therapy have been unsuccessful (*see* Depression; *and* Psychiatric treatment). A brief general anaesthetic is given during the procedure and completely prevents any tendency to fits.

ECT is sometimes remarkably successful in reversing severe depression, although the way it does this remains unknown.

Ectopic pregnancy

One which develops outside the womb (uterus). It is an abnormal site for fetal development and the fetus almost never survives. The 'error' happens at the start of pregnancy soon after fertilization of the egg (ovum). Normally the ovum passes down the Fallopian tube from the ovary and, following fertilization, implants itself into the thick, soft, inside wall of the uterus. This ensures that the early fetus is securely attached to the uterus, which in turn responds by providing it with a good blood supply, essential if the fetus is to receive adequate quantities of food and oxygen.

In an ectopic pregnancy the fertilized ovum fails to reach the uterus but gets stuck, usually in one of the Fallopian tubes. It then burrows into the thin wall of the tube and often encounters a blood vessel. Severe bleeding then occurs, mostly into the abdominal cavity. There is also a small amount of external blood loss from the vagina and a variable degree of lower abdominal pain, often accompanied by faintness. The only treatment is an emergency operation to remove the affected Fallopian tube. Provided the remaining tube is healthy, there is no reason why ova cannot continue to reach the uterus in subsequent months and for later pregnancies to occur.

Ectopic pregnancy is very rarely a cause of vaginal bleeding in early pregnancy. However, if bleeding occurring in the early weeks is accompanied by low abdominal pain, faintness or sweating, an ectopic pregnancy is likely and the mother should seek medical advice or be taken to hospital without delay.

Note Vaginal bleeding in early pregnancy is potentially serious whatever the cause, and medical advice should be obtained urgently.

Eczema
(GREEK: *EKZEIN*, TO BOIL OVER)

The word describes the blistering of the skin seen in this disorder. The terms 'eczema' and 'dermatitis' are now synonymous, and the features are discussed under dermatitis (page 76). (*See also* illustration, page 236.)

Ejaculation, premature
SEE SEXUAL PROBLEMS

Elbow joint

The elbow (*see* diagram, page 267) is mainly a hinge joint between the lower end of the humerus and the ulna.

The radius, which carries the hand at its lower end, also articulates at the elbow with the lower end of the humerus, forming a modified ball-and-socket joint. This allows rotation of the forearm and hand on the upper arm, pronation (palm down) and supination (palm up).

★Electrical injury
SEE UNDER FIRST AID (PAGE 270)

Electrocardiogram
SEE ECG

Embolus
(GREEK: *EMBOLOS*, A PLUG)

A blood clot which travels within the blood stream until it reaches a blood vessel small enough to prevent its further passage. The vessel is plugged by the embolus and the tissues served by the vessel are starved of blood. The lungs are the most common site of embolisms (pulmonary embolus, page 190), and follow the development of a thrombus or clot in a deep leg vein after abdominal surgery. Small emboli may obstruct the small vessels of the brain, to produce strokes (page 217).

Patients with emboli are treated with anticoagulants (page 23).

Emetics

Substances given to induce vomiting. They are sometimes given to children who have swallowed drugs accidentally, as an alternative to washing out their stomachs. Syrup of ipecacuanha is one of the most commonly used of the emetics, but this should only be administered under expert medical supervision. The child will in any case need to be carefully assessed following accidental drug overdose.

Emphysema

A disease of the lungs which follows severe and long-standing asthma, pneumoconiosis or chronic bronchitis, and causes varying degrees of breathlessness.

The normal lung looks like a very fine sponge but in emphysema the small air sacs (alveoli) which form the sponge are destroyed, leaving large open spaces. This means that the internal surface of the lungs available for gas exchange (oxygen in and carbon dioxide out) is greatly reduced. The blood levels of these gases become abnormal and the tissues may be starved of oxygen. Another consequence of emphysema is that the lungs become stiffer during breathing. The increased work required to get oxygen in is felt as breathlessness and this is more marked on exertion.

Smoking is the major cause of bronchitis and emphysema, though the effects on the lungs may not become apparent for 15–20 years.

Although irreversible, even well established emphysema may progress more slowly or stop if smoking is stopped.

There is no cure for emphysema. Antibiotics are given for attacks of acute bronchitis to prevent further lung damage. Anti-wheeze preparations (such as aminophylline, salbutamol by mouth or inhaler, Becotide or prednisolone) may help to decrease the breathlessness. When breathlessness is severe, oxygen can be given via a special mask from a cylinder kept at home.

★Encephalitis

Infection of the brain. The features are usually indistinguishable from meningitis (page 151).

Endocrine glands

Glands which secrete hormones (page 128) directly into the blood stream (e.g. the adrenal, thyroid and pituitary glands).

In contrast, exocrine glands secrete onto the surface of the body (sweat glands) or into the gut (salivary glands). Some glands do both (e.g. pancreas and testes).

See also Adrenal glands; Ovary; Pituitary gland; Testes; *and* Thyroid disease.

Endometriosis

SEE UNDER PERIODS: PAINFUL PERIODS

Enema

The introduction of fluid into the rectum and lower colon. Enemas are commonly used to treat severe constipation when other efforts have failed. Provided the enema can be retained in contact with the faecal material for a reasonable length of time, sufficient softening occurs and a good bowel action results. Difficulties sometimes arise if the fluid cannot be retained in the bowel. Enemas may be uncomfortable but are not painful, and the relief they provide in severe constipation justifies their use.

They are also given to clear the bowel of faeces prior to intestinal surgery. Barium is given as an enema to outline the large intestine when x-rays are taken to investigate the cause of alteration of bowel habits and rectal bleeding.

Finally, medicines to treat the lower half of the large bowel can be introduced in enema form. They are usually steroid preparations (Predsol Retention Enema) used to treat ulcerative colitis.

Enteric fever

Another name for typhoid (page 231).

Enteritis

Inflammation or infection of the small intestine, as compared with infection of the stomach (gastritis) or the large intestine (colitis). Features of enteritis are described with gastro-enteritis (page 109). (*See also* Crohn's disease.)

Enuresis

Incontinence of urine. There are many causes. Local causes include urinary infections and disorders of the bladder muscle or the muscle of the outlet sphincter (which acts like a tap). Neurological causes include dementia, stroke, and disorders of the spinal cord.

Nocturnal enuresis (bed wetting, page 37) is common in children but rarely denotes serious disease.

Epidemic

Any disease which spreads widely through a population or geographical region. Most epidemics are caused by common virus infections such as measles and influenza, but in some parts of the tropics epidemics of cholera or meningitis occur annually.

Epidural

Epidural anaesthetics are injected into the anatomical space around the lower spinal cord to block sensory nerve fibres which relay pain from the lower abdomen and legs.

Epidural anaesthesia is used most commonly to prevent pain in labour (page 184) and also for operations on the abdomen and legs in patients whose general health makes the risk of a general anaesthetic too great.

Epiglottitis

An acute infection of the epiglottis (situated at the top of the larynx). The epiglottis becomes swollen and, in children in whom the larynx is narrow, may obstruct breathing. The children develop a coarse 'growl' on inspiration and become greatly agitated and blue, and gasp for breath. This is an emergency ★ and medical advice should be obtained immediately. If not readily available, the child should be taken to hospital.

★ Epilepsy

A tendency to major (grand mal) or minor (petit mal) fits.

In a *grand mal* fit there are convulsions, usually of all the limbs, lasting for several minutes, followed by a period of deep sleep. Grand mal fits are more common and usually no specific cause is found. However, they can follow severe head injury received either in adulthood or as the result of a difficult birth. Infections such as meningitis and brain tumours are rarer causes of grand mal epilepsy.

Fits are often preceded by an 'aura' or warning, usually lasting only a second or two. There are no words to describe this sensation—perhaps 'sinking' is the commonest. The epileptic then falls unconscious

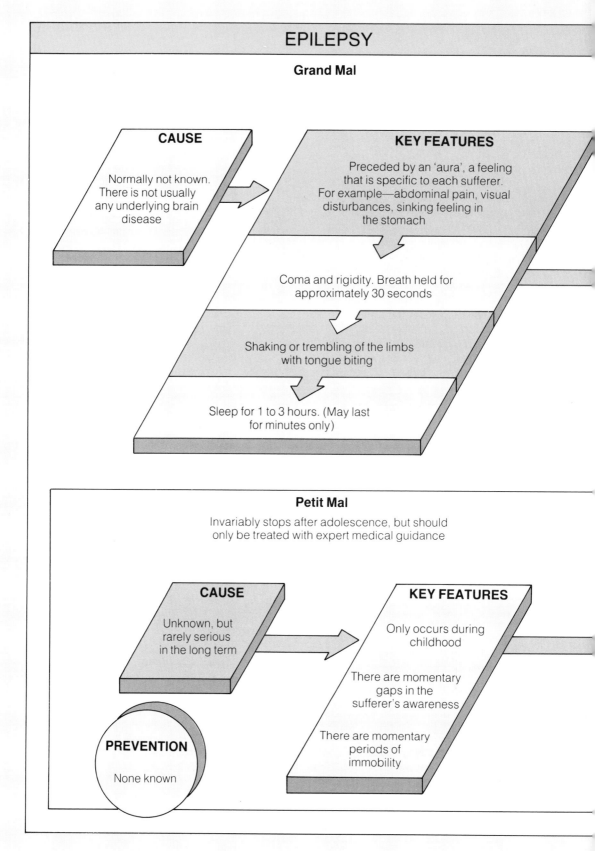

EPILEPSY

Grand Mal

CAUSE

Normally not known. There is not usually any underlying brain disease

KEY FEATURES

Preceded by an 'aura', a feeling that is specific to each sufferer. For example—abdominal pain, visual disturbances, sinking feeling in the stomach

Coma and rigidity. Breath held for approximately 30 seconds

Shaking or trembling of the limbs with tongue biting

Sleep for 1 to 3 hours. (May last for minutes only)

Petit Mal

Invariably stops after adolescence, but should only be treated with expert medical guidance

CAUSE

Unknown, but rarely serious in the long term

PREVENTION

None known

KEY FEATURES

Only occurs during childhood

There are momentary gaps in the sufferer's awareness

There are momentary periods of immobility

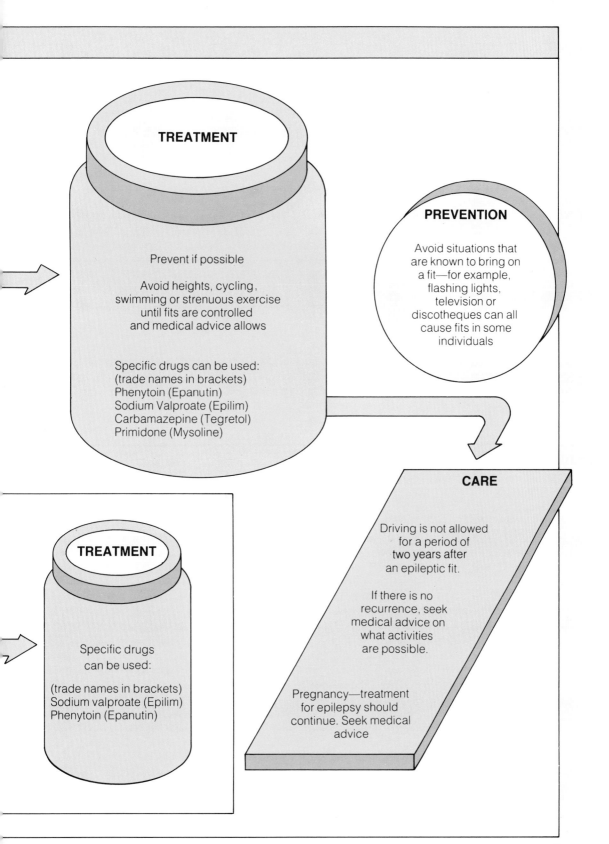

TREATMENT

Prevent if possible

Avoid heights, cycling,
swimming or strenuous exercise
until fits are controlled
and medical advice allows

Specific drugs can be used:
(trade names in brackets)
Phenytoin (Epanutin)
Sodium Valproate (Epilim)
Carbamazepine (Tegretol)
Primidone (Mysoline)

PREVENTION

Avoid situations that
are known to bring on
a fit—for example,
flashing lights,
television or
discotheques can all
cause fits in some
individuals

CARE

Driving is not allowed
for a period of
two years after
an epileptic fit.

If there is no
recurrence, seek
medical advice on
what activities
are possible.

Pregnancy—treatment
for epilepsy should
continue. Seek medical
advice

TREATMENT

Specific drugs
can be used:

(trade names in brackets)
Sodium valproate (Epilim)
Phenytoin (Epanutin)

to the ground, sometimes with a cry. It is at this stage that injury may occur, particularly if he is near a fire, at the top of a flight of stairs or crossing a busy road. The whole body becomes stiff and rigid, with clenched teeth. In a further few seconds the convulsion proper occurs, with powerful jerking movements of the limbs, trunk and jaw; often the tongue is bitten and starts to bleed, and there may be incontinence of urine. The fitting is over in a minute or two and is usually followed by a period of deep sleep, lasting for several hours.

In *petit mal* there are no convulsions but an 'absence' which lasts only a few seconds, during which time the epileptic stops whatever he is doing and becomes oblivious of his surroundings. When he recovers he has no memory of what has happened. Petit mal attacks start in childhood and disappear in adolescence, although occasionally these children develop major fits.

An epileptic fit is caused by a sudden burst of abnormal electrical activity from one area of the brain. The nerve cells in the normal brain are constantly firing off electrical impulses even during sleep. Many experts believe that the brain produces chemicals which control this electrical activity. If this substance is lacking and the brain cells are released from its constraining effects, abnormal bursts of excessive activity follow and a fit may result. The drugs used to treat epilepsy probably act by correcting the chemical deficiency.

Treatment

During a fit the major priority is to prevent the epileptic injuring himself. Any movable objects in the room, such as furniture, should be placed out of range. If he is near anything dangerous such as an open fire, there is no alternative but to drag him away. Forcible restraint of violent convulsive movements is of no value, and may even cause harm. If possible, he should be laid on his side so that if he vomits it will not drain into the lungs.

Once the convulsion is over, the epileptic can be allowed to sleep quietly in a position where there will be no danger if a further fit occurs. The fit itself may have produced a lot of sweating, so ensure he is well wrapped up to keep warm.

★ Any fit occurring unexpectedly at any age should be reported to your family physician immediately. In children a sudden fever due to viral infection, ear infection or tonsillitis may produce a single fit but this does not indicate a tendency to fits in the future. With known adult epileptics, medical help is needed only if there is an unusual feature—presuming the physician

has given instructions to you or to the patient in the past. If the fit lasts for more than 2–3 minutes you should get help anyway.

Long-term management

Many effective drugs are available for the treatment of epilepsy. Phenobarbitone has been replaced by phenytoin (Epanutin), sodium valproate (Epilim) and carbamazepine (Tegretol). Anticonvulsant drugs must be taken regularly; if the patient forgets to take even the occasional tablet the risk of a fit is increased.

School children with epilepsy should not be over-protected or labelled as 'different'. The adverse psychological consequences of being made to feel inferior at this stage far outweigh the risks of allowing young epileptics to lead a normal life.

Once the fits have been controlled there is no reason to restrict sporting activities such as physical education (including climbing frames) or horse and bicycle riding. The only important restriction is swimming, which should be done only in the presence of an adult who can swim and life-save. Schools are often unhappy about accepting this responsibility themselves, but there is no reason why a suitably qualified parent should not attend school swimming sessions.

In adults the same advice applies. Underwater swimming with breathing apparatus, or rock climbing with ropes, when other people's lives could also be endangered, is unwise. If the epilepsy is under good control, there is no reason to stop working with guarded machinery. In many ways the home is just as dangerous as the factory floor—one of the most hazardous places is the bathroom or lavatory, and the door is best left unlocked at all times.

In the United Kingdom the laws about epilepsy and driving are precise. Any fit under any circumstances means that driving will not be allowed for the next 2 years. The one exception is if the seizures have occurred only at night and have not changed in any way over the previous 2 years. Epileptics who have had no fits for 2 years, whether on or off therapy, are normally entitled to hold a driving licence.

Many people with epilepsy are worried about passing the tendency on to their children. Anyone who has a specific cause for his fits (e.g. previous head injury or meningitis) transmits no greater risk to his children. Even when there is no obvious reason, the risk of it being passed on to children is only 1–3 per cent (the prevalence in the general population is 0.5 per cent), and there are only a few families in whom epilepsy is a recurring problem.

Most drugs used to treat epilepsy render the contraceptive pill less effective.

There are few medical disorders that have attracted as many misconceptions as epilepsy. Even today there is a certain stigma attached to it, and a feeling that epileptics are different. Epilepsy can now be treated very successfully; it should not be forgotten that many very successful and highly intelligent people such as Julius Caesar, Handel and Byron suffered from epilepsy.

Episiotomy

A minor operation performed in some women immediately before the baby's head is born. Under local anaesthesia, a small incision is made at the entrance to the vagina, when delivery of the baby's head is imminent.

Episiotomy is performed to avoid tearing the skin and deeper tissue at the bottom of the vagina at the moment of delivery if the skin is over-stretched. Such tears are difficult to repair and, if extensive, may affect the normal function of the bowel and vagina. An episiotomy is much easier to stitch and heals more quickly and securely; as a result there is less likelihood of permanent soreness of the vagina which could interfere with the resumption of normal sexual relations. Stitching, again under local anaesthesia, takes 5–10 minutes, and dissolvable sutures are used.

Episiotomies are now performed only if there is a risk of serious tearing and not routinely, as small tears heal very well.

Epistaxis
SEE NOSE BLEED

Ergometrine

The chemical constituent of drugs used to induce contraction of the uterus immediately after delivery of the baby.

Erosion

Loss of small areas of cells causes small ulcers (or erosions); this affects all body tissues but commonly the skin (see Ulcer), the stomach (page 216) and the cervix of the uterus (page 55).

Erysipelas

A disease usually of old people, who develop a raised, tender, red rash of about 5–15 centimetres (2–6 inches) in diameter on the cheek or leg. Fever is present and they may have shivering and shaking attacks (rigors). The response to penicillin is invariably excellent.

Eustachian tube

The channel which connects and equalizes the pressure between the pharynx at the back of the mouth and the middle ear. Sore throats, tonsillitis and pharyngitis produce local swelling which may close the tube and cause earache (page 90).

Exercise

In heart disease strenuous exercise is best avoided; this includes competitive sports, digging, athletics and climbing. Regular non-strenuous exercise, such as walking, cycling and golf may help to prevent heart attacks. A sensible plan is to increase activity slowly until a maintenance level is achieved. For example:
1 Walk for a quarter of a mile in 15 minutes every day for 2 weeks. Increase by a quarter mile every 2 weeks to a total of 3 miles per day
2 Cycle half a mile in 5 minutes every day for 2 weeks Increase by a half mile every 2 weeks to a total of 4–6 miles per day.

It is dangerous to exercise in very cold weather if you have angina or are unfit and over 45 years old. The Royal Canadian Air Force has a well planned graded series of exercises for all ages and degrees of fitness (*Physical Fitness*, 1970, Penguin Books).

Expectorants

Drugs which aid coughing of sputum from the lungs. Most are ineffective and inhalations of steam are usually preferable.

Eye

The sight organ (see diagram, page 98). It is covered in front by a thin protective layer of transparent skin—the conjunctiva. This is continually washed by tear fluid which is naturally antiseptic. Light beams are focused by the lens in the front of the ball of the

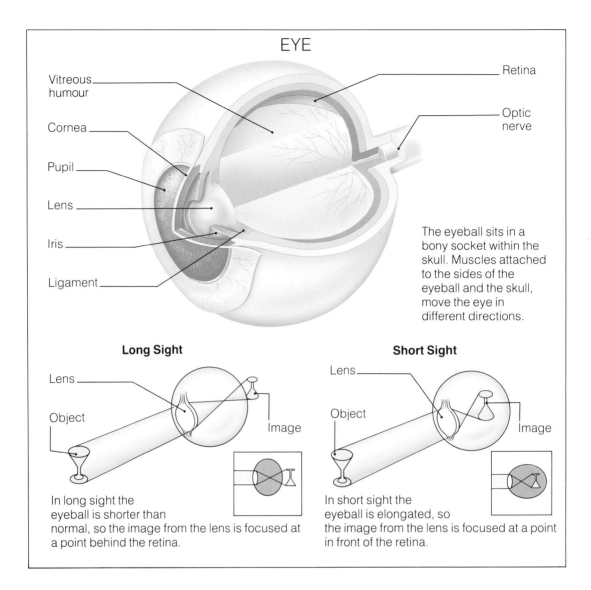

EYE

Vitreous humour

Cornea

Pupil

Lens

Iris

Ligament

Retina

Optic nerve

The eyeball sits in a bony socket within the skull. Muscles attached to the sides of the eyeball and the skull, move the eye in different directions.

Long Sight

Lens

Object

Image

In long sight the eyeball is shorter than normal, so the image from the lens is focused at a point behind the retina.

Short Sight

Lens

Object

Image

In short sight the eyeball is elongated, so the image from the lens is focused at a point in front of the retina.

eye onto the retina at the back, much as a camera lens focuses an image onto the film.

The retina consists of a layer of sensitive cells which respond to colour (cones) or low intensity light (rods) and send impulses along the optic nerves to the occipital cortex of the brain where the image is perceived.

Each eye is moved by four small muscles, and their movement is balanced together through the nerves supplying them. Damage to one of the muscles or to its controlling nerve supply causes the eyes to move in different directions, and the observed image from each eye is then seen separately and double—i.e. double vision (diplopia). Children may be born with one muscle weakened, resulting in a

squint. In these circumstances, the brain tends to suppress the image seen by the 'lazy' eye. Usually the vision in the weak eye can be improved with spectacles, or the weak muscle improved with exercises, or the squint reduced by surgery to the eye muscle.

Eye disorders are illustrated on pages 67–70 and the application of eyedrops on page 103.

Fainting

A common response to fear or excitement. It is usually momentary and has no serious significance. The head should be put between the knees or the patient should lie down.

Rarely, loss of consciousness may be caused by disorders of the brain or heart, and these should be excluded by careful medical assessment (*see* Blackouts).

Fallopian tubes

(AFTER FALLOPIUS, SIXTEENTH CENTURY ITALIAN ANATOMIST)

They transmit the eggs (ova) from the ovaries to the womb (uterus) (*see* diagram, page 263). The inner lining cells of the tube have fine hairs (cilia) which move in co-ordination, appearing under the microscope like wind blowing through a field of corn, to waft the ovum along. Infection of the tube may result in sterility (*see* Salpingitis).

Family planning

Contraception was probably first practised by nomadic tribesmen in the Middle East, who found that inserting pebbles into the wombs of their camels prevented their becoming pregnant during their long journeys across the desert—the coil is a modern method which applies the same principle.

The cap and the diaphragm
These are inserted into the top of the vagina before intercourse. They fit over the cervix, and prevent the passage of sperms into the uterus. They must always be used with a spermicidal cream or pessary.

They work effectively only if they fit correctly, and should only be used after expert medical advice. Caps and diaphragms are not as effective as the contraceptive pill and occasional failures occur.

Once in place, the woman is quite unaware of the cap, provided it is fitted correctly, and there is no interference with intercourse. The cap must be left in place for at least 8 hours after intercourse.

The coil (IUCD)
The intrauterine contraceptive device (IUCD), or coil, is favoured for older women who have had children and for whom the pill is less appropriate.

There are several types of coil. They are made of plastic; some are impregnated with copper which is slowly released inside the uterine cavity. All

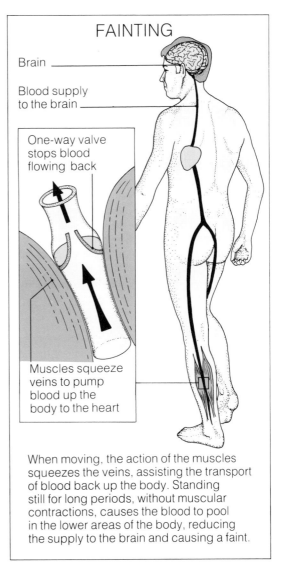

FAINTING

When moving, the action of the muscles squeezes the veins, assisting the transport of blood back up the body. Standing still for long periods, without muscular contractions, causes the blood to pool in the lower areas of the body, reducing the supply to the brain and causing a faint.

work by interfering with the attachment of the fertilized ovum to the lining of the uterus.

The coil is inserted through the cervix and passed into the uterus. The procedure is quick and relatively painless. Once in place, the coil remains in the uterus for years before being changed. (The copper varieties normally need renewing after 2 years.)

The coil may increase the heaviness of periods, although this often settles down after a few months. It may also cause vague lower abdominal pain as the uterus attempts to expel the foreign material. This, too, usually improves after a few months. Many gynaecologists feel that the IUCD should not be used in women who have had an infection in the Fallopian tubes (salpingitis, page 199) or any infection in the pelvis, for fear of recurrence.

For many older women in whom the pill is now considered too dangerous, the coil is a very acceptable alternative. Sometimes the side-effects become unacceptable and it has to be removed, but this happens in only a minority of cases. The coil is not quite as effective a contraceptive as the pill but the failure rate is small.

Coitus interruptus

This is an unsatisfactory method of contraception which is both unreliable and frustrating. At the moment of climax, the husband removes the penis from the vagina so that, in theory, sperms are not released around the cervix. However, sperms may be released long before orgasm is reached. Also, with the husband concentrating all the time on withdrawing at the right moment, the method is hardly conducive to relaxed love making.

The contraceptive pill

This is discussed in detail on page 175.

The rhythm method

This method of contraception relies on avoiding intercourse at or around the time of ovulation. Fertilization is usually possible only if intercourse takes place within 24–48 hours of ovulation. The difficulty is to determine when ovulation occurs each month, so a menstrual calendar must be kept. The time of every period is noted and, from this, the day on which ovulation occurs each month can be calculated retrospectively—it almost invariably takes place 14 days before a period (but not necessarily 14 days after). A careful record must be kept for a year because most women do not have a completely regular cycle and ovulate at slightly different times each month. The 'safe period' during which intercourse can occur with the least possible risk of pregnancy is calculated by subtracting 18 days from the shortest cycle and 11 from the longest. If, over the year, the cycle has varied between 26 and 30 days, the calculation would be:

$$26 - 18 = 8$$
$$30 - 11 = 19$$

This means that intercourse should be avoided between day 8 and day 19 (counting from the first day of the menstrual cycle which is day 1).

Many critics of the rhythm method point out that it is unreliable, and that banning intercourse for a third of each month may lead to frustration and even marital disharmony. However, this is the only method which is accepted by the Roman Catholic Church.

Another method for timing ovulation is by the use of a temperature chart. Ovulation is usually accompanied by a rise in body temperature of 0.3° C (or 0.6°F). This rise is usually maintained throughout the second half of the cycle. Immediately prior to this there is a brief fall in temperature.

A special thermometer is required to detect these small changes accurately. The temperature is measured at the same time every morning before getting out of bed (and before having a morning cup of tea). It is usually safe to have intercourse once the temperature has been raised for 3 clear days. This is a much easier method for detecting ovulation and is especially useful if the cycles are irregular. Great care must be taken in the early part of each month to avoid missing abnormally early ovulation. If the cycle is regular and ovulation easily detected, the first 6 days of the cycle are usually safe.

As a general rule, the ovum is available for fertilization 48 hours after ovulation and sperms only survive in the vagina for 24 hours. Thus, provided intercourse is avoided for the 24 hours before and 48 hours after ovulation each month, fertilization is unlikely though not impossible.

The sheath

The sheath is as reliable a contraceptive as the cap and diaphragm, but occasional failures occur if the sheath splits. It is important to use spermicidal cream or pessaries, and the sheath must be put on before intercourse begins and not just before orgasm is reached, as some sperms may be released from the penis before this. Creams and pessaries on their own are not reliable.

Advice about contraception may be obtained from a family doctor or family planning clinic who will advise and discuss the most acceptable and reliable methods available and their contra-indications.

As a rule, women over 35, and younger women with high blood pressure, epilepsy or migraine, should not take the pill.

Fats

Essential constituents of a normal diet, found in milk, butter, cheese and all oils. Within the body, fat acts as a heat insulator, a buffer between solid organs and a reserve source of energy.

Excess levels of fats within the blood predispose to angina (page 19) and heart attacks (page 120).

The levels are high in the obese and invariably return to normal after weight reduction.

Febrile convulsions

Convulsions occurring in children up to 4–5 years with very high temperatures. Usually no other cause is found and the convulsions stop as the illness subsides and the temperature abates.

Children who have convulsions should be ★ admitted to hospital, both for control and to ensure that no other disorder is present (*see below* Fever).

Femur
(LATIN: THIGH)

The thigh bone articulates with the hip at the top and the tibia at the knee joint below. (The hip is a ball-and-socket joint, and the knee is a sliding hinge joint.) (*See also* Skeleton, page 258.)

Fertility

The ability to conceive. Difficulty in conception may result from infertility of either partner, and requires careful clinical and psychological assessment and often detailed investigation (*see* Infertility).

Fever

A body temperature of above 37°C (98.4°C). Many infections produce a rise of the body temperature, which settles as the acute infection subsides.

When taking the temperature it is important first to ensure that the thread of mercury in the thermometer can be seen clearly, and that 'normal' is identified. The mercury can then be shaken down towards the bulb so that it registers well below normal. Most thermometers should remain in the mouth or under the arm for a minimum of 2 minutes. If after this time the mercury column has not moved, replace in the mouth or under the arm for a further 2 minutes.

In babies and young children the thermometer is usually placed under the arm or partially inserted into the rectum. In older children, the oral temperature is measured; hot drinks and food taken beforehand may produce an artificially high reading.

Any temperature above 37.4°C (99.5°F) in children or 37.7°C (100°F) in adults is probably due to an infection, the most frequent offender being the common cold. Children tend to develop high temperatures much more readily than adults. In the under-6 age group it is important to control the temperature if it remains raised after excessive clothing has been removed. A sudden rise in temperature may trigger a fit or seizure. Although not normally dangerous, febrile fits are extremely alarming.

If a child develops a fever, paediatric paracetamol syrup (Calpol, Febrilix) or aspirin will lower it. Avoid the natural temptation to wrap the child up; keep him in his normal nightwear in a warm but not hot room which is well ventilated. If these measures fail to bring the temperature down (or if aspirin or paracetamol are poorly tolerated because of vomiting), sponge him down with tepid water. Medical advice should always be sought if the temperature fails to fall or after a fit. When the temperature is high, considerable sweating occurs and the child must be encouraged to take regular sips of fluid, preferably cool water or squashes.

In adults, high fevers are less frequent. However, aspirin or paracetamol will bring the temperature down and relieve discomfort. Plenty of fluids are as essential for adults as for children.

There can be no hard and fast rule about when to call a doctor, and the temperature can only be taken as the roughest guide to the severity of the infection. Nevertheless, a high fever cannot be ignored. Although it may settle rapidly in children, if you are worried it is best to phone for medical advice. In adults, fevers which persist for more than 3–4 days are uncommon and suggest diseases other than infections. Recurrent or episodic fevers suggest infection in the gall bladder or kidneys, or malaria in those returning from the tropics.

See also Glandular fever; Hay fever; *and* Rheumatic fever.

Fibre

Diets high in fibre are the traditional food of the developing nations in whom certain diseases (e.g. heart attacks and cancer of the colon) are almost unknown. The Western refined diet is low in fibre so added fibre is recommended for the treatment of constipation (page 64), diverticular disease (page 85), and spastic (irritable) colon (page 212). Fibre is present in bran and wholemeal bread (for foods containing fibre, *see* Constipation). *See also* Dietary fibre.

Fibrocystic disease
SEE CYSTIC FIBROSIS

Fibroids

Simple lumps of muscle tissue which develop in the wall of the uterus. They enlarge slowly over the years and usually cause no problems. They are more common in women who have never had children and tend to occur after the age of 30 but not after the menopause. They cause heavy (menorrhagia) or painful (dysmenorrhoea) periods, pelvic discomfort or, rarely, problems with fertility.

Fibroids are best left alone unless they produce symptoms, when they can be removed. If a number of fibroids are present, it may be necessary to remove the uterus (hysterectomy).

Fibrositis
(RHEUMATISM)

Not a disease or diagnosis, but persistent aching pain in the muscles around one or more joints. It results from muscle strain and minor tears or bruising of ligaments. Simple symptomatic treatment directed to the affected area, such as local heat (i.e. hot-water bottles or products such as Algipan, Ralgex, or Deep Heat), massage and vibration, is effective. If not, analgesics (e.g. aspirin, paracetamol) will often relieve pain, which usually settles gradually over 4–6 weeks. (*See also* Arthritis *and* Rheumatism.)

Fibula

One of the bones of the shin, attached at the top to the outside of the tibia, below the knee, and forming the outside of the hinge of the ankle joint below (*see* diagram, page 259).

First aid
SEE PAGE 269

Fissure

A small tear in the inner lining of the rectum—usually the result of constipation. (*See* Anal fissure.)

Fits

An imprecise term used to describe convulsions or epilepsy (page 93), faints (page 99) and strokes (page 217).

Flat feet

The inside of the foot is usually arched. If the ligaments between the small bones of the foot are lax, the arch support is lost and the inner edge of the foot sits flatly on the ground. The cause is unknown and it is rarely a cause of severe symptoms. An arch support may relieve pain if it is present.

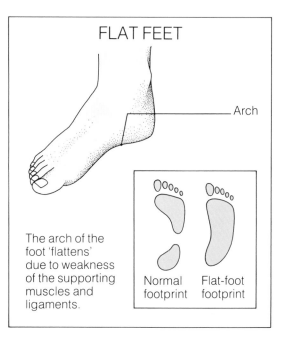

FLAT FEET

Arch

The arch of the foot 'flattens' due to weakness of the supporting muscles and ligaments.

Normal footprint

Flat-foot footprint

Flatulence

A sensation of fullness or wind at the top of the abdomen which is relieved by burping or belching. Flatulence rarely denotes serious disease and usually occurs because of air swallowing when swallowing saliva, drinks and food. The air passes into the intestine unless the quantity is large, when it collects in the stomach causing distension relieved by belching.

If flatulence is accompanied by pain in the upper abdomen then gall bladder disease or inflammation of the stomach (gastritis) may be responsible. Other possible causes include stomach ulcers (page 216), or

Eye Drops and Ointment

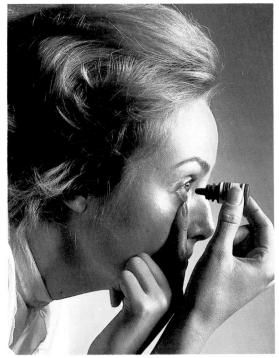

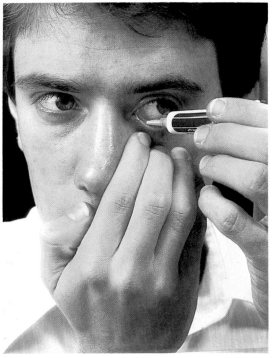

Eye drops *Sit or stand with your head tilted horizontally backwards. Pull down your lower eyelid with one hand; rest the other hand on this hand, with the dropper in position above the inner corner of the eye. Look over the back of your head and release the drops.*

Ointment *Stand in front of a mirror and pull back your lower eyelid to expose the inner surface. Hold the tube of ointment parallel to the lower eyelid and squeeze the ointment into its inner surface, starting at the inner corner and working outwards.*

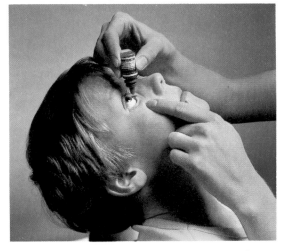

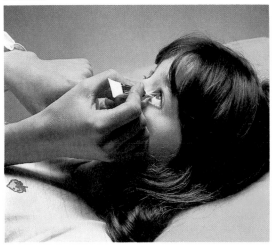

Eye drops *Sit the child down, and tilt the head backwards. Ask the child to look over the back of his or her head, then pull down the lower eyelid. Rest the hand holding the dropper on the forehead, and release the drops into the white of the inner corner of the eye.*

Ointment *Lie the child down and support the head with a pillow. Ask the child to look over the back of his or her head, then pull down the lower lid. With the tube parallel to the lower lid, squeeze the ointment along the inner lid surface, starting at the inner corner.*

Insulin Injection

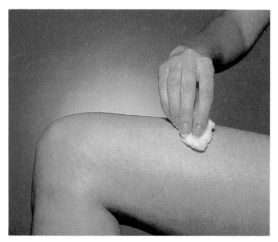

Step 1 *Choose the place where you intend to inject your dose of insulin and ensure that the area is clean and dry.*

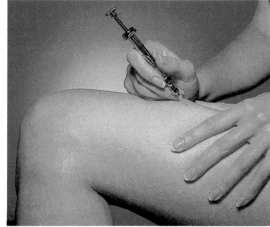

Step 2 *Pinch the skin between the thumb and forefinger of one hand, holding the syringe by its barrel in the other hand and insert the needle quickly at an angle of between 45° to 90° into the loose fatty tissue under the skin.*

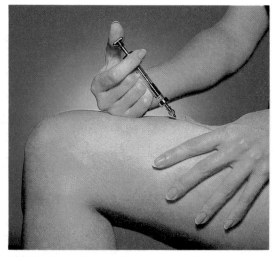

Step 3 *Before pushing the plunger in, pull it back a little to see if any blood appears in the syringe. If this happens it means that the needle is in a blood vessel and the insulin must not be injected. Withdraw the needle and make the injection in another place. If no blood appears, press the plunger all the way down to inject the insulin.*

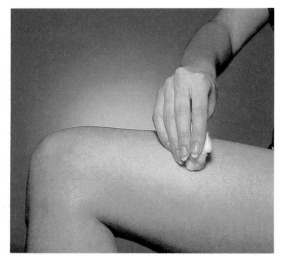

Step 4 *After giving the injection, withdraw the needle and press on the side of the injection with cotton wool to prevent any insulin from seeping out. Finally wash out the syringe and needle in industrial methylated spirit and store in the spirit proof case provided.*

a hiatus hernia (page 126) in which acid from the stomach passes up into the lower oesophagus, causing heartburn.

Treatment with milk or antacids (e.g. Milk of Magnesia, Mucaine, Asilone) relieves the symptoms. A reduction in the intake of fatty foods is often beneficial if gall bladder infection or gall stones are responsible.

Fluorides

A group of chemicals now strongly believed to decrease the incidence of dental caries in children. The evidence is sufficiently strong to support adding fluoride to water supplies deficient in it naturally. Failing this, brushing with fluoride toothpaste or taking fluoride tablets from early childhood will have the same effect.

Food poisoning

Usually caused by eating food contaminated by bacteria, usually salmonellae. Diarrhoea and sometimes vomiting and stomach cramps follow a few hours after eating. The severity varies from mild with slight diarrhoea to severe with prolonged abdominal pain, diarrhoea and vomiting leading to severe dehydration. Mild cases settle rapidly and most are better within 48 hours. If dehydration is severe, intravenous fluids are required and transfer to hospital becomes necessary. Antibiotics are virtually never necessary if dehydration is adequately corrected.

Food poisoning should be reported to the local public health authorities, who will trace the source and try to prevent further infections. Infected individuals should be meticulous about washing their hands after defecation, and not prepare food until the infection has cleared from the faeces.

The source of the infection may be a symptomless salmonella carrier who infects the food during preparation. The foods at greatest risk from salmonella poisoning include large frozen chickens or turkeys, which may be difficult to cook right through because of their size. If the middle of the bird is not cooked adequately the bacteria present will not be destroyed. A 3-pound frozen bird takes 10 hours to thaw at room temperature and 15 hours in a refrigerator. A large turkey may take 3 days to thaw in a refrigerator. An oven thermometer will show when the deepest part between the body and the thigh has reached 90–100°C (195–212°F)

If a person handling food has a septic finger, the organism (usually *Staphylococcus*) may grow in the food and produce a toxin which can cause very severe symptoms—collapse as well as vomiting and diarrhoea.

Poisoning occasionally follows the ingestion of food contaminated with chemicals. This is rare, but can happen if fruit is poorly washed after being sprayed with pesticides.

Contamination with botulism is exceedingly rare, and virtually never seen. It causes a severe infection of the nervous system and brain, which may result in respiratory failure and death. The illness is usually contracted by eating tinned meats which have not been properly sterilized during manufacture.

Forceps delivery

Forceps are used if birth is proceeding slowly because of the position of the baby's head. The head can be gently turned using the forceps and this allows labour to proceed. Forceps delivery may prevent the need for general anaesthesia and Caesarean section. (*See also* Pregnancy: labour.)

Foreskin
(PREPUCE)

The skin of the tip of the penis, removed at circumcision (page 61).

Fractures
SEE BONE FRACTURE

Frequency of micturition

Frequent urination is usually a sign of a bladder infection or irritation, and is accompanied by pain (*see* Cystitis). If accompanied by excessive thirst, diabetes (page 78) must be suspected. It occasionally occurs with prostatic enlargement in the elderly male (page 188). Medical advice should be obtained to exclude diabetes and to treat the infection.

Frigidity
SEE SEXUAL PROBLEMS

Frostbite

A rare condition occurring only in extremely cold climates and usually in mountaineers. The tips of the nose, fingers and toes, if not adequately protected, become frozen and the tissues die (i.e. gangrene). Treatment is by prevention, and adequate protective clothing should always be worn.

Frozen shoulder

A common disorder of the elderly, in whom one shoulder becomes stiff and painful. It is worse at night. Immobilization of the joint predisposes to it but often there is no known precipitating factor. The stiffness becomes progressively worse for 3–6 months, remains static for the next 6 months and then gradually improves. Physiotherapy and mild pain-killers (analgesics) such as aspirin or paracetamol improve the symptoms. If very disabling, local injection of hydrocortisone may cure a frozen shoulder almost immediately.

Fungus poisoning

The poisonous fungus (*Amanita phalloides*) is sometimes eaten in mistake for a mushroom. (The fungus can be distinguished by its green-yellow cup and white gills.) It causes nausea, vomiting, diarrhoea and sometimes shock.

★ The patient should be taken immediately to hospital for urgent treatment. If there is any delay, an attempt should be made to induce vomiting.

Gall stones

The gall bladder is a small sac the size of a small pear, which sits underneath the liver tucked up behind the rib cage on the right-hand side of the abdomen. It stores and concentrates bile produced by the liver.

Gall stones are common but only occasionally cause symptoms. Gall stones may irritate the gall bladder (cholecystitis, page 59), and this produces pain in the upper right-hand side of the abdomen, accompanied by flatulence, nausea and vomiting which may get worse after fatty meals. The symptoms vary from recurrent episodes of mild pain to episodes of acute pain and tenderness with fever, vomiting and exhaustion. This lasts for 3–5 days and settles spontaneously only to recur after an interval of 2

months to 2 years. Pain also occurs if a stone leaves the gall bladder and passes into the narrow bile duct. Muscle spasm then occurs around the stone, producing a severe intermittent colicky pain in the upper abdomen (biliary colic). Biliary colic may be accompanied by jaundice if the stone blocks the main bile duct through which bile passes from the liver to the bowel (*see also* Abdominal pain).

Gall stones are commonest in overweight women of 40–50 years (fat, fair, fertile, females of forty). People who include plenty of roughage in their diet do not suffer from gall bladder disease.

The recommended treatment for recurrent cholecystitis and gall stones is surgical removal of the gall bladder. The operation—cholecystectomy—is performed routinely in most hospitals and is usually curative because gall stones only form inside the gall bladder. The loss of the gall bladder is unimportant. Drugs are available to dissolve gall stones but their use is unsatisfactory as they have to be taken for 1–2 years and the stones tend to recur after they are stopped.

Gamma globulin

One of the protein fractions within the blood formed in response to natural infections (e.g. measles, mumps, poliomyelitis) and to protect the body against further attack. The principle of gamma globulin stimulation is used in vaccination against the common virus infections (*see* Vaccination).

Gamma globulin can be refined from blood taken at blood donor sessions, and injected to protect against infectious hepatitis. It is recommended for all travellers to the tropics of less than 35 years of age (older people are almost certainly immune); the protective effect lasts for 6 months.

Ganglion
(PLURAL: GANGLIA OR GANGLIONS)

A small benign lump which occurs under the skin around the wrist or on the back of the hand. Ganglions are very common and arise from one of the finger tendons to which they are attached. They cause few problems apart from their unsightly appearance if they become large. Pain only occurs if the ganglion is in a prominent position where it gets knocked.

They are best left alone. Surgical removal is a straight-forward procedure, employed for large ganglia particularly if they are frequently knocked and become painful or infected. Hitting them with

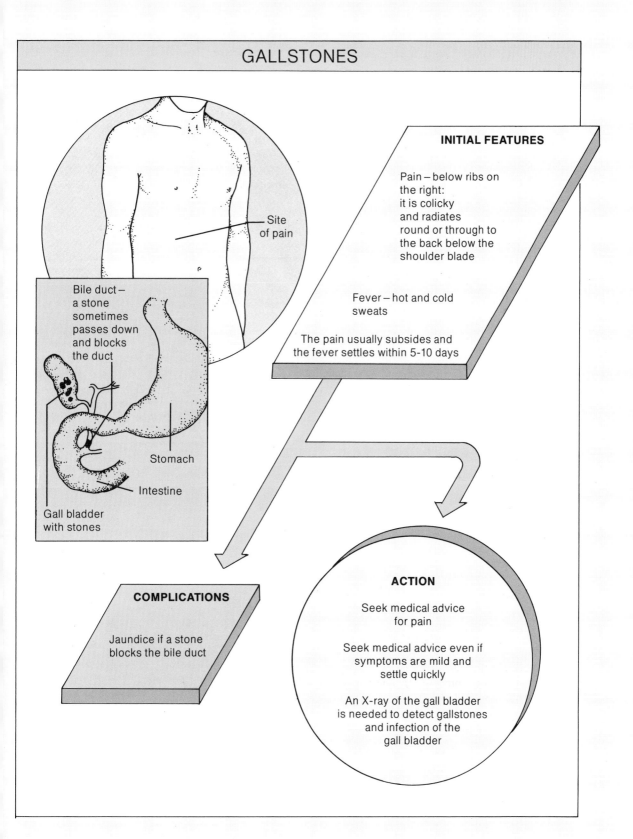

GALLSTONES

INITIAL FEATURES

Pain – below ribs on
the right:
it is colicky
and radiates
round or through to
the back below the
shoulder blade

Fever – hot and cold
sweats

The pain usually subsides and
the fever settles within 5-10 days

Site
of pain

Bile duct –
a stone
sometimes
passes down
and blocks
the duct

Stomach

Intestine

Gall bladder
with stones

COMPLICATIONS

Jaundice if a stone
blocks the bile duct

ACTION

Seek medical advice
for pain

Seek medical advice even if
symptoms are mild and
settle quickly

An X-ray of the gall bladder
is needed to detect gallstones
and infection of the
gall bladder

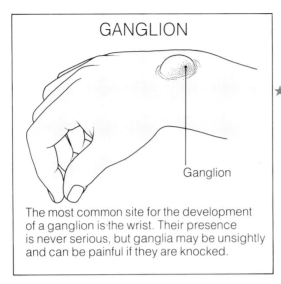

GANGLION

Ganglion

The most common site for the development of a ganglion is the wrist. Their presence is never serious, but ganglia may be unsightly and can be painful if they are knocked.

the family Bible is a traditional remedy dating from the time of enormous heavy Bibles—though not guaranteed to disperse the ganglion, the pain would certainly have taken your mind off it and very few are believed to have returned for further treatment!

Gangrene

Death of tissue. It is caused by narrowing of the arteries, usually to the feet, which become cold, pale and numb. If detected early, progress can sometimes be halted by inserting a graft to bypass the obstructed artery and restore the blood supply. The commonest cause is diabetes, and smoking the greatest risk factor (*see* Arterial disease).

Gargoylism

A very rare disorder, caused by deposition of complex sugars in the body tissues as a result of an enzyme deficit. It produces distortion of the features (hence the name) and mental retardation.

Gas poisoning

North Sea gas and the gas from portable cylinders are not themselves poisonous. However, if they are burnt with an inadequate oxygen supply or with blocked flues, carbon monoxide (a deadly gas) can be produced. Leaking gas cylinders in closed spaces, such as pleasure boat cabins, may exclude oxygen and cause asphyxia; adequate ventilation should be ensured.

Treatment is by moving the patient from the gas-filled atmosphere, and giving oxygen and artificial respiration if breathing is very slow or shallow. Domestic appliances should be regularly and expertly checked, and gas cylinders examined carefully for leaks before use, particularly if they have been stored.

Gastrectomy

The operation to remove the stomach, or part of the stomach (partial gastrectomy). The operation is performed for chronic and persistently painful stomach (page 216) or duodenal (page 86) ulcers and to remove stomach cancers

It is a major operation, safe in expert hands, and is performed under full general anaesthesia. For the first few days following surgery, fluids are given via an intravenous drip to rest the stomach and allow the wounds to heal, after which liquids and then food can be taken by mouth in gradually increasing quantities. The entire hospital stay is 14–21 days.

Gastric ulcer

Stomach ulcers are associated with excess acid and the pain results from a superficial erosion of the cells lining the inside of the stomach wall. The features are described under stomach ulcers (page 216).

Gastritis

Inflammation of the stomach, usually caused by alcoholic excess, stomach ulcers (page 216), certain drugs (e.g. aspirin) and as part of the gastro-enteritis (*see below*) of food poisoning. The pain is sore or gnawing and situated in the mid-line in the upper abdomen or behind the lower sternum. There may be associated nausea and the pain is relieved partially by milk and antacids (Rennie, Maclean's, Asilone, Gaviscon, Mucaine, etc.). It settles in 3–4 days. If there is no obvious cause such as an alcoholic binge, or if the pain is severe and is not relieved by antacids or milk and does not improve within 24 hours, medical advice should be sought.

Gastro-enteritis

Inflammation of the stomach (gastritis) and bowel (enteritis). Acute gastro-enteritis is an extremely common disease, second only in frequency to acute upper respiratory infections (i.e. coughs and colds). The symptoms vary from nausea or slight looseness of the bowels to a severe illness with fever, vomiting, and watery diarrhoea associated with abdominal colic. The acute symptoms usually settle in 24–48 hours. (*See also* Diarrhoea).

During the winter months, epidemics of diarrhoea and vomiting may sweep through families, schools and whole communities. Viruses and food poisoning cause over 95 per cent of cases.

Antibiotics are of no value as 90 per cent or more are caused by viruses, and the best treatment is to rest the stomach by drinking boiled water only with a little orange or lemon squash. Dairy products such as milk, eggs, butter, cheese and cream are best avoided until the acute symptoms have subsided. Kaolin with morphine and codeine reduce the diarrhoea and are used if symptoms persist for more than 24 hours. Aspirin or aspirin-containing preparations should be avoided if nausea or vomiting are present because they cause further stomach irritation. Alcohol is inadvisable for the same reason.

Adults usually recover from acute gastro-enteritis within 24–48 hours and it does not matter if they do not eat for a day or two, provided they maintain a good fluid intake. Great care must be taken with babies and young children, who may quickly become severely dehydrated and seriously ill following diarrhoea or vomiting. Any significant fluid loss in a baby should be reported to your doctor. If, in addition, the child has not passed much urine or is pale, limp or drowsy with a dry tongue, then the need for medical advice is urgent.

If abdominal pain or diarrhoea persists for more than 7 days, further investigation may be required—particularly in those recently returned from regions of poor sanitation and the tropics.

Gastro-intestinal tract

The digestive tract, including the stomach and the small and large intestines (*see* Digestive tract).

Gastroscopy

Literally, looking into the stomach. It is performed routinely in many hospitals if there is a strong suspicion of a gastric ulcer (*see* Stomach ulcer). It is a simple procedure, performed with the patient awake but sedated. A narrow flexible tube (a gastroscope) is passed gently down the oesophagus into the stomach. There is a light on the tip of the tube and the physician looks through a telescopic sight at the other end, and is able to clearly see and examine the stomach lining. Ulcers are easily visible. The gastroscope can be passed through the stomach into the next part of the intestine, the duodenum, to detect duodenal ulcers. The entire procedure takes about 30 minutes.

Genetic disorders

Disorders which are inherited via the genes within the parental ovum or sperm and which determine all physical characteristics. The term 'dominant' refers to a gene which will definitely produce specific characteristics in half the offspring, and 'recessive' means that it will do so only if the offspring receives two similar genes—one from each parent. Characteristics produced by 'recessive' genes are neutralized by those determined by 'dominant' genes. Well recognized examples are Huntington's chorea (page 129) which is dominantly transmitted and phenylketonuria (page 173) in which transmission is recessive.

Genes are sited within the body cells, on chromosomes, and abnormalities of these may induce transmission of disease to children. Mongolism (page 153) is the best known example. Haemophilia (page 116) is transmitted on the chromosomes which control the sex of the child.

Expert genetic counselling is strongly recommended for all who have a known genetic or chromosomal disease, or who fear they or their parents may have. This will often allay fears, but if the fears are well founded the couple may decide not to have children rather than risk transmitting the disease.

Genital tract
(LATIN: *GENITALIS*; TO BEAR, TO BEGET)

Female (*see* diagram, page 263)
This consists of the womb (uterus), the cervix, vagina and the right and left Fallopian tubes and ovaries. The egg (ovum) forms in the ovary and passes along a Fallopian tube to the body of the uterus where it may be fertilized. If fertilized, it embeds in the wall and develops further (*see* Pregnancy).

Male (*see* diagram, page 262)
This consists of the testes, vas deferens, seminiferous

GERMAN MEASLES

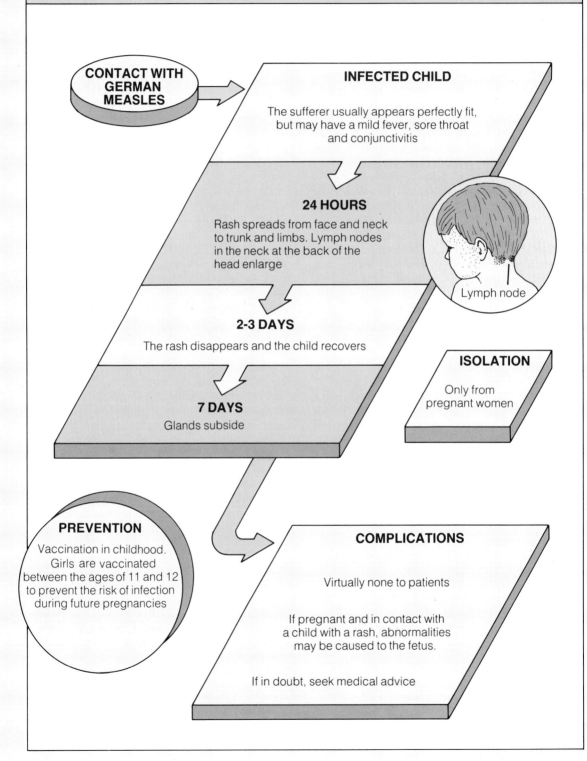

CONTACT WITH GERMAN MEASLES

INFECTED CHILD

The sufferer usually appears perfectly fit, but may have a mild fever, sore throat and conjunctivitis

24 HOURS

Rash spreads from face and neck to trunk and limbs. Lymph nodes in the neck at the back of the head enlarge

Lymph node

2-3 DAYS

The rash disappears and the child recovers

7 DAYS

Glands subside

ISOLATION

Only from pregnant women

PREVENTION

Vaccination in childhood. Girls are vaccinated between the ages of 11 and 12 to prevent the risk of infection during future pregnancies

COMPLICATIONS

Virtually none to patients

If pregnant and in contact with a child with a rash, abnormalities may be caused to the fetus.

If in doubt, seek medical advice

tubule and vesicles and the urethra of the penis. Sperm formed in the testes pass via the tubules to the vesicles, where some are stored pending ejaculation. The seminal fluid is ejected into the vagina via the erect penis, to fertilize the female ovum.

Inflammation of the testis is known as orchitis (page 162) (*see also* Urethritis).

Genito-urinary tract

The kidney, ureters, bladder, urethra, with the testes in men, and the uterus, Fallopian tubes and ovaries in women.

Genito-urinary disease is an alternative name for venereal disease (page 241).

Geriatrics
(GREEK: *GERAS*, OLD AGE; *IATREA*, TREAT-MENT)

The study and treatment of disease in old age and the elderly.

German measles
(RUBELLA)

One of the common childhood infectious illnesses which include measles, chickenpox, mumps and whooping cough. It is caused by a virus which is different from the measles virus despite their similar names.

In children
Children with German measles are rarely seriously ill and recover within a few days. Initially the illness may be indistinguishable from a cold. After 1 or 2 days' catarrh, often with a sore throat, a red rash develops. There may be enlargement of the glands (lymph nodes) in the neck. Children are infectious from the time they develop the first signs of catarrh and not merely when the rash appears. The incubation period (the time from infection to clinical illness) is usually 18 days, with extremes of as little as 10 or as much as 21 days.

In pregnant women
If a mother who has never had rubella is infected during the first 16 weeks of pregnancy there is a strong risk that the baby may be damaged and born malformed. The congenital defects which rubella causes involve the eye, heart, ear and brain. This 'congenital rubella' is completely avoidable, and all girls between the age of 11 and 12 should be vaccinated against rubella. If immunization is delayed until later, a simple blood test will show whether the woman has had rubella in the past and is immune, or whether she needs the vaccine. A blood test is the only way to be sure because the diagnosis of German measles cannot be made from the symptoms alone.

Note If you are a woman planning to have children, even if you think you have had German measles in the past, it is strongly advisable to have your blood tested to make absolutely sure, and if not be vaccinated.

Treatment
The only treatment required is aspirin or paraceta-mol syrup to reduce the temperature and ease the sore throat, and liberal fluids.

The important part of treatment is prevention, and everything possible should be done to avoid bringing any child who might have German measles into contact with a woman in early pregnancy. A pregnant woman who comes into contact with anyone with suspected German measles, or even a child with a rash, should seek medical advice within the next 24–48 hours. A blood test for rubella antibodies taken early after exposure will show whether she is or is not immune and whether the fetus is at risk from congenital infection.

Glands

SEE UNDER SPECIFIC GLANDS: ADRENAL GLANDS; LYMPH GLANDS; OVARY; PANCREAS; PAROTID GLANDS; PITUITARY GLAND; SALIV-ARY GLANDS; TESTES; AND THYROID DISEASE.

Glandular fever
(INFECTIOUS MONONUCLEOSIS)

A common virus infection which has been called the 'kissing disease'. It usually affects people in their teens or early 20s, who initially develop a sore throat and fever followed by tender enlargement of the tonsils and glands (lymph nodes) in the neck. Lethargy and depression are common features, and these may last for some weeks or even months after the acute illness subsides. Sometimes there is no acute illness at the beginning but only slowly developing malaise and lack of energy. There may be a blotchy rash which lasts 2–5 days (*see* illustration, page 237).

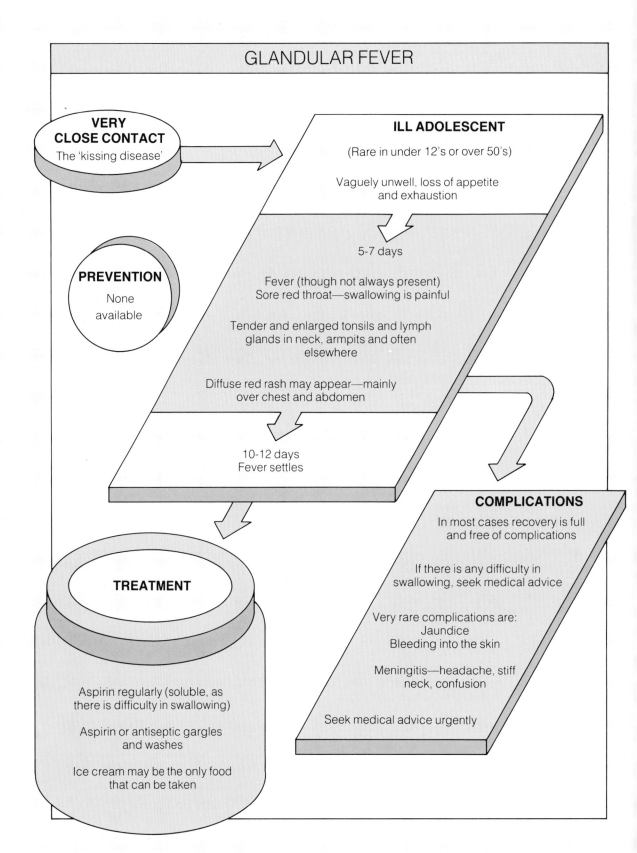

No specific treatment is needed for glandular fever and antibiotics are of no value. A simple blood test establishes the diagnosis. Very occasionally, steroids are given when the illness is particularly severe and the tonsillar enlargement sufficient to prevent swallowing.

Glandular fever is not dangerous; the persistent lethargy is more of a nuisance than anything else and will invariably improve without treatment.

Glasses
(SPECTACLES)

Used to correct refraction error of long or short sight, caused by variations in the shape of the eyeball and lens. Concave lenses correct short sight and convex lenses long sight. Contact lenses are made of inert materials and worn in contact with the eye, allowing greater visual acuity and a wider field of vision. They must be expertly fitted and may need to be worn for months before they no longer irritate the eyes.

Bifocal lenses consist of an upper large lens for distant vision and a lower smaller more convex lens for close vision. Although vision tends to deteriorate slowly with age, any alteration should be reported to an optician or the family doctor. Vision should be expertly checked every 2 years in those who wear glasses. Sudden blurring or visual loss should be reported immediately.

Glaucoma

A serious eye condition in which the pressure of the fluid in the eyeball becomes abnormally high. This damages the nerve carrying visual information back to the brain and, if left untreated, may result in blindness. (*See* illustration, page 68.)

There are two types of glaucoma: acute and chronic. The *acute* type comes on rapidly with severe aching pain in the eye which becomes red and inflamed. The vision in the eye becomes blurred and there may be an associated headache with visual haloes around lights. This is the less dangerous type of glaucoma, since the pain makes people go to their doctors immediately. Eye drops and tablets or simple surgery to the iris are used to reduce the pressure in the eye and this is usually achieved rapidly enough to avoid any further damage and before vision has been affected. After an acute attack of glaucoma, eye drops need to be continued to ensure that the pressure in the eye remains normal.

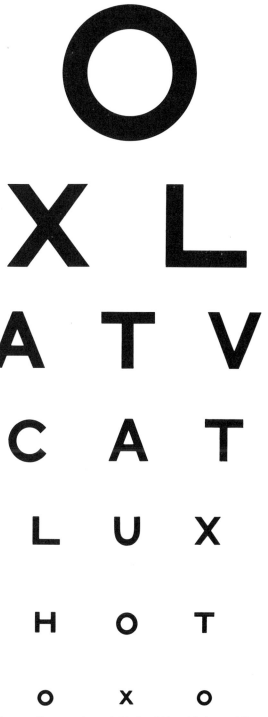

Those with normal eyesight should be able to read the smallest letters on this chart from a distance of three metres (about nine feet). The chart should be placed in a good light, and each eye tested separately, with the other covered.

The *chronic* form of glaucoma is more dangerous because it comes on insidiously. There is a gradual increase in eyeball pressure which causes slow and progressive damage but not sufficient to give rise to dramatic symptoms such as pain. The field of vision gradually diminishes and this may not be noticed until the central vision is affected, by which time considerable damage has been done. The only way to make the diagnosis of chronic glaucoma in the early stages is to measure the pressure in the eye, which is done simply and painlessly using a tonometer.

Glaucoma affects 2 per cent of the population over 40 and sometimes runs in families. Many experts believe that older people who have a closely affected relative should have their eye pressures checked.

'Glue ear'

Results from incomplete treatment of ear infection, and is a cause of deafness in children (*see* Ear infection).

Gluten sensitivity

Sensitivity of the lining of the small intestine—a fine layer of cells lining the inside wall—to gluten, a constituent of wheat. This produces diarrhoea with malabsorption of food and vitamins. The disease is also known as coeliac disease (page 62), and is cured by excluding gluten-containing foods from the diet.

Glyceryl trinitrate
(TRINITRIN, TNT)

One of the first effective drugs against angina, and it is still widely and successfully used. The tablets are placed under the tongue and allowed to dissolve slowly. They relieve the pain of angina within minutes, although they may also produce a slight headache. They are better used prophylactically (i.e. to prevent pain) by placing a tablet under the tongue before activity which is likely to produce pain (e.g. walking up hills, running, sexual intercourse).

Goitre

Any enlargement of the thyroid gland, in the neck. Some goitres are caused by a dietary deficiency of iodine, and apart from their size are of no clinical significance. If unsightly, they can be removed surgically.

Swellings of the thyroid gland also occur with both over-activity (thyrotoxicosis, page 224) and under-activity (myxoedema, page 226).

Thyroid swellings which appear over a short time are often tender and are due to an acute virus infection (thyroiditis). Very occasionally, thyroid cancers present this way and can be successfully removed if operated upon early.

Swellings of the thyroid gland are rarely serious if of long standing, but if they occur over a period of days to a few months, medical advice should be obtained.

Gonorrhoea

A common venereal disease (page 241) caused by a bacterium (*Neisseria gonorrhoeae*) which, in men, produces symptoms of burning on urination with frequency of micturition and white or yellow discharge from the urethra. In women there is a vaginal discharge in addition to cystitis (page 71) and frequency of micturition, but the infection may produce almost no symptoms and the woman may infect many men unaware that she is harbouring gonorrhoea. The disease may cause anal infection and, rarely, conjunctivitis and arthritis.

The diagnosis is made from microscopic examination of the discharge, and the disease is treated successfully by penicillin injections. All contacts should be traced and treated if infected. It is particularly important to trace female contacts even if free of symptoms.

Gonorrhoea is sometimes accompanied by other genital infections, such as syphilis (page 219) or *Trichomonas vaginalis* (*see* Vaginal discharge).

Gout

The symptoms are a sudden, excruciating pain in a single joint, which becomes red and inflamed. The joint most often affected is that at the base of the big toe, although the finger joints, ankle or wrist can be involved. In gout the level of circulating uric acid is too high. Uric acid crystals form in the joint to produce an acute attack of pain. The joint involved becomes very tender, red, warm, swollen and shiny, as well as excruciatingly painful.

The pain of an acute attack can be relieved with phenylbutazone or indomethacin or stronger pain killers. Aspirin should be avoided. If the attacks are recurrent, long-term treatment with allopurinol (Zyloric) may be advisable to keep the uric acid in the blood at normal levels.

Attacks of gout can be induced by certain drugs, which may need to be stopped. It was believed that

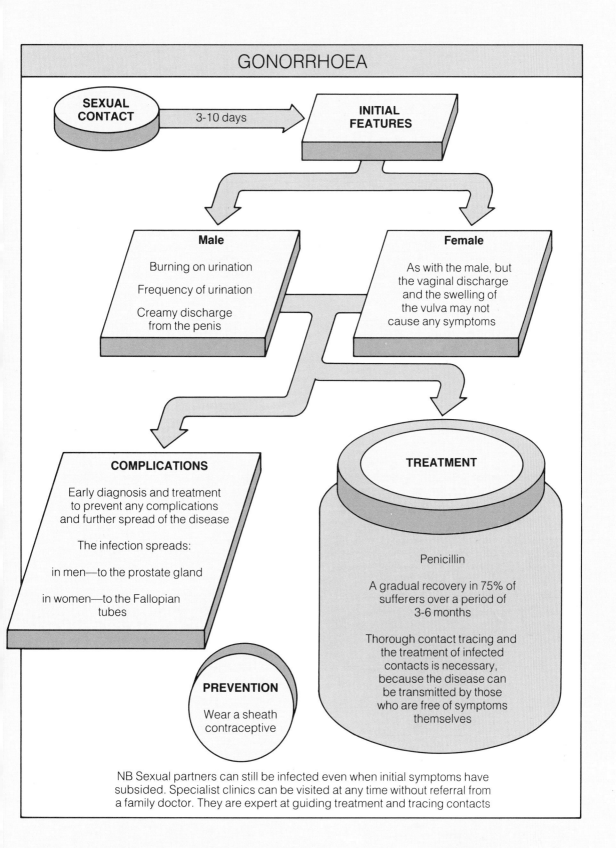

GONORRHOEA

SEXUAL CONTACT → 3–10 days → **INITIAL FEATURES**

Male

Burning on urination

Frequency of urination

Creamy discharge from the penis

Female

As with the male, but the vaginal discharge and the swelling of the vulva may not cause any symptoms

COMPLICATIONS

Early diagnosis and treatment to prevent any complications and further spread of the disease

The infection spreads:

in men—to the prostate gland

in women—to the Fallopian tubes

TREATMENT

Penicillin

A gradual recovery in 75% of sufferers over a period of 3–6 months

Thorough contact tracing and the treatment of infected contacts is necessary, because the disease can be transmitted by those who are free of symptoms themselves

PREVENTION

Wear a sheath contraceptive

NB Sexual partners can still be infected even when initial symptoms have subsided. Specialist clinics can be visited at any time without referral from a family doctor. They are expert at guiding treatment and tracing contacts

gout resulted from an over-indulgence in alcohol. This is not true. Uric acid can precipitate in the kidneys leading to the formation of stones. A liberal fluid intake is advisable if the uric acid concentration in the urine is elevated.

Graves's disease

A disease caused by over-activity of the thyroid gland (page 224), associated with large staring eyes.

Group therapy

A method of psychiatric psychotherapy (page 189).

Gullet
(LATIN: *GULA*, THROAT)

The food passage from the back of the throat to the stomach. It is also known as the oesophagus (page 264).

Guthrie test

Should be performed routinely on all newborn babies, to exclude phenylketonuria (page 173). The test involves taking a small specimen of blood from the heel and measuring the level of the chemical phenylalanine. If the level is high it may lead to mental retardation—which can be prevented, if detected early, by a diet free of phenylalanine.

Phenylketonuria is rare (about 1 in every 10,000–20,000 babies), easily detected and the complications are preventable.

Haematuria

The presence of blood in the urine. This is commonly caused by infection in the kidney or bladder but may result from a stone or a growth in the bladder or kidney. Medical advice should always be sought even if the haematuria is painless and brief.

Haemodialysis

Dialysis of the blood in the treatment of kidney failure (*see* Kidney dialysis).

Haemoglobin

The chemical constituent of the red blood cells which carries oxygen from the lungs to the body tissues. It is a compound of protein and iron. Deficiency results in anaemia (page 18).

Haemophilia

A serious blood disease which causes severe recurrent bleeding into any part of the body, but usually into large joints such as the knees, ankles and elbows, often following minor knocks and trauma. Less commonly, bleeding occurs into the gut, kidneys or muscles. The bleeding is due to the absence of a major blood-clotting constituent, known as factor VIII or the anti-haemophilic factor. The disease is carried on one of the 'X' sex chromosomes by the patient's mother who, if the other 'X' chromosome is normal, will not have a bleeding disorder. The abnormal chromosome is passed to half of her daughters or sons. It is only the sons who develop the bleeding disorder for, as XYs, they do not have a normal second X chromosome to over-ride the abnormal one. Only 50 per cent of her sons receive an abnormal X chromosome; the others are entirely normal and are not carriers.

Treatment is by transfusion of the anti-haemophilic factor and this almost invariably controls the bleeding. Any surgery, either major or minor such as tooth extraction, must be performed under careful supervision and after an injection of the anti-haemophilic factor. The disease may be very mild and cause only minor inconvenience but when severe it is life-threatening. In view of this and the absence of a cure, many believe that men with haemophilia should not have children. Their sisters may or may not be carriers and should be investigated for this and receive genetic counselling, so that they can better decide whether or not to have children.

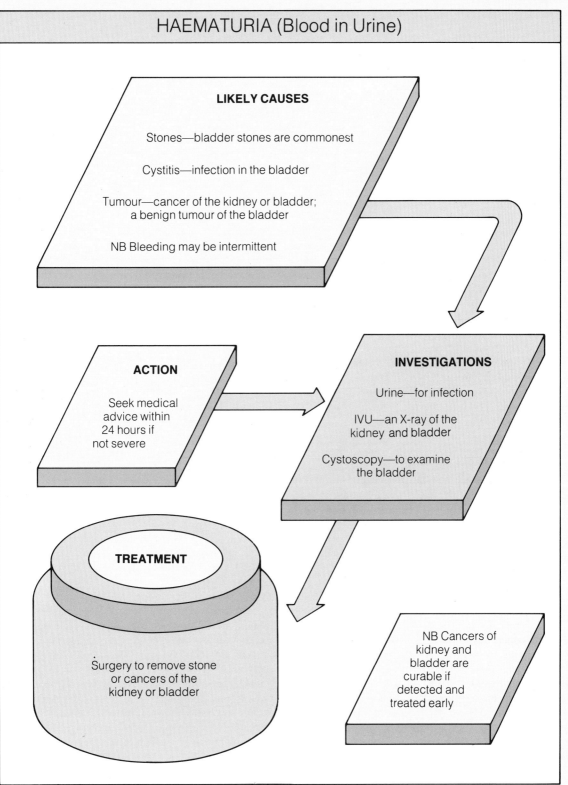

HAEMATURIA (Blood in Urine)

LIKELY CAUSES

Stones—bladder stones are commonest

Cystitis—infection in the bladder

Tumour—cancer of the kidney or bladder;
a benign tumour of the bladder

NB Bleeding may be intermittent

ACTION

Seek medical
advice within
24 hours if
not severe

INVESTIGATIONS

Urine—for infection

IVU—an X-ray of the
kidney and bladder

Cystoscopy—to examine
the bladder

TREATMENT

Surgery to remove stone
or cancers of the
kidney or bladder

NB Cancers of
kidney and
bladder are
curable if
detected and
treated early

Haemorrhage
SEE BLEEDING *AND UNDER* FIRST AID, PAGE 269

Haemorrhoids
SEE PILES

Hair growth

Each hair grows from a root in a hair follicle. The hair, once it has emerged from the skin, is a 'lifeless' structure and has no nerve or blood supply. Hairs are lubricated by a greasy substance known as sebum, which is secreted by sebaceous glands adjacent to each follicle and prevents it becoming brittle.

Hair grows at the rate of 1 millimetre (0.039 inch) a day but it is not a continuous process. Each individual hair passes through a series of phases, beginning with a growth phase lasting 2–3 years, followed by a period of about 2 weeks when growth slows down. Finally a resting phase is reached, during which there is no further elongation of the hair. The cycle returns to the beginning again when a new hair grows out from the follicle and the old hair naturally falls out. There are around 100,000 hairs on the scalp and at any one time 85–95 per cent are in active growth phase. It is normal for about 50–75 hairs to be lost every day.

Baldness can result if large numbers of hairs all go into a resting phase at the same time. This occasionally follows pregnancy or a high fever, and occasionally after stopping the contraceptive pill. While most upsetting at the time, hair grows again without any treatment although this may not begin for several months.

Hair loss

In men
The 'male pattern' of hair loss is caused by sensitivity of the hair follicles to male sex hormones (androgens). Some follicles seem particularly sensitive to androgens so that hair growth from them stops and the hair falls out. Recession of the hair line characteristically begins each side of the mid-line at first and spreads centrally. Then there is thinning over the crown area followed by total loss of hair over the top of the head, leaving only the back and sides covered.

There are many patent cures for male baldness, but none of them has been proven to be effective. They are usually very expensive and absolutely worthless. If baldness does cause excessive anxiety, a wig is the simplest remedy.

In women
The hair gradually becomes thinner as women become middle aged. This can produce great anxiety but hair loss is rarely excessive, and baldness extremely rare. Hair loss is a common feature of myxoedema, when there is deficiency of the hormone thyroxine. If detected early and adequately corrected, hair loss will stop and the hair regrow.

In children
Babies often develop bald patches on the sides or back of the head, by rubbing the hair off on the sides of their cots.

Older children sometimes develop the habit of twisting their hair round their fingers, exerting considerable traction on the roots and the hair may fall out in patches. It grows again once the habit is cured. It is called trichotillomania, and in an adult may be a symptom of an underlying mental disorder.

Other cause of hair loss
Alopecia areata
A skin disorder in which the hair tends to fall out in small areas, leaving round bald patches. Regrowth usually begins in 2–3 months.

Halitosis
SEE BAD BREATH

Hallucinations

The perception of imagined objects which may be seen, heard, or tasted. The visions are usually unpleasant and may be terrifying, and the voices may give the patient the feeling of being persecuted. A typical example is seen in alcoholism when hallucinations often take the form of terrifying animals such as birds, spiders or insects. The concept of an aggressive butterfly is difficult to grasp but it is not infrequently a major cause of anxiety to an alcoholic. Hallucinations occur in acute alcoholism, alcohol withdrawal (delirium tremens), in disorders such as schizophrenia and in acute infections of the brain (e.g. meningitis). Hallucinations may be caused by brain damage following falls, road accidents, strokes, tumours of the brain and shock.

Hallux valgus

A deformity of the joint at the base of the big toe, which becomes prominent. It rubs against footwear and a bunion inevitably forms on its surface. If severe and painful, the joint can be straightened surgically (*see also* Chiropody: bunion).

Hammer toe
SEE UNDER CHIROPODY

Hang nail
SEE NAIL

Hangover

The after-effects of excessive alcohol or sedative drugs. The typical features are exhaustion, woolly-headedness, and banging headaches with nausea and sometimes vomiting. The cause is unknown but may be a combination of the direct action of alcohol on the brain with the added effects of the dehydration resulting from the increased urine output produced by alcohol and perhaps from other chemical compounds in red wine, port, brandy and sherry. The nausea may be due to the direct toxic effect of alcohol on the stomach lining.

There are many cures but prevention is the best, though sometimes difficult to achieve. The effects of drinking the hangover away—drinking 'the hair of the dog that bit him'—usually makes the symptoms worse. Rapid rehydration immediately after alcohol with 1–2 pints of water may help but few can contemplate the additional fluid volume required. Two tablets of soluble aspirin for the headache plus a few hours' sleep are as good as anything.

Hare lip

A birth deformity which produces a vertical gap in the upper lip, resembling the lip of a hare. The deformity is not usually serious but occasionally is associated with a cleft in the palate. This may prevent the newborn baby sucking. Both hare lip and cleft palate can be repaired by plastic surgery, leaving only minor scars which are virtually unrecognizable.

Hashish
SEE CANNABIS

Hay fever

An allergic disease (*see* Allergy) which usually begins in the spring when the pollen count starts to rise. It is named after the flowery grass or hay which appears in late spring, though other pollens may be responsible. The features are a running and stuffy nose, with irritation and sneezing, and sore red eyes. Attacks may be intermittent but in a few very sensitive subjects the symptoms may persist without break throughout the spring and summer. Skin tests will show which pollens are responsible. Some sufferers are sensitive to only one pollen but most people with hay fever are sensitive to a multitude of them.

Treatment
It is sensible to avoid country districts at times of high pollen counts but this is often more easily said than done. Antihistamine drugs may suppress the symptoms but most of them cause some degree of tiredness or even drowsiness. Nasal sprays containing ephedrine act by constricting the nasal blood vessels and thereby decrease congestion. They are used successfully by many sufferers. Recently, anti-allergic drugs have been produced (e.g. sodium cromoglycate, Rynacrom) which can be given by inhalation into the nose and work by suppressing the local reaction to the sensitizing pollens. This drug is also effective in asthma caused by hypersensitivity.

Desensitization injections can be given if skin tests show that a sufferer is sensitive to only one or perhaps two pollens. Sadly this is rarely the case and most patients are sensitive to 10 or more pollens.

Hay fever may range from very mild with occasional attacks, to very severe when daily life can be virtually ruined. Newer drugs offer great hope and sufferers of severe hay fever are strongly advised to seek expert help.

Head injuries

Usually caused by road traffic accidents, falls or blows to the head. The brain has a texture of thick porridge and is supported by a supporting membrane—the meninges. The inner layer of the meninges (the arachnoid) is enclosed in a strong fibrous bag (the dura). The cerebrospinal fluid (within the dura) bathes the brain and absorbs shocks. The skull protects the brain from severe trauma, and the cerebrospinal fluid and meninges allow the brain almost to float within the skull—which acts as another buffer against damage. Head injuries may be open or closed.

With open injuries, the skull is fractured and the skin over it broken. Bone, a weapon, or part of a car may enter the brain, and the amount of damage depends upon the nature of the weapon and the degree of damage. With bullet wounds the entire brain may be disrupted by the speed of the bullet.

With closed head injuries, the skull shape is not altered although there may be narrow undisplaced fracture of the skull. Closed injuries are caused by falls or blunt instruments. Damage to the brain will not occur if the protective buffer of the cerebral fluid is sufficient to absorb the blow, but with greater trauma the brain substance tends to become bruised by twisting upon itself. This results in confusion or even loss of consciousness, but as recovery proceeds over hours or weeks (or even months if the trauma is severe), confusion decreases and intellectual ability returns. Memory for the period of illness rarely returns, and the events immediately preceding the injury when the patient was still normally conscious are often forgotten. This fascinating but fortunate memory loss is known as 'retrograde amnesia'.

If the initial injury is very severe, full intellectual recovery may not occur. This can only be assessed accurately after many months, as many patients recover completely months and even years after the initial accident.

Headaches

One of the more common symptoms which take people to their doctors. In the vast majority of cases, the pains over the front and top of the head are related to tension at home or work and settle spontaneously after a few days or after taking one or two analgesic tablets, such as aspirin or paracetamol.

If there is serious underlying anxiety or depression, the headaches tend to persist.

Pain behind the eyes may be a result of poor eyesight or the strain of reading in dim light. It is particularly common in students during periods of intense study before examinations, when tension is also a factor. Pain behind the cheek bones often follows colds and infections of the nasal air sinuses and takes the form of a dull, persistent ache, often with pain in the teeth of the upper jaw. Pain at the back of the head and at the top of the neck are often caused by muscle strain and, in the middle aged or elderly, arthritis of the vertebral bones of the neck.

Severe acute headaches occur in migraine (page 152), meningitis (page 151) and after head injuries, but there are usually other symptoms as well; such headaches rarely occur in isolation. Many people

fear that a headache means that they have a tumour of the brain. Brain tumours are exceedingly rare but headache is extremely common. Nevertheless, if a headache is a new symptom and if it persists for more than a few days it is reasonable to seek medical advice and reassurance.

Hearing
SEE DEAFNESS

Heart

The pump which circulates the blood round the body (*see* diagram, page 253). It is really two pumps bound together side by side, with valves in each which prevent back-flow. There are two chambers on each side: a low-pressure *atrium* (Latin: entrance hall of a villa), which receives blood and passes it through a valve to a *ventricle* which pumps it through another valve to a large artery. In the right heart, the right atrium passes blood through the tricuspid (three cups) valve to the right ventricle which pumps it through the pulmonary valve to the lungs. Here the blood receives oxygen, and this oxygenated blood passes into the left atrium and thence through the mitral valve (shaped like a bishop's mitre but upside down) to the left ventricle.

The wall of the left ventricle is very muscular and thick, and it pumps the blood at high pressure (120–160 mmHg) via the aorta to the rest of the body. If the valves are damaged by disease, they may become too narrow (stenosis) or may leak (regurgitate) blood backwards. If the heart's pumping efficiency is seriously affected (congestive heart failure) there may be congestion of blood in the lungs, producing breathlessness or poor circulatory flow in the tissues—resulting in swelling of the ankles. In most situations the valve can be successfully replaced or repaired by open-heart surgery. Rarely, children are born with a hole in the septum between the right and left atria (atrial septal defect) or in the septum between the two ventricles (ventricular septal defect) (*see* Hole in the heart).

Heart attack
(CORONARY)

An episode of damage to part of the muscle of the heart. It is sometimes referred to as a coronary because the arteries which are affected in the attack are called coronary arteries (page 252). Narrowing of

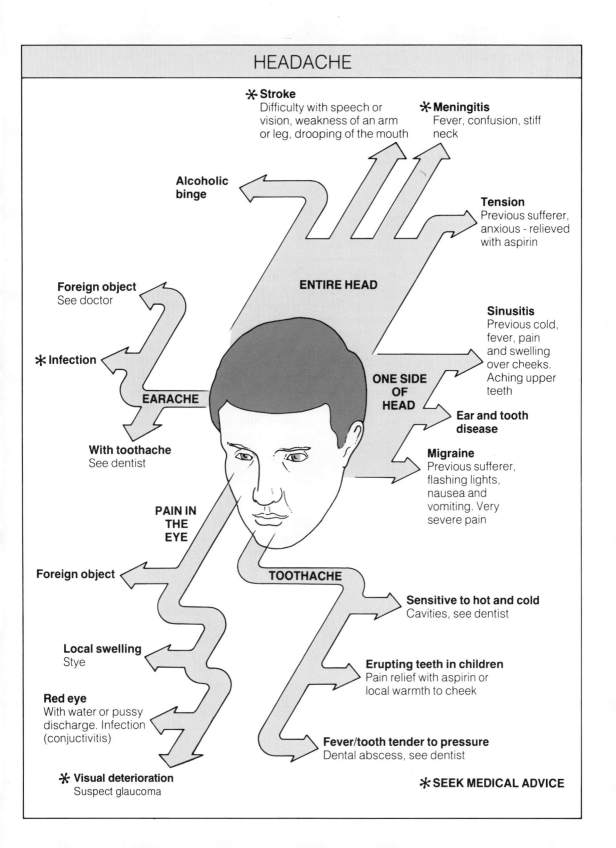

HEADACHE

✳ Stroke
Difficulty with speech or vision, weakness of an arm or leg, drooping of the mouth

✳ Meningitis
Fever, confusion, stiff neck

Alcoholic binge

Tension
Previous sufferer, anxious - relieved with aspirin

ENTIRE HEAD

Foreign object
See doctor

Sinusitis
Previous cold, fever, pain and swelling over cheeks. Aching upper teeth

✳ Infection

ONE SIDE OF HEAD

Ear and tooth disease

EARACHE

Migraine
Previous sufferer, flashing lights, nausea and vomiting. Very severe pain

With toothache
See dentist

PAIN IN THE EYE

Foreign object

TOOTHACHE

Sensitive to hot and cold
Cavities, see dentist

Local swelling
Stye

Erupting teeth in children
Pain relief with aspirin or local warmth to cheek

Red eye
With water or pussy discharge. Infection (conjuctivitis)

Fever/tooth tender to pressure
Dental abscess, see dentist

✳ Visual deterioration
Suspect glaucoma

✳ SEEK MEDICAL ADVICE

121

these arteries by atheroma, a substance produced partly from ingested animal fats (*see* Arterial disease), reduces the blood supply to the heart muscle. If the reduction falls below a critical level or the narrowed artery becomes blocked, the oxygen supply to that portion of the heart is cut off and the muscle is damaged or may even die.

Usually only a small amount of muscle is damaged, whilst the rest of the heart, which is unaffected, continues to beat and easily compensates for the muscle lost.

Symptoms

Pain is the main symptom and is usually experienced as a crushing sensation or tightness in the centre of the chest. Sometimes pain can also be felt in the neck, jaws or arms. If severe, the pain may cause nausea and sometimes shock, with a fall in blood pressure which in turn results in a rapid shallow pulse, sweating and pallor. Breathlessness may be a more obvious symptom, particularly in the elderly. Recurrent episodes of pain of this character may occur on exercise in patients whose coronary arteries are narrow.

In these circumstances the oxygen supply to the heart muscle is sufficient for normal function at rest but exercise puts greater strain on the heart and increases its oxygen demand to a level which the narrow arteries are unable to supply. This is angina and is similar to cramp in the calves. Patients who develop features suggesting a heart attack or angina should lie down and rest to reduce strain on the heart by minimizing its work—medical advice should be sought immediately. Angina (page 19) usually responds very well to treatment.

Heart transplantation

Following the success of kidney and liver transplants, there was considerable hope that severely diseased hearts could be replaced. Although the surgery is technically feasible in expert hands, the problems of rejection and infection which follow have not yet been fully overcome. Heart transplantation has not become a routine medical procedure, though it is still performed under very careful observation in a few specialized hospitals.

Heart valves

The heart has four valves: the tricuspid, mitral, pulmonary and aortic valves (*see* diagram, page 253).

These can be damaged during attacks of rheumatic fever, but this is now very rare in the developed countries. Severe damage to the valves greatly reduces the ability of the heart to pump blood round the circulation. If this occurs, blood may pool in the veins of the lungs, causing breathlessness, and in the legs, causing ankle swelling.

Artificial heart valves can be used to replace damaged valves. If the heart muscle is healthy and has not been involved in the original infection, the results are often perfect.

Heartburn

The burning pain felt behind the breast bone (sternum), caused by reflux of acid from the stomach into the oesophagus—also called reflux oesophagitis (page 194). (*See also* Indigestion *and* Hiatus hernia.)

Heat stroke
(*SEE ALSO* SUN STROKE)

A rare but dangerous acute illness caused by working in a very hot environment. Normally the body loses excess heat by sweating and by increasing respiration. Heat stroke occurs if the heat gained from the environment exceeds the maximum loss. The features are confusion, very rapid respiration, a rapid thready pulse and collapse. If the person is not moved to a cooler environment, his temperature continues to rise and he eventually begins to 'fit' and finally collapses into a coma. Even if moved early, the outcome may be fatal because the body's heat regulator mechanisms may be lost if the temperature has risen to very high levels. Treatment must be carried out under expert supervision and is aimed at keeping the temperature below 40°C (104°F) and dealing with the complications of shock and coma. It may take up to 7-10 days for the body to regain its ability to control temperature.

Hemp
SEE CANNABIS

Hepatitis

Inflammation of the liver due to infection, chemicals or drugs. The features are pain and tenderness below the ribs on the right side, due to expansion of the inflamed liver within its capsule. Jaundice colours the

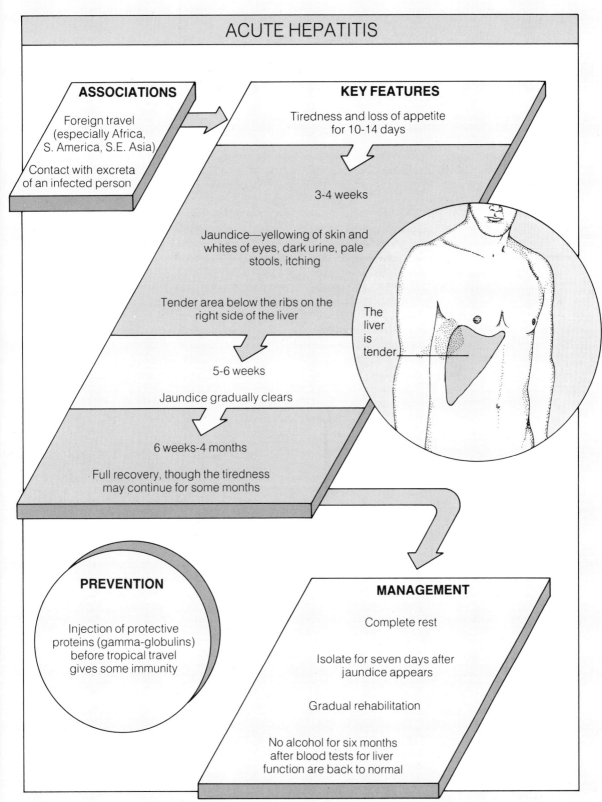

ACUTE HEPATITIS

ASSOCIATIONS

Foreign travel (especially Africa, S. America, S.E. Asia)

Contact with excreta of an infected person

KEY FEATURES

Tiredness and loss of appetite for 10-14 days

3-4 weeks

Jaundice—yellowing of skin and whites of eyes, dark urine, pale stools, itching

Tender area below the ribs on the right side of the liver

The liver is tender

5-6 weeks

Jaundice gradually clears

6 weeks-4 months

Full recovery, though the tiredness may continue for some months

PREVENTION

Injection of protective proteins (gamma-globulins) before tropical travel gives some immunity

MANAGEMENT

Complete rest

Isolate for seven days after jaundice appears

Gradual rehabilitation

No alcohol for six months after blood tests for liver function are back to normal

whites of the eyes yellow and follows an increase in the concentration of bile in the blood. The bile spills into the urine and makes it a darker yellow colour than usual. Other common features are fever, nausea, vomiting with loss of appetite and weight.

The commonest cause of hepatitis is infection caused by viruses though many chemicals, particularly fat solvents such as dry cleaning fluid and some drugs if taken by mouth either accidently or during attempted suicide, may cause severe inflammation of the liver.

Virus hepatitis

The illness begins with a vague feeling of ill health which resembles mild influenza, followed by loss of appetite, nausea and a distaste for cigarettes and sometimes alcohol. A few days later, tenderness may be felt below the ribs on the right side, rapidly followed by jaundice. Many patients start to feel better as the jaundice appears, and a small number return to full fitness in a few days. Most remain tired to some degree for 3 weeks to 3 months. Treatment consists of rest during the acute phase, after which the patient can get up and go out if he wishes. Alteration of diet plays no part in recovery, though the patient may remain nauseated for some time, particularly with fatty foods—or even the thought of them. Alchohol is directly damaging to the already diseased liver, and should be avoided for 6 months after full recovery.

There are two types of virus—one spread by contamination of food by faeces, and the other by blood (serum hepatitis). It is very important that patients wash their hands thoroughly after going to the lavatory, to prevent spread of the disease to their families. Doctors need to be extremely careful when they take blood from patients with hepatitis.

Virus hepatitis is very common in the tropics and subtropics, and travellers can be protected by an injection of serum containing antibodies to the virus. An injection gives immunity for about 6 months.

Hernia
(RUPTURE)

The internal body organs are held in place by the muscles of the body and by the skeleton. Any weakness or damage to these may result in parts of underlying organs coming through them. This is known as herniation, and the herniated tissues can usually be felt beneath the unbroken skin. The term 'internal hernia' also describes a similar occurrence within the body and most commonly is seen in

herniation of the upper part of the stomach into the chest (*see* Hiatus hernia).

Hernias commonly occur at points of natural weakness in the muscles, commonly in the groins or inguinal regions of the male abdomen. Developmentally, the movement of the testes down into the scrotum leaves a potential pathway through the muscles of the lower abdomen. With age, the muscles and tissues tend to weaken, and any cause of increased pressure within the abdomen such as persistent coughing or straining due to constipation may force a small portion of the intestine outwards and open up the pathway through the muscles.

The herniated bowel may cause a bulge in the groin which produces a visible and palpable impulse on coughing. Occasionally, the bowel within the hernial canal is pinched off by the muscles through which the hernia passes. If the blood supply is cut off, the hernia becomes 'strangulated' and extremely painful and tender. Surgery is then necessary to prevent gangrene.

Occasionally a sudden increase in pressure within the abdominal cavity forces the muscles apart momentarily and the bowel into the hernial canal. If the pressure is released, the muscle may return to its previous position, nipping the bowel and preventing the passage of food. This intestinal obstruction sometimes reverses without help, but surgery is often necessary. (*See also* Intestinal obstruction.)

Heroin

A very potent analgesic or pain killing drug derived from morphine (page 154). It is more powerful than morphine on a weight-for-weight basis but it is doubtful whether it has any advantages as a pain killer. Its reputation as being more potent has made it a favourite of drug addicts and for this reason its manufacture was banned in the USA. Sadly this had little effect on illicit traffic in drugs.

The actions of heroin, and the features of overdose, addiction and withdrawal are similar to those of morphine.

Herpes

The family name of the viruses which cause cold sores (*Herpes simplex,* page 62) and shingles (*Herpes zoster,* page 205). 'Herpes' is from the Greek 'to creep' which describes the way in which the blisters spread from an initial single lesion. 'Zoster' means 'a girdle', describing the way the blisters of shingles

HERNIA REPAIR (Inguinal Hernia)

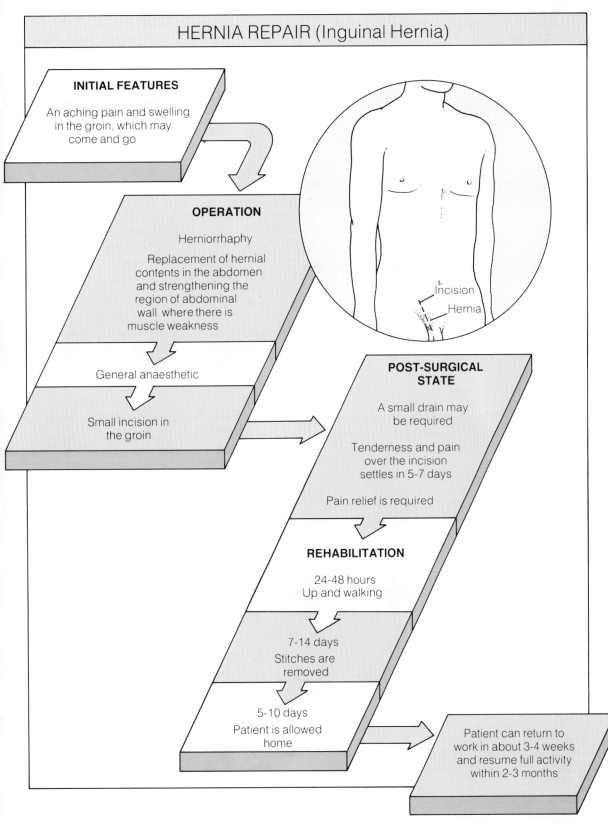

INITIAL FEATURES

An aching pain and swelling in the groin, which may come and go

OPERATION

Herniorrhaphy

Replacement of hernial contents in the abdomen and strengthening the region of abdominal wall where there is muscle weakness

General anaesthetic

Small incision in the groin

Incision

Hernia

POST-SURGICAL STATE

A small drain may be required

Tenderness and pain over the incision settles in 5-7 days

Pain relief is required

REHABILITATION

24-48 hours
Up and walking

7-14 days
Stitches are removed

5-10 days
Patient is allowed home

Patient can return to work in about 3-4 weeks and resume full activity within 2-3 months

appear around the body in the position of a belt.

The zoster virus is the same as the chickenpox virus. The fluid from the zoster blisters can cause chickenpox in those who have not previously had the disease.

Herpes genitalis is a sexually transmitted virus infection caused by the *Herpes simplex* virus. The features are of single or multiple small blisters which are irritant and usually painful on the penis or the cervix, vagina and surrounding skin. Any tissues in contact with the sex organs can be infected.

Most recover without treatment but a small number recur and few remain free of symptoms while continuing to be infectious to their partners. Expert advice should always be sought both for treatment and to prevent spread.

Hiatus hernia

A common condition where the lower oesophagus and upper end of the stomach rise up through the diaphragm (*see* diagram page 194). The oesophagus leaves the chest and passes down into the abdomen through a hole or 'hiatus' in the muscular diaphragm. Any increase in the abdominal pressure from coughing, corsets or constipation tends to force the upper stomach up through the hiatus in the diaphragm; if the diaphragm is weakened as commonly occurs with increasing age, and particularly when the patient stoops, the upper stomach herniates through.

Acid from the stomach regurgitates (refluxes) into the oesophagus, producing a burning or gnawing sensation behind the breast bone (sternum), rising sometimes up to the throat and leaving an acid taste in the mouth (heartburn, page 122). This is induced by stooping or lying flat and occurs commonly whilst gardening or on going to bed. The pain is relieved by antacids (page 22), and if it is worse at night, can be partially relieved by sleeping propped up on pillows.

Hiccup
(HICCOUGH)

Hiccups are caused by pressure upon, or irritation of, the diaphragm which contracts repeatedly in response. They commonly occur after large meals when the full stomach presses against the diaphragm. The hiccups last for a few minutes to a few hours and settle spontaneously. There are many folk remedies for treating hiccups—including breath holding for 1 minute, quickly drinking a tablespoon of vinegar and drinking from the opposite of a full tumbler of

water—but none is guaranteed to work. Occasionally disease of the lungs may irritate the diaphragm and cause hiccups; if it persists for more than 12–24 hours, medical advice should be sought to ensure that the lungs are healthy and to obtain relief.

High blood pressure
SEE BLOOD PRESSURE

Hip Joint

A ball-and-socket joint between the socket (acetabulum) of the pelvis and the ball-shaped head of the femur (*see* diagram, page 267). This arrangement allows movement in all directions. The head of the femur is attached by a narrow neck to the main body of the femur; it is this part which is particularly prone to fracture in the elderly.

See Arthritis; *and* Dislocation: congenital dislocation of the hip.

Hoarseness

Caused by damage or irritation to the vocal cords in the larynx. Infection due to viruses is the commonest cause, and cigarette smoke may contribute. Cancer of the larynx is a rare cause. Rarely, hoarseness is an early feature of thyroid under-activity (hypothyroidism, page 224). If hoarseness occurs with a cold, sore throat and a fever, it can be safely assumed that nothing more serious than an acute virus infection is present. Treatment consists of stopping smoking and taking simple analgesics such as paracetamol or aspirin to suppress the pain if present. Steam inhalations may also help in pain relief.

If the hoarseness fails to improve after 7–10 days, and particularly if the fever and general symptoms of infection have settled, advice should be sought.

Laryngeal cancer presenting with hoarseness is easy to diagnose, and curable if detected early.

Hodgkin's disease

A cancerous condition of the lymph glands. It results from multiplication of the cells within the glands which therefore enlarge. The glands of the neck are often the first to swell, and are usually painless. If they continue to enlarge or fail to decrease in size after 10–14 days, particularly if there is no obvious sign of infection in the face or on the head, expert advice should be sought. Glands which swell in response to infection are usually tender and start to decrease in size by 7–14 days.

HIP REPLACEMENT

INDICATIONS

Severe and disabling pain and deformity, which is usually caused by osteo-arthritis

Pelvis

Damaged joint surface

Head of femur

Femur

OPERATION

Replacement of the head of the femur and insertion of a new cup into the pelvis

General anaesthetic

Incision over the hip joint

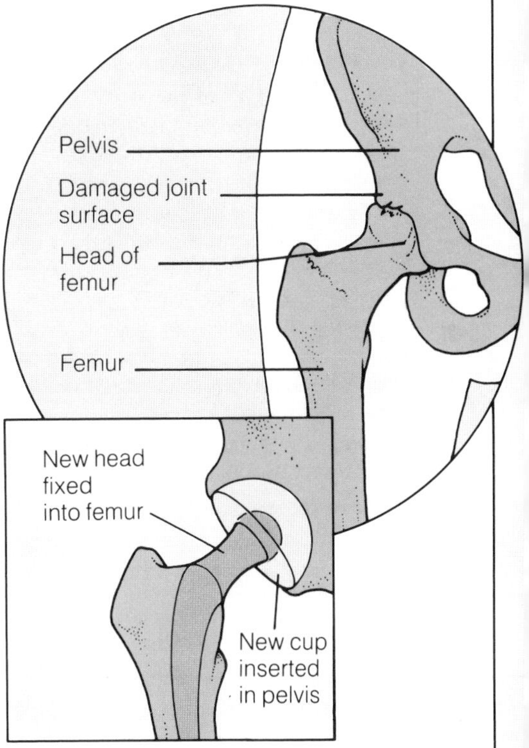

New head fixed into femur

New cup inserted in pelvis

POST-SURGICAL STATE

Pain-relieving drugs are needed for 2-4 days

REHABILITATION

24-28 hours walking

7-10 days removal of stitches

2-3 weeks patient is allowed home

3-4 months return to work (depending on occupation)

Hodgkin's disease is one of the cancers which can be completely cured if detected early.

Hole in the heart

Abnormality of the heart, present at birth (congenital). Normally a dividing membrane exists between the left and right atria, and the right and left ventricles (*see* diagram). During fetal development the divisions, or septa, may not close completely—leaving holes between the two atrial (or two ventricular) walls. These are known as, respectively, atrial and ventricular septal defects. Often these are small and cause no major changes of pressure within the chambers of the heart and no clinical illness. If the holes are large, blood may flow through them from the left to the right of the heart. This leaves less blood to go to the aorta and round the main circulation. In this case, it is essential to close the holes before the excess volume of blood flowing through the lungs produces irreversible damage.

If operation is performed early, the results are

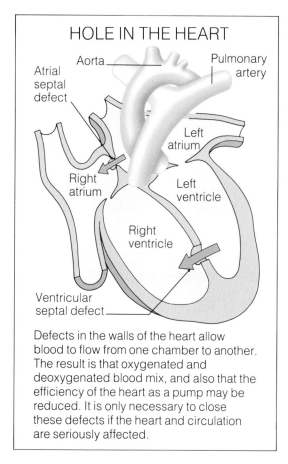

HOLE IN THE HEART

Aorta

Pulmonary artery

Atrial septal defect

Left atrium

Right atrium

Left ventricle

Right ventricle

Ventricular septal defect

Defects in the walls of the heart allow blood to flow from one chamber to another. The result is that oxygenated and deoxygenated blood mix, and also that the efficiency of the heart as a pump may be reduced. It is only necessary to close these defects if the heart and circulation are seriously affected.

excellent and the patient is able to continue a perfectly normal existence. 'Blue babies' occur when there is a birth defect which causes blood to flow from the right to the left side of the heart without passing through the lungs; i.e. oxygen-deficient (blue) blood flows into the general circulation.

Homoeopathy

A practice of medical treatment devised in the late eighteenth and early nineteenth centuries in Germany. It is based on the principle that 'like should be cured by like'—that is, a substance which can produce symptoms in a healthy person will, in minute doses, cure a sick person showing the same symptoms (hence the Greek *homoeopathy*: the same—disease). It is claimed that the method of preparing the small doses is important: in 'potentization' the substance is diluted 1 in 100 and shaken vigorously (succussion) and this is repeated up to 30 times. Though little or none of the original substance may be left, the 'medicinal power' and 'latent curative energy' are said to be enhanced. Another aim of homoeopathy is to treat the whole patient rather than specific complaints alone.

Homoeopathy was devised before modern scientific discoveries opened the fields of biology and chemistry and related them to medicine. The cause of many illnesses is now known, and orthodox medicine aims to treat specific disorders; e.g. chloroquine for malaria, vitamin B_{12} in pernicious anaemia. Nevertheless, homoeopathy is widely practised and, as with orthodox medicine, can produce good results when carefully used by experienced medical practitioners.

Hormones

Chemicals produced by the adrenal, pituitary and thyroid glands (pages 13, 177, 224) and by the ovaries (page 163) and testes (page 222). The hormones produced and secreted by these glands are described under their separate headings. (*See also* Menopause *and* Family planning.)

Hot flushes

During the female menopause (page 151) intermittent transient flushing of the face is very common.

Housemaid's knee

A small delicate cushion, or bursa, sits just in front of the upper tibia at the point of contact with the ground when kneeling. Inflammation of this cushion, either

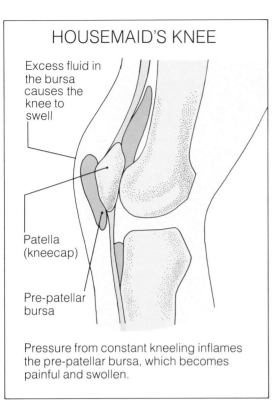

HOUSEMAID'S KNEE

Excess fluid in the bursa causes the knee to swell

Patella (kneecap)

Pre-patellar bursa

Pressure from constant kneeling inflames the pre-patellar bursa, which becomes painful and swollen.

from no obvious cause or from the frequent irritation when kneeling excessively, inflames the bursa which enlarges and becomes red, tense and tender.

For obvious reasons this is known as housemaid's knee (or prepatellar bursitis). Treatment is by rest, the application of warm or cold packs whichever gives more relief, and simple pain-killing drugs such as aspirin or paracetamol.

Humerus
(LATIN: *HUMERUS*, SHOULDER)

The bone of the upper arm, which articulates with the shoulder blade (scapula) at the shoulder joint—a modified ball-and-socket joint—and with the ulna and radius at the elbow—a modified hinge joint. (*See* diagrams, pages 259 and 267.)

Huntington's chorea

An inherited (genetic) disorder which causes mental deficiency and abnormal jerking movements of the limbs beyond voluntary control (chorea). It begins at 20–40 years of age and progresses slowly. There is no known cure, but sufferers are recommended to

obtain expert advice before having children, who will have a 50 per cent chance of developing the disease.

Hydrocele

The accumulation of fluid around the testicle within the scrotum. The cause is unknown.

If discomfort is marked, the fluid can be drained by inserting a small needle under local anaesthetic. The process is simple and painless apart from the needle used to give the anaesthetic, but the fluid tends to recur. Other causes of swelling in the scrotum are discussed on page 203.

Hydrocephalus

This means 'water-head', and describes an illness of infants who have excessive cerebral fluid which causes the head to enlarge. The pressure within the head tends to increase and this may, if untreated, lead to permanent brain damage. It is associated with and described under spina bifida.

Hypertension
SEE BLOOD PRESSURE

Hyperthyroidism

Excess secretion of thyroxine from the thyroid gland (*see* Thyroid disease).

Hypnosis

In clinical practice, hypnosis is of most value in treatment of psychiatric disorders induced by emotional factors. When hynotized, patients are receptive to suggestion and this may reduce or abolish their symptoms if caused by emotional stress, and this persists after waking. Hypnosis has also been used to treat asthma, high blood pressure and some skin diseases, and in place of anaesthetics for tooth extraction.

Hypnosis for medical purposes should be performed only by expert medically qualified practitioners.

Hypochondriasis

A disability caused by the belief that one has a serious illness for which no cause can be found. The common fears are of bowel or lung cancer, brain tumour and heart disease. Most people, and particularly doctors and nurses, have these fears from time to time, but usually a careful clinical examination will exclude serious disease, reassure the sufferer and remove the symptoms.

Very occasionally, the fears either persist or disappear to be replaced by another fear. This may continue for months or years, and understandably can totally disrupt people's lives. If this occurs, expert psychiatric help is needed.

Hypothermia

Occurs when the body temperature falls below normal. Serious symptoms occur below 35°C (95°F), and death is common at body temperatures below 32°C (89.6°F). Apart from mountaineers and polar explorers, hypothermia is virtually restricted to the very old and the very ill. Sedative drugs, including alcohol, may potentiate the fall in temperature. The very old often live alone in poorly heated houses and eat little—partly from inclination but often as a result of poverty. Their ageing temperature-regulating systems are unable to maintain body temperatures and they become more dependent on external heat. In severe winters there is a great danger of their body temperature dropping as the night temperature falls. This results first in confusion and finally complete loss of consciousness, and if they are not found soon after this, death follows.

Treatment consists of slowly warming them by putting them in a warm but not hot room, and covering them with a blanket. The aim is to raise the temperature by 0.6°C (1°F) per hour. If the temperature rises too rapidly the blood vessels in the skin dilate and cause a fall in pressure to the arteries to the brain, kidneys and heart. Treatment is therefore usually best carried out under careful supervision in hospital.

Hysterectomy

Removal of the uterus (womb), including the cervix (neck of the womb)—performed for fibroids and in cases of suspected benign or malignant tumour. It is less commonly performed to relieve symptoms of irregular or heavy periods, discomfort due to prolapse or low abdominal pain sometimes made worse by sexual intercourse. It is not a dangerous operation and about 60,000 are carried out every year in England and Wales.

Because the vagina is not removed, a normal sex life can be expected after the operation. The ovaries may be removed at the same operation.

The uterus is usually removed through an incision made in the lower abdominal wall. In the elderly and if there is also a prolapse present, the uterus can be removed through the vagina. The patient is usually up and about within a few days and leaves hospital in 7–10 days.

Normal physical activity can usually be resumed 2 or 3 months after the operation. There are many 'old wives' tales about hysterectomy but there is no truth in the rumours that it makes people depressed, overweight or takes away their sex drive or enjoyment.

Hysteria

'Hysteria' is used to describe two groups of people. In lay terms, hysteria denotes an excessive reaction to some usually unpleasant or worrying event, and implies gross excitability. In psychiatric terms, hysterical illness means the development of definite features of illness (e.g. weakness or paralysis of a limb) in the absence of any underlying disease. Hysterical features are often a response to stress, though the trigger may never be found.

The patient is unaware of what he is doing, but may well be focusing on one part of his body or on a specific illness in an attempt to escape or divert his own attention from his real problem. Hysteria may mimic any recognized clinical illness and it may be difficult to be certain that no organic illness is present. The classic features are sudden blindness, deafness or weakness of one or more limbs, total paralysis, loss of speech, tremors and unsteady gait. Throughout the sufferer appears to be totally unconcerned about what in most people's mind is a serious disability. Usually the abnormality settles spontaneously or after carefully supervised psychiatric treatment.

I

Ileitis
SEE CROHN'S DISEASE

HYSTERECTOMY

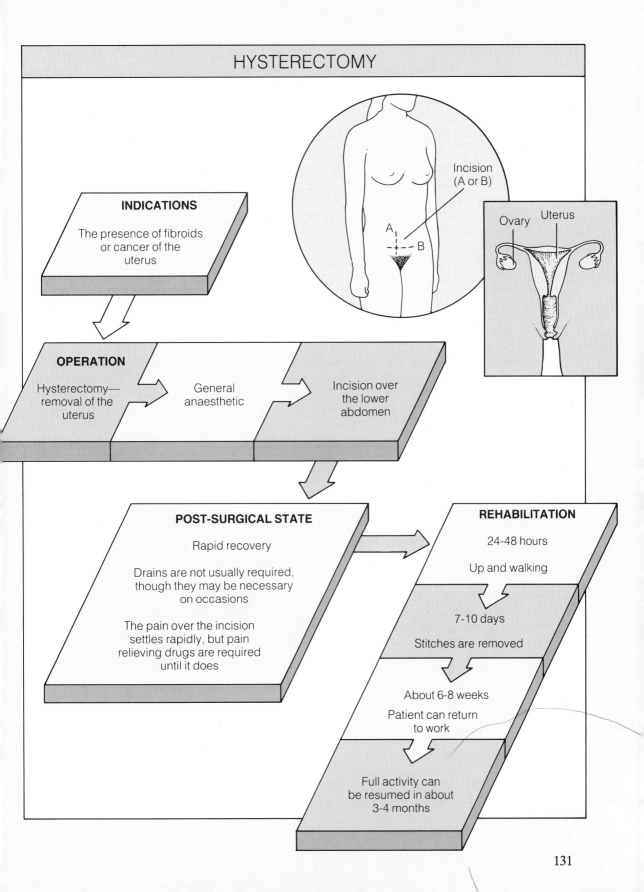

INDICATIONS

The presence of fibroids or cancer of the uterus

Incision (A or B)

Ovary Uterus

A
B

OPERATION

Hysterectomy—removal of the uterus

General anaesthetic

Incision over the lower abdomen

POST-SURGICAL STATE

Rapid recovery

Drains are not usually required, though they may be necessary on occasions

The pain over the incision settles rapidly, but pain relieving drugs are required until it does

REHABILITATION

24-48 hours

Up and walking

7-10 days

Stitches are removed

About 6-8 weeks

Patient can return to work

Full activity can be resumed in about 3-4 months

Ileostomy

A surgically made artificial outlet from the intestines, in which the ileum is attached to an opening in the anterior abdominal wall. This is performed if the colon is removed to treat acute ulcerative colitis (page 232) and occasionally to rest the colon before later removal of a colonic cancer.

Ileum

The last part of the small intestine (page 136), connecting the jejunum to the caecum. The ileum is the major site for absorption of food, water, essential chemicals and vitamins; it is extremely long (approximately 4–5 metres) and convoluted, allowing an enormous area for absorption (*see* diagram, page 265).

Immunization

It is now possible to immunize successfully against many natural infections, to the extent that smallpox has been totally eradicated and poliomyelitis is virtually non-existent in the Western world. The available vaccines, including those for travellers to the tropics, are discussed on page 233.

Impetigo

A skin infection, usually of children, caused by two groups of bacteria. The infection may affect only a small area of skin which becomes red, tender, hot and swollen and over which crusts form. In more severe cases, and particularly in infants, large areas of skin may be infected, causing a severe illness with high fever, shivering attacks and shock due to infection spreading to the blood stream from the skin. In minor infections, local washing with antiseptics (e.g. chlorhexidine, betahistine) may be sufficient. Occasionally, and always with more serious infections, antibiotics are required and can be life-saving.

Impotence

The inability of the male to develop an erection of the penis, or to ejaculate during intercourse (*see* Sexual problems).

Incontinence

A very distressing condition, caused by loss of voluntary control of the muscle sphincters either at the base of the bladder or around the lower rectum and anus. The result is spontaneous and uncontrolled passage of urine or faeces. Incontinence is common in the very old where there is also a large element of confusion or forgetfulness. Transient incontinence often follows minor strokes or head injuries, but this usually improves as the brain damage settles. Bed wetting at night is common in young children, and they invariably grow out of it (*see* Bed wetting).

Incontinence is very rare in other age groups but may follow damage to the spinal cord (page 214) when there is disruption to the controlling nerves which run from the brain to the sacral plexus of nerves and thence to the muscles of the bladder and anus.

The outlook in children who wet the bed is excellent, but adults who have spinal damage may not recover full control. Following strokes, continence usually returns but incontinence developing in the very old is likely to persist. This causes great problems of nursing care in ensuring that the patient remains clean and does not develop sores, particularly if bed-ridden. Incontinence places a great strain on the family caring for an elderly parent, who for practical purposes has returned to the stage of infancy, and will from then on require constant and skilled attention often by night as well as by day.

Fortunately for the old, incontinence usually occurs with loss of mental awareness, and the terrible disabilities may not cause the patient great concern, though this is not always so. If it is too distressing, a permanent catheter can be inserted to drain the urine from the bladder into a disposable bag.

Incubation period

The time between contact with an acute infectious disease and the appearance of symptoms. The incubation periods of the common childhood illnesses are:

Chickenpox	14–21 days
German measles	14–21 days
Measles	10–14 days
Mumps	14–21 days
Whooping cough	14–21 days

For the period of time children with infections should remain away from school, *see* page 290.

Indigestion
(DYSPEPSIA, FLATULENT DYSPEPSIA, ACID RE-GURGITATION, ACID REFLUX, PEPTIC OESOPHAGITIS, HEARTBURN)

A term used to describe symptoms—usually discomfort or pain but also nausea, vomiting, flatulence, heartburn or feelings of distension—which occur after taking food. Very often the cause is emotional (*see* Anxiety) or the symptoms may be due to abnormal movements of the alimentary tract. Avoidance of foods which induce symptoms may completely prevent them—most people who have indigestion know which foods are bad for them and have to weigh the known pleasures against the risk of symptoms which, although unpleasant, are not dangerous.

The pain is usually relieved by simple antacid preparations (e.g. Rennie, Maclean's, Asilone) although these may not improve associated flatulence.

Indigestion may be produced by many specific disorders, such as peptic ulcer (page 216), gall stones (page 106) or hiatus hernia (page 126), or by rarer conditions such as pancreatitis (page 166) or liver disease. If indigestion lasts for more than a week or attacks recur over regular intervals, medical help should be sought.

Induction of labour
SEE PREGNANCY: LABOUR

Industrial diseases

The most common diseases of occupation are caused by the inhalation of irritant particles into the lung, usually of coal miners (*see* Pneumoconiosis). Other well recognized conditions are: decompression sickness in deep-sea divers (page 38), contact dermatitis in workers in the chemical and petroleum industries, lead poisoning in makers of lead batteries and accumulators (page 144), anthrax in those working with animal skins (page 22) and brucellosis in farm workers in contact with cattle and goats (page 50).

Infant feeding

The majority of experts now believe that breast feeding is preferable to bottle feeding. Breast feeding not only assures strong psychological bonding between the baby and mother but also breast milk is better absorbed and contains specific proteins which protect the child against infant gastro-enteritis.

In fact, gastro-enteritis is very rare in breast-fed babies.

Bottle feeding is necessary if the mother has a breast infection, a breast abscess or a slowly healing cracked nipple. Some drugs given to the mother are excreted in breast milk and may become a potential hazard to the baby. Some mothers prefer not to breast feed for personal reasons.

Feeding is best begun 'on demand'—i.e. when the baby cries, usually every 2–3 hours initially. This interval slowly increases and most babies sleep through the night (i.e. from midnight to 5–6 a.m.) within 2–3 months. A baby which does not settle is rarely unwell but merely showing its own personal character. None the less, medical advice should be obtained if the baby starts to wake more frequently than previously or if it cries after feeding. The doctor will check that the baby is developing normally and that its weight is increasing at a suitable rate. Remember that babies usually lose a little weight immediately after birth but regain this in 7–10 days, and thereafter gain on average 25–40 grams (1–2 ounces) per day for the next 100 days. As a guide, bottle-fed babies require about 30 millilitres (1 ounce) per kilogram body weight (or ½ ounce per pound) on the first day, increasing by 25 millilitres per kilogram per day up to 150 millilitres per kilogram (2½ ounces per pound body weight) on the seventh day.

However, like adults, different babies have different demands and the important thing to notice is that they appear healthy and are gaining weight at a satisfactory rate. Bottle-fed babies require regular vitamin supplements, and particularly vitamin D to ensure healthy bone development. It is equally important not to give too many vitamins to babies (or indeed adults), because some, particularly vitamins A and D, can give rise to toxic effects in excess. Expert advice about feeding is given to all mothers before they leave hospital. After that, medical advice should be sought if the baby appears unwell, fails to gain weight or appears unwilling to drink.

Infantile eczema
SEE DERMATITIS

Infantile paralysis
USUALLY CALLED POLIOMYELITIS (PAGE 180)

Infectious diseases

The common diseases which are transmitted as the result of close contact are chickenpox (page 56), measles (page 149), German measles (page 111), mumps (page 155) and whooping cough (page 248).

Typhoid (page 231) and paratyphoid (page 167) are uncommon in the developed countries, as is diphtheria (page 83). Scarlet fever (page 199) is exceedingly uncommon and smallpox (page 208) has now been eliminated.

Children with these diseases should be kept away from school until no longer infectious (page 290).

Infectious mononucleosis
SEE GLANDULAR FEVER

Infertility

The inability to conceive affects up to 10 per cent of couples. Although the cause often remains unknown, it is important to seek expert advice because a number of disorders can be successfully remedied. Conception depends upon active male sperm fertilizing the female egg (ovum), which travels from the ovary along the Fallopian tube towards the body of the uterus (*see* diagram, page 263). Infertility can occur if the sperm are too few in number or their activity is reduced. The ovary may not produce an ovum or, more often, the Fallopian tubes are narrowed or blocked by previous infection.

Despite intensive testing it may not be possible to find any anatomical or biochemical abnormality in either the male or female partner, yet they remain unable to conceive. Interestingly, there are a number of couples who, having adopted children, then conceive.

Recent advances in knowledge have shown that excess prolactin, a hormone produced by the pituitary gland, may be one of the commonest causes of impotence in men and infertility in women. It can now be accurately measured in the blood.

Artificial insemination involves the insertion of sperm either from a donor or from the husband into the uterus of the wife of an infertile or impotent husband. This is generally available for infertile couples but only after careful investigation has indicated that this approach is the best from both physical and psychological points of view for both the man and the woman.

Experimental work in progress has allowed conception outside the uterus ('test tube babies') using the couple's own ovum and sperm, thus excluding the need to use sperm from an unknown donor. This is not routinely available, but may become so.

Influenza

The influenza viruses cause an acute illness with high fever, sweating and aching in the muscles and sometimes the joints. The infection may begin as a simple cold, but the virus multiplies in the cells of the upper respiratory tract and spills over into the blood stream to cause the more severe symptoms.

Influenza is a very unpleasant illness but healthy children and adults almost invariably recover completely within 7–10 days. A general feeling of debility and exhaustion may persist and post-influenzal depression is not uncommon and may last for up to 3 months.

The severity of the illness varies from person to person but most prefer to stay in bed. The temperature can be reduced by aspirin taken regularly as recommended by a medical practitioner, and it is important to drink plenty of fluids to prevent dehydration. An adult should take between 2 and 3 litres (4–6 pints) per day of water, fruit juice or anything he wishes. Eating is not important initially and the appetite returns as the acute illness subsides—usually by the third or fourth day. After this he should be able to start getting about and should be allowed to do what he feels he can do. Many are able to return to full activity within 7 days but it may take longer.

Influenza is more serious in the very young, the very old and those with heart or lung disease (e.g. chronic bronchitis). Such people are more likely to develop other infections in addition to the 'flu'. These groups need more careful medical supervision from the outset.

Asian 'flu
One group of influenza viruses which causes world-wide epidemics every 2–3 years. The epidemics start in Asia and vary widely in size and severity. Treatment is the same as for the common forms of influenza.

Gastric 'flu
Many viruses infect the stomach and intestines to cause nausea, vomiting and diarrhoea. In addition, they enter the blood stream, causing fever and muscle aches identical with influenza—hence the confusion (*see* Gastro-enteritis).

Ingrowing toe nail
SEE UNDER NAIL

INFLUENZA

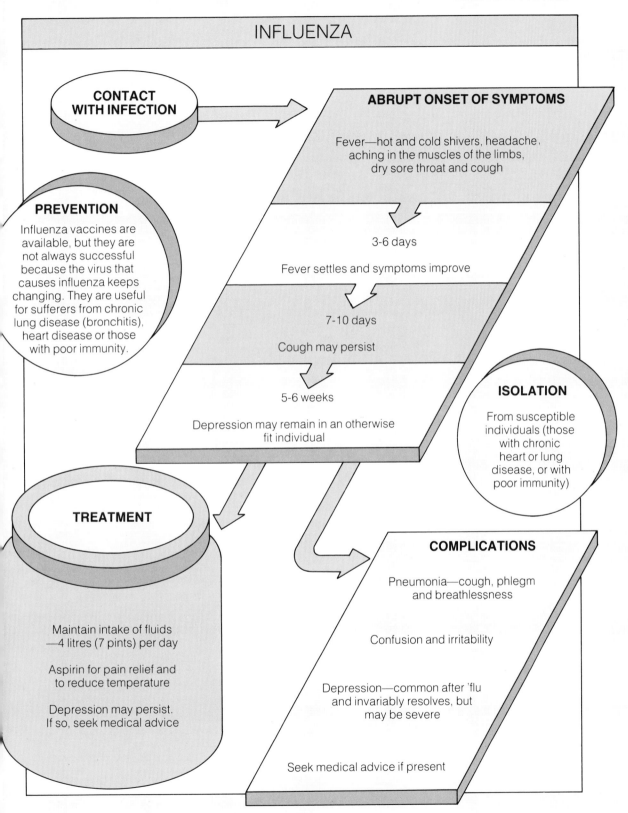

CONTACT WITH INFECTION

ABRUPT ONSET OF SYMPTOMS

Fever—hot and cold shivers, headache, aching in the muscles of the limbs, dry sore throat and cough

3-6 days

Fever settles and symptoms improve

7-10 days

Cough may persist

5-6 weeks

Depression may remain in an otherwise fit individual

PREVENTION

Influenza vaccines are available, but they are not always successful because the virus that causes influenza keeps changing. They are useful for sufferers from chronic lung disease (bronchitis), heart disease or those with poor immunity.

ISOLATION

From susceptible individuals (those with chronic heart or lung disease, or with poor immunity)

TREATMENT

Maintain intake of fluids —4 litres (7 pints) per day

Aspirin for pain relief and to reduce temperature

Depression may persist. If so, seek medical advice

COMPLICATIONS

Pneumonia—cough, phlegm and breathlessness

Confusion and irritability

Depression—common after 'flu and invariably resolves, but may be severe

Seek medical advice if present

Inguinal hernia

This is caused by weakness in the muscles of the abdominal wall in the inguinal region or groin. The mechanism and features of hernias are described under hernia (page 124).

Insemination, artificial
SEE ARTIFICIAL INSEMINATION

Insomnia

Difficulty in getting to sleep and early waking are common features in mild anxiety, and everyone has insomnia on odd days from time to time (*see* Sleep disturbance).

Insulin

A hormone produced by specialized 'islet cells' in the pancreas (page 166), which lowers the concentration of sugar in the blood. Lack of effective insulin leads to diabetes mellitus. Injections of insulin are often used in treatment and there are many proprietary preparations; these are described under diabetes (page 78).

Intercourse

Problems relating to intercourse are considered with sexual problems (page 204).

Intermittent claudication

Cramp in the calf during exercise. The pain tends to settle with rest but recurs after a recognized effort (e.g. walking 100 yards). Claudication is caused by narrowing of the main artery to the leg, and can be successfully reversed by inserting an arterial graft to bypass the obstruction (*see* Arterial disease).

Intervertebral disc
SEE DISC

Intestinal infection
SEE GASTRO-ENTERITIS

Intestinal obstruction

A rare cause of severe abdominal pain. In obstruction, the usually smooth rippling muscular activity of the bowel wall—peristalsis—increases greatly in an attempt to overcome the obstruction. The intense intermittent contractions are felt as colic. The pain, which is the major feature, is severe and intermittent and tends to make the sufferer roll about in agony. If the obstruction is not relieved, back-pressure up the bowel eventually leads to vomiting and, later, dehydration from loss of fluids from the stomach. The bowel expands above the obstruction and the abdomen becomes greatly distended. Constipation and an absence of faeces are usual in complete obstruction.

Intestinal obstruction in infants and children is caused by pyloric stenosis (page 191) intussusception (*see below*) and, very rarely, by large fruit stones · though surprisingly these usually pass through without obstructing despite their size relative to the diameter of the bowel. In adults pyloric stenosis may follow inflammation around a peptic ulcer but this is not common. In the older age groups, obstruction may follow incarceration of a hernia (page 124) or blockage by a cancer of the colon.

Surgical relief is required urgently for all forms of obstruction.

Intestine
(LATIN: *INTESTINUS*, WITHIN)

That part of the digestive system which leads from the stomach to the rectum (*see* diagram, page 265). It is divided into the small and the large intestine. The small intestine consists of three anatomical parts: the duodenum (page 86) which leads from the stomach to the jejunum and thence to the ileum which ends at the caecum (to which the appendix is attached). It produces enzymes which digest the food and thus make it absorbable.

The large intestine (colon) arises from the caecum and ends at the rectum. Much of the food value has been extracted by the small intestine. The large intestine collects the solid residue and adjusts its water content.

Intussusception

A disorder of young infants in which a small length of intestine slips inside a nearby piece which sits as a collar around it. This causes narrowing of the bowel ★ and intestinal obstruction, with colicky abdominal

INTERMITTENT CLAUDICATION

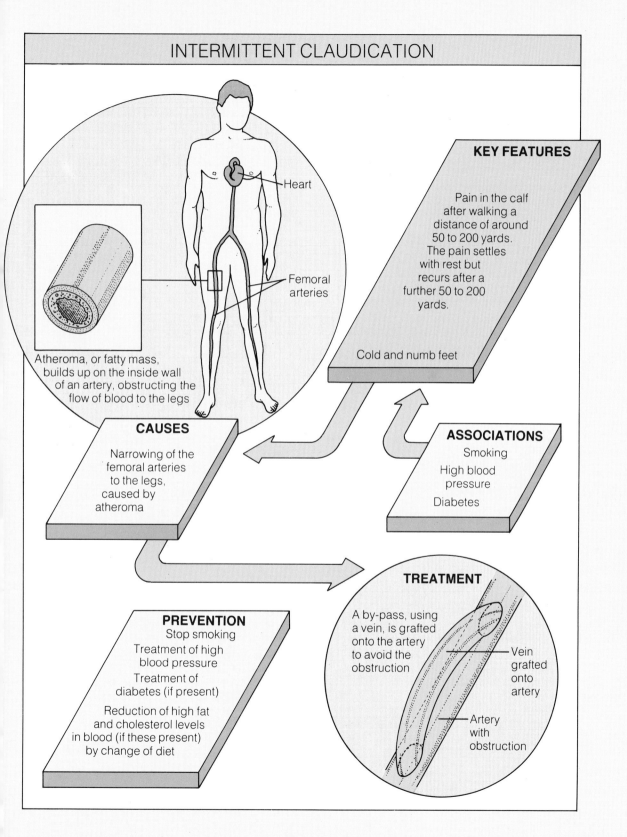

Atheroma, or fatty mass, builds up on the inside wall of an artery, obstructing the flow of blood to the legs

Heart

Femoral arteries

KEY FEATURES

Pain in the calf after walking a distance of around 50 to 200 yards. The pain settles with rest but recurs after a further 50 to 200 yards.

Cold and numb feet

CAUSES

Narrowing of the femoral arteries to the legs, caused by atheroma

ASSOCIATIONS

Smoking

High blood pressure

Diabetes

PREVENTION

Stop smoking

Treatment of high blood pressure

Treatment of diabetes (if present)

Reduction of high fat and cholesterol levels in blood (if these present) by change of diet

TREATMENT

A by-pass, using a vein, is grafted onto the artery to avoid the obstruction

Vein grafted onto artery

Artery with obstruction

pain and sometimes the passage of a small amount of blood.

Surgery is required to relieve the obstruction and to ensure that the blood supply to the intussuscepted bowel has remained intact. It is sometimes necessary to remove a small length of intestine if its blood supply has been restricted for too long.

Iron

An essential component of all tissues, and is found in small quantities in every cell—where it forms part of the enzyme system which controls energy production and hence cellular function. It is of particular importance in the formulation of red blood cells and is incorporated into haemoglobin (page 116), the compound which carries oxygen around the body.

Iron is present in meat, shellfish, beans, nuts and many breads, and it is absorbed into the body from the small intestine. The commonest cause of anaemia is iron deficiency and this is more commonly due to bleeding than to poor dietary iron intake. Red blood cells are rich in iron and every 1 millilitre (0.04 fluid ounce) of blood contains 0.5 milligram (0.006 grain) of iron; although minimal blood loss occurs normally from the wall of the intestine, the quantity is minute (about 0.5–2 millilitres, 0.02–0.08 fluid ounce, per day) and not noticeable as the lost iron is easily replenished from food.

Any bleeding greater than the normal minute loss causes a fall in the body's iron stores and results in anaemia (page 18). The common causes are bleeding haemorrhoids, peptic ulcers, heavy periods and some drugs, particularly aspirin if taken in excess in sensitive persons.

Less commonly, cancers of the intestine cause loss of iron by bleeding, sometimes over many months. This is why people with iron deficiency anaemia which has not responded to iron tablets, need careful investigation. The anaemia of iron deficiency is rarely serious; it is easy to diagnose and usually responds well to iron tablets.

Irritable bowel
SEE SPASTIC COLON

Itching
(PRURITUS)

Everyone itches on occasion, usually from insect bites. The itching is usually localized to a small area of skin and goes away rapidly either on its own or after scratching. Why the skin should become irritable without an obvious cause is unknown. Local irritation (e.g. by stinging nettles or sunburn) releases histamine and other chemicals into the skin from surrounding cells and this may produce intense itching. A similar mechanism is responsible for the itching and the dermatitis occurring in people sensitive to rubber, certain soaps and detergents. Many skin diseases itch, particularly infections with fungi such as thrush (page 223) and parasitic infestations such as scabies (page 199). These are very common, particularly around the anus or vagina, in the groins and under the breasts.

Some internal diseases such as jaundice and kidney failure are associated with itching.

In the absence of other symptoms, itching, though most unpleasant, is not serious and responds to simple remedies such as calamine. A simple barrier cream may prevent irritation. Antihistamine tablets may be prescribed if the itching persists for more than 2 or 3 days.

-Itis

This means infection or inflammation; e.g. appendicitis, cystitis (of the bladder), nephritis (of the kidney).

J

Jaundice

The word comes from the French (*jaune*, yellow) and describes the colour of the whites of the eyes in this condition (*see* page 70). The yellow colour is due to excess of the pigment, bilirubin, which circulates in the blood and is deposited in the tissues.

Bilirubin comes from the haemoglobin in red blood cells, which only survive for about 120 days. The pigment from the old and broken down red cells is converted to bilirubin in the liver. Under normal circumstances the small amounts of bilirubin released by the liver leave via the bile duct, enter the intestine and are then ejected from the body in the stools (*see* diagram, opposite).

Jaundice can occur if:
1   The red cells are broken down in excess.

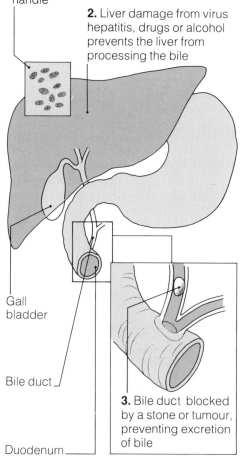

JAUNDICE

1. Increased breakdown of red blood cells releases excess bile which the liver cannot handle

2. Liver damage from virus hepatitis, drugs or alcohol prevents the liver from processing the bile

Gall bladder

Bile duct

Duodenum

3. Bile duct blocked by a stone or tumour, preventing excretion of bile

2 The liver is damaged and cannot make or excrete bilirubin (virus hepatitis or drug damage).

3 If the bile duct is blocked and excretion of bile from the liver prevented. There is a build-up of bilirubin in the blood, with progressively increasing jaundice.

When (3) happens the bile cannot enter the stools, which therefore become very pale. It then builds up in the blood and passes out in the urine, which becomes very dark. This obstruction suggests that there is a gall stone at the end of the bile duct and this may have to be removed surgically.

The commonest cause of jaundice is virus hepatitis, and the jaundice disappears as the infection within the liver settles—which it invariably does.

Everyone who becomes jaundiced should obtain medical advice, particularly if they are over 40 (when virus hepatitis is less common) or if the jaundice persists or increases.

Joint pain

Any damage to the joint from injury or infection or arthritis causes pain if the nerves are intact. Treatment is described under arthritis (page 27).

Joints

There are two major types of joint: the hinge joint (e.g. the knee, ankle, elbow and fingers) allows movement in only one plane—e.g. in a backward and forward direction; ball-and-socket joints (e.g. the shoulder and hip) allow movements in nearly all directions and also allow rotation. (*See* diagram, page 267.)

Most joints do not fit exactly into these two groups, but are slightly modified to allow some additional range of movement—e.g. the wrist is a modified hinge joint (page 250), and the elbow combines a hinge with a modified ball-and-socket joint (page 92).

The stability of the joints is maintained by the surrounding muscles. The ligaments tend to limit the range of movement and prevent displacement.

Kala-azar
(LEISHMANIASIS)

A tropical disease caused by parasites of the genus *Leishmania*. The parasite is transmitted to man by the sandfly, and multiplies in and causes enlargement of the lymph glands, the liver and the spleen. Death results if untreated.

Cutaneous leishmaniasis is a less serious form which infects a small area of skin. This usually heals spontaneously without treatment.

Kaolin

Potter's clay (aluminium silicate). When purified for medical use it is an excellent and safe preparation taken as a liquid mixture for the treatment of diarrhoea. In some countries, a small amount of morphine is added (kaolin and morphine). Morphine and related drugs (codeine) themselves cause constipation if taken in larger doses.

Kidney

The two kidneys are bean-shaped, and about 13 centimetres (4 inches) long. They are situated one on each side of the spine on the back wall of the abdomen, just beneath the diaphragm (*see* diagram, page 261). The blood which passes into the kidneys contains the impurities produced by the body cells as they utilize oxygen and nutrients. The blood is filtered in glomeruli which are small networks of vessels, so that the impurities in solution are passed through the kidney substance in small tubes, and the purified blood is passed back into the circulation. In these tubes water and some chemicals are reabsorbed or secreted in amounts necessary to maintain a steady level within the body. The most important of these are the acid hydrogen and alkaline bicarbonate, sodium, potassium, calcium and glucose. What is left passes from the kidneys via the ureter to the bladder.

See also Kidney dialysis; Kidney failure; Kidney infection; Kidney stones; *and* Kidney transplantation.

Kidney dialysis
(RENAL DIALYSIS)

Before renal dialysis was developed, almost all patients with chronic progressive kidney disease died. Now that it is possible to dialyse a patient's blood, such premature death can frequently be postponed or prevented. There are two dialysis techniques and both use the principle of bringing the patient's 'poisoned' blood into contact with a

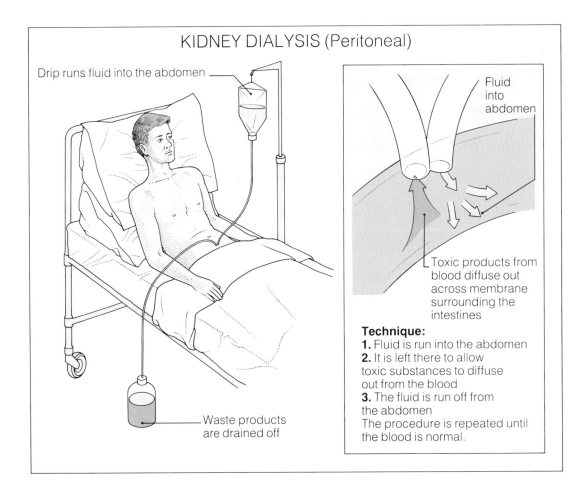

KIDNEY DIALYSIS (Peritoneal)

Drip runs fluid into the abdomen

Waste products are drained off

Fluid into abdomen

Toxic products from blood diffuse out across membrane surrounding the intestines

Technique:
1. Fluid is run into the abdomen
2. It is left there to allow toxic substances to diffuse out from the blood
3. The fluid is run off from the abdomen
The procedure is repeated until the blood is normal.

specially prepared 'clean' fluid across a semi-permeable membrane through which accumulated 'poisons' such as urea can pass, but larger particles such as proteins and blood cells cannot.

In *haemodialysis*, blood is taken from an artery, passed over a cellophane (or similar) membrane in a machine and returned to a vein. On the other side of the membrane there is a constant stream of warmed dialysis fluid which contains the correct proportion of the various salts and substances normally present in the blood. These substances present in an increased concentration in the patient's blood (such as urea, ammonia, creatinine and potassium), then diffuse through the membrane and pass out into the drain in the used dialysis fluid.

In *peritoneal dialysis*, the fluid is passed in and out of the peritoneal cavity—which is the abdominal cavity surrounding the intestines. It is through this outer gut membrane that dialysis with blood takes place. If the renal failure is due to short-term damage (e.g. following the shock of bleeding from a road accident), only one or two dialyses may be necessary to maintain health until the patient's own kidneys recover sufficiently to function again. If kidney disease is irreversible, maintenance dialysis is necessary once or twice weekly. This can now be performed either in hospital or, if the conditions allow it, at home under the direction of the local kidney specialist. With careful management of renal failure, and enthusiasm from the patients, it should be possible to allow those who previously would have died to continue a full and enjoyable life both at work and at leisure.

Kidney failure

The function of the kidneys is to excrete the unwanted waste chemicals produced by the body as a result of metabolism. In normal concentration some of these chemicals are essential to normal life but they become dangerous if they accumulate. The special function of the kidneys is to exclude these whilst at the same time retaining essential blood constituents such as protein, water and sodium in the correct proportions and quantities (*see* Kidney). If the function of the kidneys is severely reduced, waste products and acids accumulate and their concentration in the blood rises. All the body tissues are affected but the effects are most severe on the bone marrow, causing severe anaemia, and on the brain, causing confusion, irritability, coma and death if the renal failure is progressive and untreated. There are many causes of kidney failure, some temporary and acute, others progressive and chronic. Severe dehydration or shock alone may so reduce blood flow to the kidneys that the waste products cannot be removed in sufficient quantity. Blockage of the urine flow in the ureter, bladder or urethra may result in renal failure. Damage to the tissues of the kidneys themselves is rare. Renal damage of any degree requires careful investigation:

1   To assess and monitor kidney function.
2   To exclude dehydration and obstruction.

Sometimes a renal biopsy (page 38) is necessary to obtain a specimen of kidney tissue for examination under the microscope so that a definite diagnosis can be made before choosing the correct treatment.

Kidney infection

Infection is rare in the kidneys (*see* Pyelitis) but common in the lower renal tract (*see* Cystitis).

Kidney stones

Calcium stones form when a high concentration of calcium is passed into the urine. This occurs when there is excess calcium in the blood and with dehydration, both of which produce these high concentrations. Similarly, excess uric acid, the cause of gout, may precipitate in the urine to form stones.

Kidney stones (calculi) are fairly common. The cause is frequently not determined, but the commonest association is long-standing severe infection. This usually produces 'staghorn' stones, so called because of their branching shape.

The stones may stay in the kidney and cause no symptoms whatsoever, except an occasional aching sensation in the loin. If the stone leaves the kidney and passes down the ureter, there is frequently severe spasm which causes the pain of renal colic.

Renal colic

This excruciating pain shoots from the small of the back overlying the kidney, down and around the abdomen and into the groin, and, in men, the testes. The pain is intermittent, corresponding with the timing of the spasm in the ureter, and the shafts of colicky pain make the sufferer roll about in agony.

The stones are usually small and eventually pass out of the ureter and into the bladder, with relief of pain. If it becomes stuck in the ureter, urine flow is obstructed and surgical removal becomes necessary to relieve both the symptoms and the obstruction which, if left, results in back-pressure and damage to the kidney.

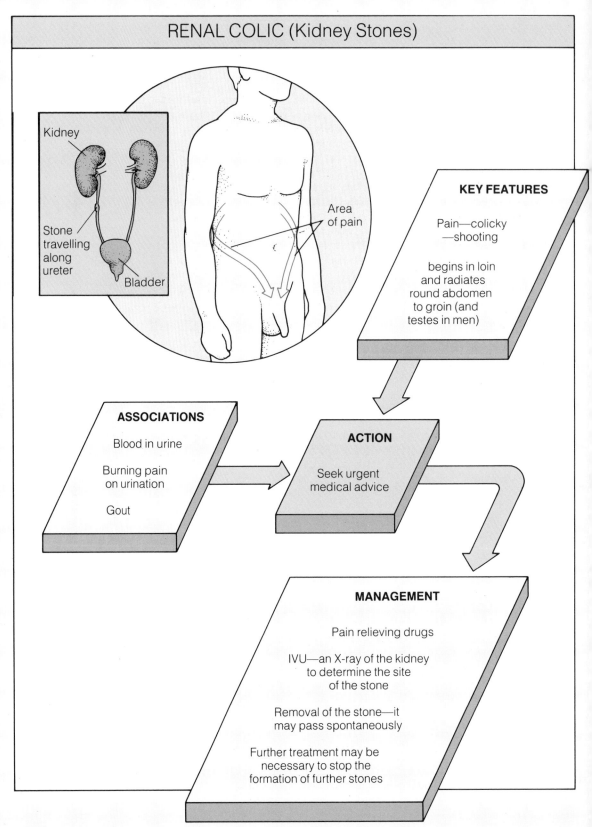

RENAL COLIC (Kidney Stones)

Kidney

Stone travelling along ureter

Bladder

Area of pain

KEY FEATURES

Pain—colicky
—shooting

begins in loin
and radiates
round abdomen
to groin (and
testes in men)

ASSOCIATIONS

Blood in urine

Burning pain
on urination

Gout

ACTION

Seek urgent
medical advice

MANAGEMENT

Pain relieving drugs

IVU—an X-ray of the kidney
to determine the site
of the stone

Removal of the stone—it
may pass spontaneously

Further treatment may be
necessary to stop the
formation of further stones

Treatment of colic requires powerful pain-killing drugs such as pethidine and, when necessary, surgical removal. All patients with kidney stones should be investigated carefully to exclude the presence of excess calcium or uric acid in the blood and urine and to assess kidney function. If these values are normal the patient is instructed to drink 3–3.5 litres (5–6 pints) of water daily. In hard-water districts this should be softened and of course the dietary intake of calcium controlled, with particular attention to restricting milk and bread.

Bladder stones

These form in the same way. They usually cause aching over the front of the lower adomen, burning on passing water, or blood in the urine. Careful investigation is required to assess kidney and bladder function and to exclude other causes of blood in the urine. Bladder stones are larger than stones in the kidney and ureter and usually have to be removed surgically through a cystoscope (page 72).

Kidney transplantation

In a small number of people with severe renal failure, it is possible to replace the kidneys with one from a healthy kidney donor. This is not always possible because so few people offer their kidneys in the event of their death. Moreover, the transplanted donor kidney must be of a similar tissue type (as with blood transfusion grouping) to the patient's or recipient's tissue. Advice may be obtained from a local Renal Dialysis Association, who will also supply kidney donor cards.

Kissing disease
SEE GLANDULAR FEVER

Knee joint

A hinge joint connecting the femur above to the tibia below (see diagram, page 267). The bones have a cartilage plate (page 53) between them, which sometimes tears during sport when the body twists on a leg firmly placed on the ground.

Kwashiorkor

A tropical disorder caused by gross malnutrition and especially a deficiency in dietary protein. The typical features are exhaustion, diarrhoea, weight loss, dry skin, thin brittle hair, and susceptibility to infections. Death is inevitable if untreated, but the response to a good diet containing protein is excellent.

Labour

The process of delivering the baby from the womb (uterus) via the birth canal to the outside world (see Pregnancy: labour).

Labyrinthitis
SEE VERTIGO

Lacrimal gland

A small gland under the upper outer eyelid, which secretes fluid containing the antibacterial substance lysozyme, which keeps the eye moist and free from infection.

Lactation

Milk production (see Infant feeding).

Laparoscopy

Examination, under anaesthesia, of the tissues and organs within the abdomen by the introduction of a fine fibre-optic telescope. This may be inserted through the front of the abdomen into the pelvis to examine the uterus, Fallopian tubes and the ovaries, commonly during investigation for infertility.

Laparotomy

The surgical procedure of opening the abdomen either to examine the enclosed organs or to remove or repair diseased tissues.

Large intestine
(COLON)

The part of the digestive tract from the ileum at the end of the small intestine to the rectum (*see* diagram, page 265). In the abdomen the colon assumes the position of a picture frame around the abdomen. It is divided anatomically in the ascending, transverse and descending colon.

Laryngitis

Infection of the larynx and the vocal cords (page 246) produces soreness, coughing and a hoarse voice. Sometimes the voice may be lost completely during the phase of acute inflammation. Laryngitis rarely occurs alone, and is usually associated with infection of either the pharynx above or the trachea below (laryngo-tracheo-bronchitis) producing a sore throat and a burning sensation behind the breast bone (sternum) on breathing in.

Laryngitis is very common and is due to infection by the same viruses which cause colds and influenza. Very occasionally, severe irritation of the vocal cords follows inhalation of noxious chemical gases, and cigarette smoke is to some extent a special and common example of this. Acute laryngitis lasts for 3–10 days and recovers completely. The symptoms can be partially relieved by inhalations of steam, and by simple analgesics such as soluble aspirin. A cough linctus taken at night, with or without a sleeping tablet, can help to give a good night's sleep during the early acute phase.

In infants and young children, acute laryngitis is potentially more serious because the airways are narrow and obstruction is more likely to occur following the tissue swelling of acute infection (*see* Bronchitis).

Larynx

The upper part of the main airway (*see* diagram, page 255). The larynx lies between the back of the mouth and the upper end of the trachea (page 228). It has a firm shell of cartilage which keeps it rigid. The two vocal cords within it run front to back, and movements of them alter the pitch of the voice; the tighter they are and the closer they come together, the higher the pitch.

Lassa fever

A recently discovered and extremely rare virus infection named after the town in northern Nigeria where it was first detected. It is transmitted to man by the bite of a rat, and should be suspected in anyone who develops a fever within 3 weeks of returning from tropical Africa. The other features are sore throat, headache, muscle aches and pains, and, if it progresses, haemorrhage into the skin. Similar features occur with green monkey disease (Marburg disease), which is also exceedingly rare, and usually fatal.

Laxatives
(LATIN: *LAXARE*, TO LOOSEN)

Drugs used to treat constipation. There are hundreds of preparations and the most commonly used are listed on page 285.

Recently it has been realized that the bowel can become constipated because we eat insufficient foods which form bulky soft stools. These produce a physiological or normal response from the muscle in the bowel wall. Unprocessed bran and similar products have become a very popular method of treating constipation. A dessertspoonful of miller's bran daily added to the diet helps many people towards more normal bowel function. (*See also* Dietary fibre.)

Lead poisoning

This very serious disorder has become very rare since the exclusion of lead from paint, toys and water pipes. There is a growing awareness of the increased concentration of lead in the atmosphere from the fumes of car exhausts, and fears have been expressed about the level of lead in the blood of children who live close to busy road junctions. Disagreement continues between authorities on the importance of these observations. There is still a risk of lead intoxication for infants who live in old buildings where old lead paint has been used because some children tend to eat or lick the paint. Workers in industries which use lead (such as petroleum manufacture, smelting, printing and battery factories) are at risk from inhalation of lead fumes, and special limits are set for the concentration in the air.

Acute poisoning requires the ingestion of a large quantity of lead and is thus very rare. The features are severe abdominal cramps, muscular paralysis, and acute confusion and coma. Chronic poisoning results in slowly progressive exhaustion and lethargy, anaemia, constipation, muscle weakness and mental deterioration. The diagnosis is confirmed by finding excess lead levels in the blood and urine. The sufferer must be removed from further exposure and the source fully investigated to prevent others developing similar trouble.

Leg ulcers

Ulcers on the shin just above the ankle are common in association with varicose veins (page 239), and are caused by a combination of poor blood circulation and the pooling of blood at the ankles due to gravity. Other causes of leg ulcers are rare and include injuries and atherosclerosis (which causes narrowing of arteries supplying the distant parts of the leg around the ankles, feet and toes which then become deficient in oxygen and essential nutrients).

Treatment consists of keeping the ulcers clean, free from infection and protected from injury. A dry piece of lint will prevent rubbing and local damage. Superficial infection is best treated with an antiseptic solution such as chlorhexidine. If varicose veins are present, the leg should be elevated during the day for ½–1 hour to decrease any swelling around the ankle; 'stretch' tights or elastic stockings also are usually of help. Varicose veins may have to be treated surgically. If the blood supply to the shin and foot is severely reduced by a short block in an artery higher up the leg, it may be possible to improve the blood flow by inserting a graft. (*See also* Arterial disease.)

Legionnaire's disease

A rare form of pneumonia caused by the bacterium *Legionella pneumophila*. It was first detected following an outbreak of pneumonia in a group of American army veterans attending a legionnaires' congress. The disease begins with 'flu-like symptoms of fever with muscle and joint pains, followed by cough and breathlessness. Diarrhoea is common.

It must be distinguished from other forms of pneumonia (page 179) and, if detected early, responds rapidly to antibiotics.

Leprosy

A common disease widespread throughout the developing world and caused by a bacterium (*Mycobacterium leprae*) related to the organism which causes tuberculosis. The disease begins commonly as a patch of whiteness on the skin which becomes anaesthetic (i.e. insensitive to touch). Other features which may be present at the same time include nodules in the skin, and thickening of and damage to nerves which may result in paralysis at the wrist or ankle and eventually deformity. Blindness commonly follows involvement of the eye.

The size of the problem in terms of numbers is gigantic, and there may be 15–20 million people affected by leprosy. Once detected, treatment is with dapsone (a drug related to the sulphonamides), and this may prevent progressive blindness, nerve damage, paralysis and deformity if treatment is started early. Expert orthopaedic surgery can greatly improve any deformities which develop.

Despite common belief, leprosy is only minimally contagious.

Leptospirosis
(WEIL'S DISEASE)

An occupational disease of sewage workers who are infected after being bitten by an infected rat. It also affects swimmers in rat-infested streams. The disease begins with 'flu-like symptoms of fever and muscle pains, but involves the liver, kidneys and brain to cause jaundice (page 138), bleeding from the kidneys and meningitis (page 151).

It responds rapidly to penicillin given in high doses by injection.

Leucotomy

An operation to sever the connection between the frontal lobe and the remainder of the brain. The frontal lobe controls feelings of guilt and worry, and the operation was performed to treat severe depression (*see* Depression).

Leukaemias
(GREEK: *LEUKOS*, WHITE; *HAIMA*, BLOOD)

There are a number of types of leukaemia, which are all malignant disorders affecting the white cells of the bone marrow where most of the cells of the blood are formed (*see* Blood). Some of the marrow white cells become malignant and, like malignant solid tumours elsewhere in the body, grow in excessive numbers at the expense of the red cells (leading to anaemia) and the platelets (leading to a tendency to bleed and bruise easily). Although the number of white cells is greatly increased, they function poorly and this leads to an increased risk of infection. In some leukaemias there may be generalized enlargement of the lymph nodes, or a distension of the abdomen by enlarged spleen and liver or, rarely, bone tenderness.

Leukaemia can be confirmed by examination of the blood and the bone marrow.

The idea of suffering from leukaemia is nerve-racking and many people who become tired or develop a few big lymph glands become unnecessarily anxious. Fortunately, the leukaemias are all rare and microscopic examination of the blood will quickly allay fears. Furthermore, some leukaemias, particularly in the elderly, can be entirely symptomless and cause no decrease in life expectancy. With modern drug therapy and the use of powerful antibiotics to combat infections, many patients with leukaemia are now cured.

Lice
SEE NIT

Ligaments
(LATIN: *LIGARE*, TO BIND)

The hard fibrous bands which form the attachments of muscle to bone. They are frequently overstretched or torn by unusual or vigorous muscular activity (*see* Sprains).

Lithium

A chemical from the same group as sodium and potassium, which is used for treating patients with mania or depression. (*See* Depression *and* Psychiatric treatment.)

Liver

The liver is the largest organ of the body, measuring approximately 30 cm (12 inches) across and 15 cm (6 inches) from front to back. It weighs 1.5 kg (3–4 lb) and sits on the right side of the upper abdomen against the diaphragm. It is protected by the vertebrae behind and the lower seven or eight ribs on the right as they curve round from the spine to the breast bone (sternum). It has a large blood supply from the aorta via the hepatic artery, and from the portal vein which carries blood from the intestine containing the absorbed products of digestion. In life the liver can be likened to a blood filled sponge. It receives the products of intestinal digestion—i.e. fats, carbohydrates (sugars) and amino-acids (the basic components of protein)—and stores these for later use. The liver is also the main store of vitamin D, essential for bone growth and repair. From the amino-acids it manufactures proteins for tissue health and repair. Bile is also produced in the liver and passed via the bile duct into the intestine for fat digestion. A further important role of the liver is to convert toxic products in the blood to neutral urea, for removal from the body through the kidneys.

The commonest diseases of the liver are acute virus infections (acute hepatitis) and alcoholic damage which, if severe and persistent, leads to cirrhosis.

See also Digestive tract (page 264).

Local anaesthetics
SEE ANAESTHETICS

Lockjaw

The (appropriate) name applied to the effect produced by spasm of the chewing muscles in tetanus (page 222).

Long sight
SEE GLASSES

Louse
SEE NIT

LSD
(LYSERGIC ACID DIETHYLAMIDE)

One of the drugs of addiction. It is taken by drug addicts to produce hallucinations and a loss of awareness of time with altered perception of sound and vision. There is a peculiar feeling of light-headedness and weightlessness. A number of addicts have died from accidents while under the influence of the drug.

The effects of the drug are not always pleasant and some users report severe anxiety, irritability, fear and depression. In view of the serious and potentially lethal effects of the drug it is unwise as well as illegal either to possess or take it. (*See also* Addiction.)

Lumbago
(LATIN: *LUMBUS*, LOIN)

The term used to describe strains or tears in the muscles and ligaments of the lower back, in which the sufferer may find himself suddenly seized with severe backache and unable to rise from the bending position. (*See also* Backache.)

Lumbar puncture

A special investigation to obtain a specimen of the cerebrospinal fluid (CSF), which bathes the brain and spinal cord. Examination of this fluid helps with the diagnosis of various diseases of the central nervous system and is particularly useful in patients with suspected meningitis (page 151).

Lungs

The organs of the body where oxygen is transferred from the atmosphere to the blood, and the waste gas carbon dioxide moved in the opposite direction. This rapid exchange of large amounts of gas is made possible by the enormous surface area of the inside of the lungs and the thinness of the alveolar lung tissue which is the only immediate separation between the blood in the blood vessels and the gases in the alveolus. (*See* diagram, page 254.)

Atmospheric inspired air is about one-fifth (21 per cent) oxygen. The other four-fifths is almost entirely nitrogen which the body does not use. There is a very minimal amount of carbon dioxide (0.03 per cent). When air is breathed in it is transported to the very smallest air sacs (alveoli) and gas exchange of oxygen and carbon dioxide can take place. Occasionally, as in some anaesthetics, other gases such as ether and nitrous oxide may also pass across this membrane. The oxygen is joined onto the haemoglobin molecules in the blood which then turns from a dusky blue to red, and is circulated around the body. If for one reason or another this process does not occur correctly, the patient will tend to look blue rather than pink where the skin is normally thin such as the inside of the lower eyelid, the tongue, lips and nail beds. This blueness is called 'cyanosis'. The body tissues use up the oxygen and in the process (very similar to a coal fire, for instance) produce the carbon dioxide waste gas and some heat. This is why blood in veins, which is going back to the heart from the tissues, is always bluer than the blood being sent out by the heart in the arteries.

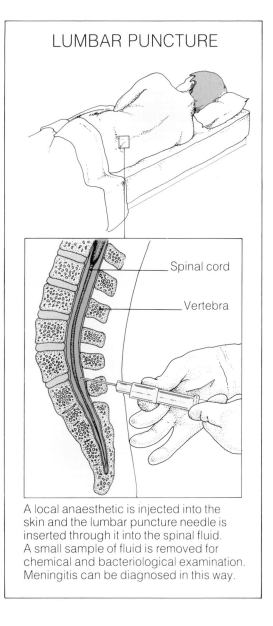

LUMBAR PUNCTURE

Spinal cord

Vertebra

A local anaesthetic is injected into the skin and the lumbar puncture needle is inserted through it into the spinal fluid. A small sample of fluid is removed for chemical and bacteriological examination. Meningitis can be diagnosed in this way.

See also Asbestosis; Asthma; Bronchitis; Emphysema; Pneumonia; Pneumoconiosis; Smoking; *and* Tumour.

Lymph glands

The lymph glands and the lymphatic ducts which both supply and drain them with lymph are part of the body's defence system against infection. Lymph drains from every part of the skin and every organ of the body. It carries those infecting organisms, such as bacteria and viruses, together with the white cells which have attacked them at the site of infection, ★ back to the local lymph glands. Thus infection in the face may result in enlargement of the neck glands on the same side of the neck, and infection between the toes can cause the glands of the groin to swell. These regional lymph nodes destroy and filter most of the infecting organisms, and the remaining debris in fluid form is passed via larger lymphatic ducts to more central lymph glands (for instance those near the large veins in the abdomen). The fluid lymph then passes back into the circulation to the spleen where final processing is performed. During this process the antibodies necessary to reject the infecting organisms are identified and manufacture of them is started.

Enlargement of local and regional lymph nodes in the neck and groin is very common because there is often superficial infection in the scalp, throat, sinuses, face and feet. Enlargement of more than one group of lymph nodes is usually seen in virus infections such as German measles, measles and glandular fever. The lymph glands in these conditions return to their normal size within 10–14 days after the acute illness, though occasionally they may remain enlarged for longer. Very rarely, enlargement of glands denotes a more serious illness such as leukaemia (page 145) or Hodgkin's disease (page 126). If enlarged glands do not return to normal in 2 weeks, and particularly if they are painless or there is no obvious infectious cause, medical advice should be sought.

M

Malaria

This important disease occurs in the tropics and subtropics, and is one of the most common disorders to affect man. It accounts for millions of deaths per year. The disease is caused by a parasite carried by the anopheles mosquito. These insects tend to bite human beings in the evening and at night, injecting parasites into the blood stream which then travel to the liver. There they multiply rapidly within the cells and these subsequently burst, to release more malarial parasites into the blood stream where they enter the red blood cells. This causes the clinical features of a marked swinging fever, associated with cold sweats and shivers, or rigors. Anyone with these symptoms should seek medical advice.

One of the malarial species—*Plasmodium falciparum*—also occasionally causes widespread destruction of the red cells which then block the kidney vessels, to produce renal failure. Very occasionally, this form of malaria may infect the brain, causing confusion, coma and death. If malaria is inadequately treated or left untreated and the patient survives, it tends to recur, causing intermittent fevers, general ill health and anaemia. The diagnosis of malaria must be considered in everyone with a fever who has recently returned from a malarial zone.

The diagnosis is confirmed by looking at a stained film of the patient's blood through a microscope. Malarial parasites appear within the red cells.

Treatment should be started immediately with chloroquine by mouth. This brings the temperature down, usually within 24 hours, though occasionally the patient does not respond because the malarial parasite is resistant to chloroquine. In these few cases oral quinine is curative.

Malaria is best prevented by:
1 Destroying the mosquitoes in their breeding grounds.
2 Giving adequate prophylactic drugs to all travellers to and from malarial zones.

Unfortunately, attempts to attack the breeding grounds have not been successful due to their wide distribution and their ability to repopulate an area very quickly from the few survivors of most eradication programmes. DDT (dichlorodiphenyl trichloroethane) also has ecological dangers, especially when used on a wide scale.

Advice about anti-malarial tablets is best obtained via your family physician from an expert in tropical diseases who will be able to determine the appropriate drug for the countries being visited. Currently, proguanil (Paludrine) or chloroquine taken daily, and pyrimethamine (Daraprim) taken weekly are the most commonly prescribed. Whichever is chosen, the drug should be started on the day of departure and continued for 6 weeks after return from the malarial zones. It is continued for this long because parasites which have entered the body on a day when you forgot the prophylactic drug can be killed as they emerge from the liver.

Malignancy

A term synonymous with cancer (page 51).

Malta fever

Brucellosis (page 50) caused by the bacteria *Brucella melitensis*.

Mammogram
(LATIN: *MAMMA*, BREAST)

An x-ray of the breast which is used to help distinguish simple breast lumps from cancers. Since this technique is not 100 per cent diagnostically accurate, it may be necessary to proceed to surgery to remove a breast lump.

Manic depression

'Mania' is often used to describe madness of any description, and it is particularly loved by producers of American and English murder films ('homicidal maniac'). In medicine, however, 'mania' refers to a state in which the patient is detached from reality and hyperactive to a degree which interferes with normal life. The hyperactivity may be so marked that it is impossible for the sufferer to finish one thing before moving on to the next, and thus never completes anything. Occasionally this reaches such a pitch that he cannot stay still long enough to eat or drink and never sleeps. Visions may also be seen in extreme cases. It is very uncommon in its pure form, but to a minor degree is part of the manic-depressive state when there is marked and intermittent alteration of mood. Initial treatment is sedation, which allows the patient to eat and drink (or to be fed). Psychiatric assessment may then define the basic illness and long-term care within the community or very occasionally (and sadly) in a hospital.

Manipulation
(LATIN: *MANIPULARE*, TO HANDLE)

A term used chiefly to describe any handling of the muscles or joints of the body—a technique employed extensively by physiotherapists in an attempt to remove swellings and increase motility within damaged or inflamed muscles and joints. Osteopaths use manipulation in an attempt to repair or realign misplaced muscles, ligaments and joints. Chiropractors manipulate the spine with a similar purpose.

The word 'manipulation' is also used to describe that form of behaviour universal in children at some time, and in everyone from time to time, when other people's emotions (e.g. parents) are played upon to achieve a desired result.

Marburg disease

A very rare virus disease which produces a severe illness with fever and multiple bleeds into the skin. The outlook is very poor and similar to Lassa fever (page 144).

Marihuana
(MARIJUANA)

The Spanish name for cannabis (page 51).

Mastectomy

An operation to remove a breast, or a portion of it—usually to examine and remove an underlying cyst or cancer. The operation is now considered technically a minor procedure, though it requires general anaesthesia. (*See also* Breast disorders.)

Radical mastectomy is a more extensive deeper removal of tissue and is now performed much less frequently.

Mastitis

Inflammation or infection of the breast, which becomes tender, red and swollen. The most common cause is a breast abscess, which is common in pregnancy and interferes with breast feeding (*see* Infant feeding).

Measles

A very common acute illness of children, which begins 10–14 days after contact with an infected child. The disease begins acutely with a fever and features resembling a severe cold: running eyes, running nose, cough and sneezing. About 4 or 5 days later, a widespread bloody red rash (*see* illustration, page 235) appears, which often begins behind the ears and spreads downwards over the face, chest, abdomen and limbs. Following this the temperature slowly falls and the child recovers.

The outlook is invariably excellent but very occasionally measles is complicated by pneumonia or infection of the middle ear (*see* Otitis media). There

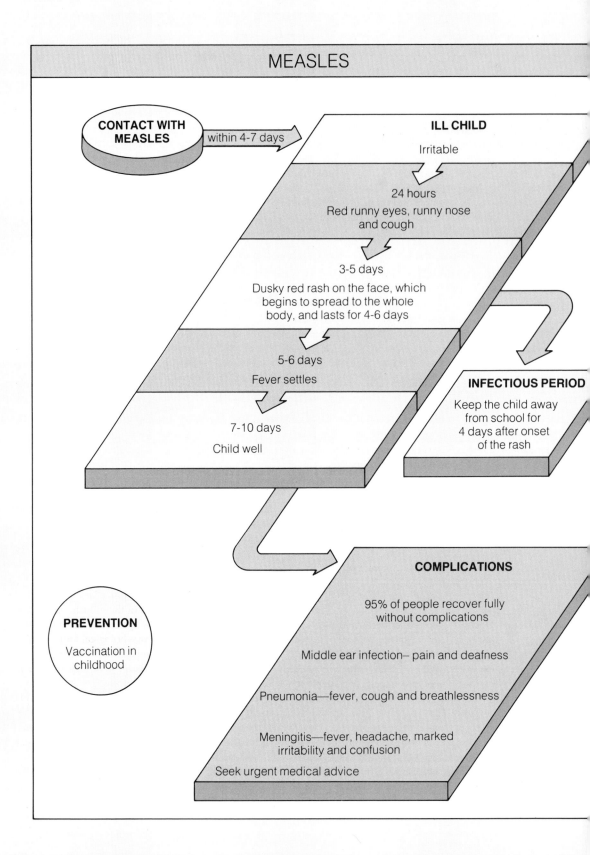

MEASLES

CONTACT WITH MEASLES

within 4-7 days

ILL CHILD

Irritable

24 hours

Red runny eyes, runny nose and cough

3-5 days

Dusky red rash on the face, which begins to spread to the whole body, and lasts for 4-6 days

5-6 days

Fever settles

7-10 days

Child well

INFECTIOUS PERIOD

Keep the child away from school for 4 days after onset of the rash

PREVENTION

Vaccination in childhood

COMPLICATIONS

95% of people recover fully without complications

Middle ear infection– pain and deafness

Pneumonia—fever, cough and breathlessness

Meningitis—fever, headache, marked irritability and confusion

Seek urgent medical advice

is no specific treatment for measles which, because it is caused by a virus, does not respond to the usual antibiotics. Immunization against measles is recommended during the first years of life, when immunization is also given against diphtheria, tetanus, whooping cough and poliomyelitis. Children with measles should be kept away from school for 14 days after the appearance of the rash.

Melanoma

A small spot or mole on the skin, coloured by a black pigment called melanin. Most moles are dark brown or pink and everyone has a few. If the mole is jet black and in a site which is often damaged (e.g. the shaving area of the face, under a finger or toe nail, in the collar region of the neck, etc.), it can enlarge and possibly bleed. If moles are present in these sites, or if they enlarge or bleed, they should be removed.

Menarche
(GREEK: *MENSIS*, MONTH; *ARCHAIOS*, THE BEGINNING)

The beginning of monthly periods in a young girl. The age varies widely and the menarche may begin usually between 10 and 16 years. The psychological problems associated may be considerable but, except in a small number of girls, they are rapidly overcome with reassurance from one or both parents or guardians. Too many girls still arrive at menarche without preparation.

Ménière's disease

Named after Ménière, a Paris physician of the late eighteenth century, who described severe acute attacks of vertigo, nausea, vomiting, with ringing in one ear which becomes increasingly deaf. Eventually, when the ear is completely deaf, the attacks cease. The illness is caused by an excess of fluid within the semicircular canals of the ear which control balance.

Treatment during acute attacks requires drugs, to prevent nausea and vomiting, combined with sedatives. If the attacks are very frequent or severe, or if they are interfering excessively with the patient's life style, it may be necessary to destroy the labyrinth or the supplying nerve surgically—this completely stops the symptoms but leaves the patient deaf on that side.

Meningitis

The meninges are the membranes surrounding and supporting the brain. They can become inflamed as the result of infections caused by various viruses or a small number of bacteria. The infection, as elsewhere in the body, produces a swelling of local tissues and dilation of local blood vessels. This results in the symptoms of severe headache, and stiffness in the neck muscles develops as if to prevent painful movement of the underlying meninges. Inflammation of the brain tissue next to the meninges may produce discomfort in the eyes when looking at bright light (photophobia) and, if more extensive, nausea, vomiting and confusion. If any of these is present, seek medical advice.

Meningitis is usually caused by one of a number of viruses; recovery is invariably rapid and complete in 5–6 days although it may leave the patient lacking in energy and in powers of mental concentration for some weeks or even months.

Meningitis caused by bacteria is much less common and more dangerous, and frequently fatal if untreated. The clinical distinction between the early stages of bacterial or viral meningitis can be virtually impossible. The diagnosis is established by lumbar puncture (page 147). A fine hollow needle is passed, under local anaesthetic, into the fluid around the spinal cord. A small volume of this cerebrospinal fluid is removed and examined microscopically for bacteria, and the white cells produced in reaction to the infection. On the basis of the findings, the correct antibiotic can be given immediately; in such instances, the outlook is very good, and recovery, though slow, eventually complete.

Menopause

The end of the reproductive phase of life in women, and denoted by termination of the monthly periods. This occurs normally at any age from 35 to 55 years.

A few women develop psychological and organic symptoms which are due in part to a decrease in the quantity of circulating oestrogens secreted by the ovaries. The typical features are headache, irritability and episodic 'hot flushes' in the face and sometimes the entire body. There may be anxiety and depression, which can occasionally be severe. Some think that the symptoms are related to a feeling of diminished femininity combined with a further realization of increasing age.

The menopause is a natural and inevitable stage of development and does not indicate a cessation of attractiveness or sexual awareness. If symptoms are severe, a small dose of oestrogens will usually decrease their severity and frequency. Fortunately, the symptoms settle completely irrespective of their initial severity.

For vaginal bleeding after the menopause, see page 239.

Menorrhagia

Heavy monthly periods. *See under* Periods.

Menstruation

(LATIN: *MENSTRUALIS*, MONTHLY) *SEE* PERIODS

Mental handicap and subnormality

Mental subnormality in children may result from genetic and biochemical disorders which affect the developing child from conception to birth. Mongolism (*see opposite)* and phenylketonuria (page 173), now tested for routinely at birth, are important examples. Brain damage very rarely can occur at birth. It is usually prevented by comprehensive ante-natal care, and optimum conditions during labour and immediately after birth. It is for this reason that many authorities consider that it is much safer both for the mother and, particularly, for the newborn baby if all children are born in hospital.

A normal child may suffer brain damage in the early years from acute meningitis which may leave him mentally handicapped. This is, fortunately, extremely rare.

The best approach to mental handicap is prevention. If a couple are known to possess a genetic predisposition to produce a mentally handicapped child, careful and thorough genetic counselling is essential. The damage to a developing fetus from rubella (German measles, page 111) can be prevented by immunization of school girls before they reach reproductive age. If mongolism is a real possibility, examination of amniotic fluid which surrounds the developing baby in the uterus (amniocentesis) can give the diagnosis in very early pregnancy.

There has recently been a much greater awareness of 'apparent' mental subnormality in normal children whose intellectual and environmental stimulation has been poor, or who have chronic ear disease ('glue ear') which makes them deaf and hence slow learners, or who have a specific reading block (*see* Dyslexia). These deficiencies must be identified as early as possible because late correction may not be complete. Well Baby Clinics will allow suspected mental handicap to be detected very early and result in immediate attempts at correction when a reversible disorder is present.

In the majority of children with mental subnormality the cause remains unknown. If the degree of handicap is small these children are usually best looked after at home and educated in normal schools. Special schooling is available for children with greater degrees of subnormality and, if extremely marked and particularly if associated with anti-social behavioural problems, it may be necessary to bring the child up in specialist boarding schools.

The decisions about where and how best to educate children with mental handicap are often extremely difficult and complex. Careful discussion from all aspects—medical, nursing, educational and psychological—must include the parents and take their feelings and views into the greatest consideration. Theirs is the greatest worry and their sadness the most intense.

Mental illness
SEE PSYCHIATRIC ILLNESSES

Migraine

A well recognized and common type of headache, which runs in families. It is typically one-sided, preceded by abdominal discomfort or spots before the eyes, and associated with sensitivity to light (photophobia) and severe nausea, sometimes with vomiting. Very occasionally there is partial loss of vision and numbness or weakness in the arm or leg of one side. The severity varies widely from attacks lasting a few hours to those lasting 1–2 days, during which the sufferer may be forced to go to bed.

There are a number of proprietary drugs available, and most contain ergot (e.g. Migril, Orgraine)—which acts to constrict the cerebral blood vessels and reverse the cause of the pain. It is not possible to predict which drug will be effective, and many may have to be tried before finding a successful remedy. The addition of drugs which prevent nausea (e.g. metoclopramide, Maxolon; promethazine, Phenergan) may dramatically improve the symptoms. If attacks are frequent and severe, they may be prevented by regular use of clonidine.

Migraine is sometimes precipitated by specific foods, and, once recognized, these should be avoided. The contraceptive pill may induce migraine, and is not recommended for women with a known history.

Miscarriage

The loss of a developing fetus from the uterus early in pregnancy is often associated with some abnormality in the fetus or in its implantation within the uterine wall. This thought may be some consolation to the prospective parent, who, but for the miscarriage, might have had an abnormal child. (*See also* Abortion.)

Mites
SEE SCABIES

Moles

Small pink or brown blemishes usually present at birth, and rarely of significance (*see* Birthmark) unless they are melanomas (page 151) which are black.

Mongolism
(DOWN'S SYNDROME)

A congenital disorder present from birth. The children are affected both physically and mentally. They have a characteristic facial appearance with deep skin folds over the middle ends of the eyes on each side of the bridge of the nose. The ears are often set low, and they tend to have short, stubby hands with abnormal skin creases. Internal abnormalities and heart defects may also occur.

These children are usually of limited intelligence but often very affectionate. Many parents find that this compensates for the lack of intelligence even though they usually need constant supervision.

Mongolism is caused by a defect in the genes. In every living cell, genes are carried on small anatomical structures (chromosomes), and in the human there are 46 chromosomes arranged in 23 pairs. In the mongol there is an extra chromosome identical to the 21st pair—i.e. these children have one chromosome too many.

The common type of mongolism occurs more often in babies born to older mothers as the result of a biological 'mistake' in the early development of the

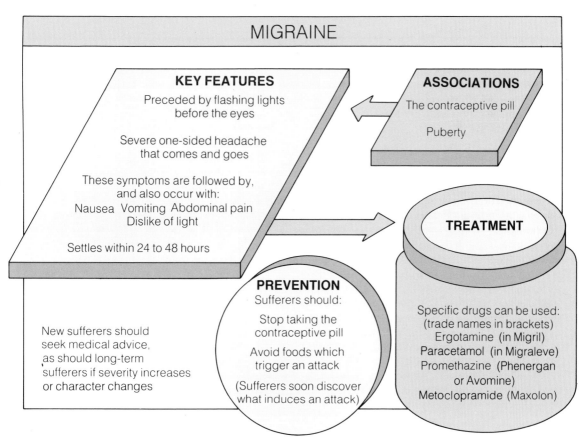

MIGRAINE

KEY FEATURES

Preceded by flashing lights before the eyes

Severe one-sided headache that comes and goes

These symptoms are followed by, and also occur with:
Nausea Vomiting Abdominal pain
Dislike of light

Settles within 24 to 48 hours

New sufferers should seek medical advice, as should long-term sufferers if severity increases or character changes

ASSOCIATIONS

The contraceptive pill

Puberty

PREVENTION
Sufferers should:

Stop taking the contraceptive pill

Avoid foods which trigger an attack

(Sufferers soon discover what induces an attack)

TREATMENT

Specific drugs can be used:
(trade names in brackets)
Ergotamine (in Migril)
Paracetamol (in Migraleve)
Promethazine (Phenergan or Avomine)
Metoclopramide (Maxolon)

egg (ovum). The risk of this happening increases steadily with the age of the mother, and about half of all the mongols born are to women over 40. Examination of the amniotic fluid (*see* Amniocentesis) during pregnancy can diagnose mongolism while the baby is developing in the uterus; older mothers may decide to have this test performed so that their pregnancy can be terminated if they are carrying an affected child.

A second type of mongolism occurs in which there is an abnormality in the genes of either the mother or the father. In this situation there is a risk that other children born to these parents will also be mongols.

After a mongol baby is born, it is routine for both parents to be tested to discover whether they carry the abnormal gene. If the parents are genetically normal they can be reassured that there is no extra chance of their having an abnormal baby next time.

Monilia

The old name for the fungus which causes thrush in the mouth, skin and vagina (*see* Thrush). It is now called *Candida* (*see Candida albicans*).

Morning sickness

Nausea with or without sickness is extremely common in the first months of pregnancy. It is probably caused by the sudden increase in circulating oestrogenic and progestogenic hormones associated with the pregnancy. Treatment is considered under pregnancy (page 181).

Morphine

A powerful pain-relieving drug derived from poppy opium. Its additional clinical advantage is the production of a feeling of detachment which is beneficial in severe and acute illness where there is an extreme degree of anxiety irrespective of any pain. It is widely used by drug addicts because it gives them an extreme sensation of detachment and elation, although how much of this is the effect of the drug is uncertain. Morphine is a very carefully controlled and monitored drug both because in slight overdose it may stop respiration and because of the added problem of addiction. Addicts who are officially registered and under constant psychiatric supervision can obtain morphine on prescription from special drug clinics (*see* Addiction).

Mouth ulcers

Ulcers in the mouth are very common and painful, sometimes sufficiently so to prevent eating. The fine surface lining of the tongue and inside the cheeks and lips is easily damaged by sharp objects such as a jagged tooth or a bone, but healing is rapid.

Infections in the mouth are common, and some viruses (e.g. *Herpes simplex* virus) produce small ulcers about 3–10 millimetres (0.12–0.39 inch) across which are extremely painful. These sometimes respond to treatment with hydrocortisone lozenges. If eating and drinking is difficult, application of anaesthetic gels to the ulcer will stop the pain for a short time and allow the sufferer to eat. A similar effect can be achieved with ice or ice cream held against the ulcers. Patients with severe illnesses, such as established acute leukaemia, may develop small ulcers in the mouth which require specific therapy under expert guidance. If ulcers are small and painful and disappear within 10 days they can be treated as described and generally ignored. If ulcers are painless, recur in one site and do not disappear, medical advice should be sought.

Multiple sclerosis (MS)
(FORMERLY CALLED DISSEMINATED SCLEROSIS, DS)

A disorder of the nervous system which affects people of both sexes, usually between the ages of 20 and 50. Although the common view of the disease is of rapid deterioration and muscular paralysis, this tragic occurrence is fortunately not so common and about half of those affected have no disability up to 10 years after the initial symptoms, and 25 per cent are only moderately affected.

The typical features are of intermittent disorder which affects different parts of the nervous system in turn. It commonly begins with blurring of vision due to inflammation of one of the optic nerves. This symptom usually resolves without specific treatment and since it may not be associated with MS there may never be another attack. Less commonly, the major nerve tracts from the brain to the limbs may be affected, resulting in partial and usually transient paralysis of a limb. Recovery is often complete.

If the cerebellum is involved, there may be an inability to co-ordinate movements, causing slurring speech and unsteadiness on walking. Numbness and tingling in a limb is often misinterpreted as a first sign of MS but is almost always due to pinching of a nerve while asleep or by spinal arthritis.

In severe cases, the episodes tend to recur after short intervals and recovery becomes progressively less complete, with muscular paralysis, persistent unsteadiness, a tendency to incontinence and a wheelchair existence. Treatment is aimed at strong reassurance, explaining that only a few people who have the initial symptoms will become severely disabled. Also, even if disability is marked, it is usually restricted to one part of the body and the combination of a strong will, good personal support and sometimes the addition of mechanical aids will allow a useful and enjoyable life.

The cause of multiple sclerosis remains unknown, although it may be caused by a slow-growing virus; the disease of scrapie in sheep is very similar and known to be caused by such a virus. There is tremendous support for research into the cause and treatment and a breakthrough must be close.

Mumps

A common virus infection which affects children of school age and young adults. The illness begins with lethargy, fever and usually pain at the angle of the jaw, accentuated by chewing. This is soon followed by swelling of one or more of the salivary glands—usually parotids situated just below and in front of the ears over the angles of the jaw. The enlarged, tender, infected parotids settle in 3–4 days and recovery is then rapid and uneventful. Unlike most common virus infections, there is no rash in mumps. (*See* chart, page 156.)

The major worry is the well known danger of infection of the testicles (orchitis) and of subsequent sterility. This is fortunately uncommon because mumps orchitis is usually only severe on one side and occurs in only about 10 per cent of males who have passed puberty. Of these, only about 10 per cent may become sterile.

Treatment is aimed at relieving symptoms. If the mouth is very dry, antiseptic washes can be soothing. Occasionally the pain on opening the mouth may be so severe that only fluids can be taken, and this is most easily achieved by using a straw until the acute parotid tenderness subsides. The infection is spread by coughing and children should be kept at home until the parotid swelling has subsided.

Muscle

Consists of bands of contractile filaments which shorten when stimulated by nerve impulses. Large groups of the filamentous bands form the major muscles such as the biceps. These are attached to a bone each side of a joint; contraction of the muscle moves the bones each side of the joint. Thus, at the elbow joint, the biceps muscle is attached to the humerus above and the ulna below; contraction of the biceps will shorten the muscle and bend (flex) the elbow.

Muscular activity uses up about three-quarters of the body's energy. (*See also* Muscle and joints, page 266.)

Muscular dystrophy

A group of hereditary disorders in which there is slow but progressive degeneration of muscles, usually in the region of the thighs, calves or shoulders. Despite great research activity, the cause of these disorders remains unknown. The rate of muscle damage is frequently very slow and with some forms of muscular dystrophy a long and full life can be expected with only minor abnormalities of gait.

Genetic counselling for prospective parents with one of the diseases is generally available.

Muscular rheumatism

Aches and pains in damaged and bruised muscles and ligaments are common in sportsmen and the elderly (and particularly in elderly sportsmen). Despite the name, this has nothing to do with rheumatic fever (page 195) or rheumatoid arthritis (page 197) and most muscular aches rapidly settle after a few days. Immediate if transient relief often follows a warm bath or local warmth and massage.

Myasthenia gravis

A muscle disease affecting the muscles controlling the eyes and, less commonly, speech, swallowing and the shoulders and arms. The muscles become progressively weaker with increased use, but recover when subsequently rested. Myasthenia is caused by lack of acetylcholine, a chemical which is essential for transmission of impulses from nerves to muscle.

Treatment is with neostigmine or pyridostigmine which destroy the enzyme which neutralizes acetylcholine in the nerve endings, and is usually very successful.

Myocardial infarction

A medical name for a heart attack (page 120). Obstruction to the blood supply (thrombosis) of part

MUMPS

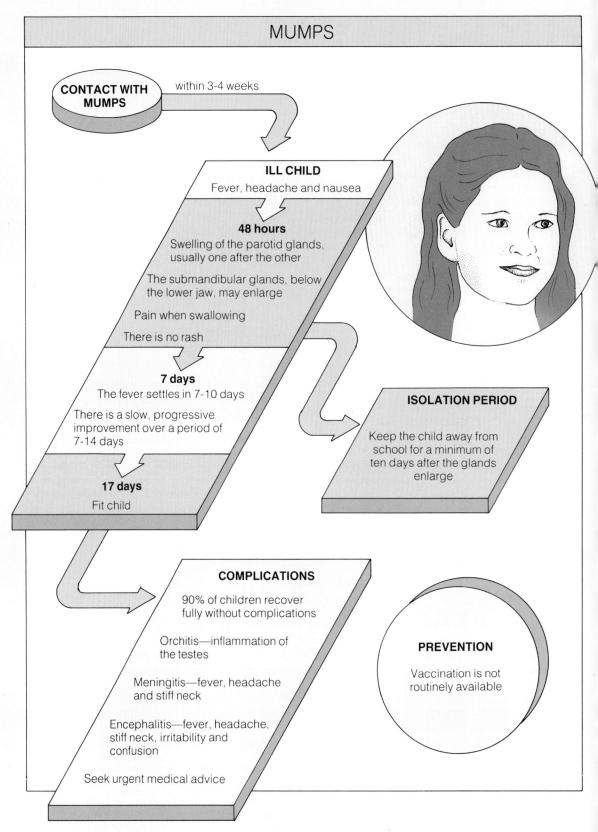

CONTACT WITH MUMPS

within 3-4 weeks

ILL CHILD

Fever, headache and nausea

48 hours

Swelling of the parotid glands, usually one after the other

The submandibular glands, below the lower jaw, may enlarge

Pain when swallowing

There is no rash

7 days

The fever settles in 7-10 days

There is a slow, progressive improvement over a period of 7-14 days

17 days

Fit child

ISOLATION PERIOD

Keep the child away from school for a minimum of ten days after the glands enlarge

COMPLICATIONS

90% of children recover fully without complications

Orchitis—inflammation of the testes

Meningitis—fever, headache and stiff neck

Encephalitis—fever, headache, stiff neck, irritability and confusion

Seek urgent medical advice

PREVENTION

Vaccination is not routinely available

of the muscle (*myo*), of the heart (*cardia*) results in destruction (infarction) of some heart muscle.

Myopia

This means short sight (*see* Glasses).

Naevus
SEE BIRTHMARK

Nail

The nails grow forward from the nail bed at a slow rate which is constant in health. Any severe illness may slow the rate, leaving a transverse ridge across the nail which grows forward as health is restored and nail growth returns to normal.

Hangnail is the name applied to a broken slip of skin at the side of the nail, which should not be pulled off as this may result in a long tear which becomes infected. The skin should be cut carefully with scissors.

Ingrowing nails occur if a sharp edge is left by cutting. This edge may pierce the skin, which becomes infected and red, tender and swollen. The help of a chiropodist and antibiotics may be required. (*See also* Whitlow.)

Splitting of the nails is common, but not related to any known underlying disease. It is possible that frequent washing may be contributory and it is well worth trying the effect of wearing gloves when washing and laundering.

Spooning of the nails occurs in severe iron deficiency anaemia (page 18).

The nails may be affected in a number of skin disorders such as psoriasis (page 188), and infection with the ringworm fungus (page 198) and thrush (page 223) is common. The half moons, which are normally absent in a small percentage of the population, tend to disappear in severe anaemia.

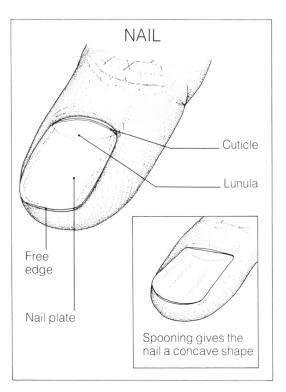

NAIL

Cuticle
Lunula
Free edge
Nail plate

Spooning gives the nail a concave shape

Nail biting

A nervous tic common in young children. It has no serious significance and nearly all children grow out of it, though some adults retain the habit.

Children's nails can be painted with bitter preparations to help break the habit but it is usually successful only in those with determination to stop without such help.

Nappy rash

The commonest form of nappy rash is ammonia dermatitis, and nearly all babies are affected. Bacteria on the skin break down urine to produce chemical products (such as ammonia) which irritate the skin, causing inflammation and even ulceration.

Treatment is aimed at preventing prolonged skin contact with ammonia products. Frequent nappy changes should be encouraged, and the nappies should be washed well and rinsed very well. (Boiling the nappies kills the bacteria which produce the ammonia.) If necessary, a nappy liner should be used. When the rash is severe, the use of plastic pants should be restricted as they promote a damp hot environment inside the nappy.

The skin should be gently cleaned and dried well between changes, and a barrier cream such as zinc and castor oil or a silicone-based cream applied. A nappy-free period during the day is often beneficial.

Sometimes nappy rashes are caused by infection which may be secondary to ammonia dermatitis. Treatment requires the above measures and the use of a bactericidal or fungicidal cream (see Thrush).

A rash in the nappy area is occasionally caused by an eczematous dermatitis, and this may also become infected. Treatment is more complicated because antibiotics or anti-fungal creams are required in addition to creams containing steroids, and is therefore best planned with medical help.

Narcotics
(GREEK: *NARKE*, STUPOR)

Strictly these are drugs which induce sleep or stupor. The term is also more commonly and inaccurately applied to all drugs taken by addicts, including heroin, amphetamines and LSD.

Nasal sinuses

Air-filled spaces surrounding the nose and pharynx. The largest of these are the antra behind the cheeks, and the frontal sinuses just behind the inner end of the eyebrows. They lighten the weight of the skull, and also make the voice resonant when speaking or singing. (*See also* Sinusitis.)

Nausea
SEE PREGNANCY: VOMITING; TRAVEL SICKNESS; *AND* VOMITING.

Navel
SEE UMBILICUS

Nephritis
(GREEK: *NEPHROS*, KIDNEY; *-ITIS*, INFLAMMATION)

Inflammation of the kidneys. Damage to these tissues may be caused by infection (page 141) and by some analgesic drugs such as phenacetin if taken in excessive quantities. Most forms of nephritis recover completely but very occasionally the inflammation persists, leading to kidney failure (page 141).

Nerves

Thin fibres which transmit electrical impulses. These impulses may travel in two directions. The sensory nerves transmit information from the skin or body organs, travel to the spinal cord and thence to the central nervous system. In the other direction, impulses originating in the brain pass via the spinal cord and motor nerves to the muscles.

Sensory nerves tell the brain about pain, temperature changes, touch and alteration in the positions of joints. A typical nervous reflex follows a burn to the hand: pain sensation passes along the sensory nerve to the spinal cord; connections between nerves at this level in the spinal cord then send an impulse along the motor nerve to the arm muscles, which contract to move the hand away from the painful stimulus. This 'reflex arc' is very rapid and the response takes only a tenth of a second. (*See also* Brain and nervous system, page 256.)

Nettle rash
SEE URTICARIA

Neuralgia
(GREEK: *NEURON*, NERVE; *ALGOS*, PAIN)

A term used to describe various pains due to pressure on a nerve or to disordered function. The common forms are listed below.

Brachial neuralgia
Follows pressure on or damage to the brachial or upper limb network (plexus) of nerves. The damage is often at the site of exit of the nerve from between the vertebrae in the neck due to osteoarthritis of the joints; this causes numbness and pins and needles along the nerve in the arm, sometimes with pain which may be dragging or shooting.

Post-herpetic neuralgia
Nerve pain which occurs during and occasionally following shingles or *Herpes zoster*. The pain is felt at the site of the rash (see Shingles).

Sciatica
A form of neuralgia which affects the sciatic nerve as it leaves the lumbar vertebrae to pass down the leg (see Sciatica).

Trigeminal neuralgia
Severe piercing pain which shoots along the middle branches of the fifth cranial nerve (the trigeminal

nerve), causing pain over the cheek and in the upper jaw. The pain is set off by stimulation of the nerve by chewing, brushing the teeth, shaving or even a gust of cold air. The cause is unknown, though it can be stimulated by dental infection and root abscesses. The pain is spasmodic but extremely severe, and may not respond to potent pain-killing drugs. In such a case, cutting the nerve surgically may be the only means of stopping the pain.

Neurosis and neurotic illness

Although these terms are generally used to describe people who are easily excitable or perhaps unpredictable, they are used medically to describe a number of specific psychiatric illnesses such as anxiety state, depression, hysteria and the phobias (e.g. agoraphobia and claustrophobia). (*See* Psychiatric illnesses; *and* Psychiatric treatment.)

Nightmares

Bad dreams are very common in both adults and children. In children particularly, the fears are very real and, since they cannot rationalize their thoughts on waking, they may have long outbursts of crying even after they have stopped dreaming.

The cause of nightmares remains unknown but they are easily forgotten by the next morning and do not indicate anything other than a normal imagination. Some medicines, including those given to promote sleep, cause nightmares in susceptible people.

Although rapidly comforted by their parents, children may be scared of going to sleep because of the fear of nightmares, and simple measures such as leaving a small light on and the bedroom door ajar will usually be sufficient to calm them.

Recurrent nightmares in children and adults may result from previous horrifying experiences. They are common, for instance, in ex-prisoners of war. In such people it is well worth seeking expert psychiatric advice.

Nipple disorders

Uncommon but should always be taken seriously. Breast cancer is common and successfully treated if detected early. Changes in the nipple shape or discharge from it, may be the first indication (*see also* Breast disorders, page 45).

Discharge from a nipple other than during pregnancy and the period of breast feeding must always be regarded seriously. Pus suggests an underlying infection or abscess, and blood indicates trauma, infection, an underlying cyst or cancer.

Rarely, milk will discharge from the breast of a man or a non-pregnant woman; this may be the result of excess prolactin, a hormone secreted by the pituitary gland (page 177), and sometimes is caused by drug therapy.

If there is a discharge from the breast, advice should be sought quickly so that the cause can be determined and the understandable anxiety caused by it relieved.

Retraction of one or both nipples is common and rarely of dangerous significance though it will prevent breast feeding. However, a normal nipple which then becomes retracted indicates underlying disease such as infection or cancer.

Sore or cracked nipples are common during breast feeding (*see* Infant feeding), and improve if the child is fed away from the involved breast for 7–14 days.

Nit

Nits are the eggs of lice. Nits and lice affect the head, body or genital areas, and live either on the skin or in the clothing. They are transmitted by close personal contact, often during sexual intercourse (crab lice). They cause irritation with itching. Scratch marks are often present and may become infected.

Once suspected, careful inspection of the affected skin with a lens usually reveals the small, oval, greyish nits attached to the hairs and which cannot easily be dislodged. Lice may also be present. Once diagnosed, treatment is easy. Clothing and bedding should be thoroughly laundered and boiled and the affected skin treated with a preparation containing gamma benzene hexachloride (under medical supervision because the application can result in dermatitis).

Nitrazepam

One of the most commonly used sleeping tablets (hypnotics) in the UK. It belongs to a group of drugs called benzodiazepines. Nitrazepam is produced by several manufacturers under different trade names (e.g. Mogadon, Nitrados, Somnased, Somnite).

The benzodiazepines are now used in preference to barbiturates as hypnotics because they do not cause the same degree of physical dependence. There is also less chance of interacting with other drugs, which barbiturates do commonly. However, there is a degree of psychological dependence, and withdrawal causes a temporary disturbance of sleep pattern. Newer drugs in this group such as temazepam (Normison, Euhypnos) are shorter acting and cause less hangover in the morning.

Nitrous oxide

A safe anaesthetic gas, well known as 'laughing gas'. It is used with a mixture of oxygen and other anaesthetic agents to maintain general anaesthesia during surgical operations. It is also commonly employed in dental practice.

Nitrous oxide with oxygen (Entonox) is used during childbirth as a self-administered analgesic, giving effective and safe pain relief without anaesthesia.

Nocturnal enuresis

Enuresis means incontinence and nocturnal enuresis refers to incontinence at night in children. (*See* Bed wetting.)

Nose bleed
(EPISTAXIS)

Nose bleeds in children, adolescents and young adults may occur spontaneously or follow minor trauma when blowing and picking dry crusts or with cold and hay fever.

Treatment involves placing the casualty in a sitting position with the head held slightly forwards, whilst pinching the soft part of the nose for about 10 minutes; the mouth should be kept open and swallowing forbidden. Once the bleeding has stopped, the nose should not be handled or blown for a few hours in case the clot is disturbed.

Nose bleeds generally stop using this technique. In the young, a second and third attempt is worth trying if bleeding recurs. In the elderly, particularly if they feel faint, medical advice should be obtained if there is rebleeding.

See also under First aid, page 269.

Nose disorders

Blocked noses are very common in association with colds, sinusitis and any infection involving the upper respiratory tract, and they clear as the acute infection subsides. Recurrent nasal discharge is the most uncomfortable feature of nasal allergies and hay fever (*see* Hay fever). Persistent discharge suggests a chronic sinusitis or the presence of a nasal polyp which may have to be removed surgically. Bleeding from the nose (epistaxis) usually follows acute trauma, but if chronic or recurrent, can indicate a weak small blood vessel or a chronic infection. Expert advice should be obtained. Children tend to push objects up their noses and these can produce persistent discharge and bleeding.

Broken nose
Features of a broken nose are tenderness, swelling and discoloration of the overlying soft tissue, with mobility and deformity of the nose.

The first-aid treatment is to control any bleeding, but for subsequent treatment medical advice should be sought. Where there is no significant deformity, no treatment may be required. If the nose is deformed, readjustment of the nasal bones is performed under general anaesthetic. This procedure is not performed immediately because of the soft tissue swelling, but must be done before the broken bones begin to unite; the optimum time is usually 3–5 days after the injury.

Loss of sense of smell
Usually occurs when air and its contained odours cannot pass up to the olfactory nerve endings which

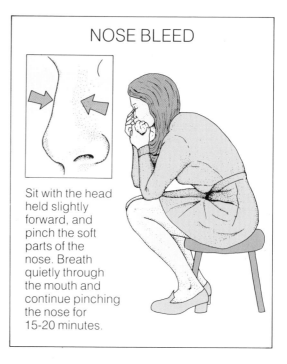

NOSE BLEED

Sit with the head held slightly forward, and pinch the soft parts of the nose. Breath quietly through the mouth and continue pinching the nose for 15-20 minutes.

lie in a groove in the skull just below the frontal air sinuses. This is common with acute sinusitis and improves as the infection subsides.

Rarely, permanent loss of smell occurs in chronic sinus infection, or following skull fracture when the nerve is damaged as it passes through the skull. Very occasionally, it occurs when a cyst or tumour presses on the olfactory nerve.

Sinusitis *see* page 207

Notifiable disease

The occurrence of certain infectious diseases must be reported to the health authorities. (This law dates from 1899 and is revised under the Public Health Regulations 1968.) Notification serves two purposes: the first is to control serious infections and the second is to provide information on the changing incidence of the disease.

The notifiable diseases are:

Anthrax	Plague
Cholera	Acute poliomyelitis
Diphtheria	Relapsing fever
Dysentery	Scarlet fever
Acute encephalitis	Smallpox
Food poisoning	Tetanus
Infective jaundice	Tuberculosis
Leprosy	Typhoid and
Leptospirosis	paratyphoid fevers
Malaria	Typhus fever
Measles	Whooping cough
Ophthalmia	Yellow fever
neonatorum	

Numbness

Anaesthesia of the finger tips and toes most commonly follows exposure to cold, and soon recovers after entering the warm. Everyone develops episodes of transient numbness from time to time after pressing on a nerve, as for example when crossing the legs or resting an arm over the back of a chair. It may be associated with pins and needles (page 177), often as the limb recovers. Other examples of numbness caused by nerve pressure are the numbness of the part of the foot and leg where the sciatic nerve is compressed between the lumbar vertebrae (*see* Sciatica), and when the median nerve is compressed at the wrist producing numbness in the thumb, index and middle fingers of the hand (*see* Carpal tunnel syndrome).

Narrowing of blood vessels may so decrease the oxygen supply to peripheral nerves that they become damaged, which in turn causes numbness. This almost invariably affects the nerves of the feet, and follows arteriosclerosis of the femoral arteries, the major vessels to the legs (*see* Arterial disease). This may occur as an isolated event or as part of a more generalized vascular disease (e.g. diabetes, page 78).

Transient numbness is rarely a cause for concern but if it continues to recur or it persists, medical advice should be sought.

Nystatin

A drug used to treat thrush (page 223). This infection is caused by the fungus *Candida albicans* which may affect the mouth, cause nappy rash in babies, and skin and vaginal infection in adults. Nystatin may be given as drops when there is mouth infection, as a cream in skin infections and as pessaries in vaginal infection. Nystatin tablets may be given to reduce the bowel reservoir of *Candida albicans* which is a source of re-infection if there is recurrent vaginal thrush.

Obesity
SEE OVERWEIGHT

Obsessional personality

Obsessional features are very common—e.g. ensuring that the kitchen or desk is tidy, or double checking that the car is locked—and are a part of most people's character. Many are perfectly normal and do not indicate any underlying psychological disorder. Obsession becomes a matter of concern when the obsessive acts become so frequently repeated that they interfere with normal life and thought. In the most severe cases the personalities are characterized by being rigid, perfectionist, morbidly scrupulous, prone to self-reproach and in a state of doubt and indecision. There may be a disturbance of sexual life with a turbulent sexuality underlying a prim and over-correct demeanour. These are features of nervous psychiatric disease and should be managed with help from a psychiatrist.

Occupational diseases
SEE INDUSTRIAL DISEASES

Oedema
(GREEK: *OIDEMA*, SWELLING)

Swelling of tissues due to an increase in fluid within them. This commonly occurs following soft-tissue injury.

Oedema is most often seen at the ankles. Ankle oedema may occur in elderly people due to immobility with the legs maintained in a dependent position for long periods; e.g. following prolonged car or air travel. The commonest cause of ankle swelling in middle age is varicose veins (page 239).

More seriously it may be a sign of a failing heart which increases the back-pressure in the veins. If this happens, oedema may also occur in the lungs (pulmonary oedema) to cause shortness of breath, which is worse on exertion and lying flat.

Oesophagitis

Inflammation of the oesophagus (gullet), through which food passes to the stomach. There is a complex valve system between the lower end of the oesophagus and the stomach which prevents stomach contents regurgitating (refluxing) up the oesophagus (*see* diagram, page 194). When this valve system fails in the presence of a hiatus hernia (page 126), the stomach contents reflux into the oesophagus. The acid irritates the oesophagus, causing oesophagitis resulting in a burning or sore pain in the middle of the upper abdomen, which spreads upward behind the sternum (heartburn, page 122). The bitter tasting acid may regurgitate up to the back of the mouth.

Oesophagitis is relieved by substances which neutralize or dilute the stomach contents (e.g. milk, magnesium sulphate, Rennie, Milk of Magnesia, Maclean's, Asilone).

Onchocerciasis

A common disease of tropical Africa and South America, caused by a worm (*Onchocerca*). This inhabits the skin, which reacts by forming nodules wherever the worm travels. Occasionally the cornea of the eye is affected, resulting in blindness (African river blindness).

Opium

Extracted from the dried capsule of the poppy, opium is the source of morphine and heroin and is amongst the most powerful pain relievers in medical use. It is a strongly addictive drug (*see* Addiction), so its use must be reserved for the treatment of severe pain, and then only under medical supervision.

Oral contraception

The most commonly used form of oral contraception is the combined pill which contains two hormones—an oestrogen and a progestogen. This pill is taken cyclically to allow a withdrawal bleed, or period. The strength of the pill is determined by the oestrogen content, and most pills now contain only 30 micrograms. (*See* Pill.)

Orchitis

Infection of the testis, which is painful and swollen; the scrotum is red and swollen, and general constitutional symptoms with a raised temperature and nausea (and sometimes vomiting) are frequent. Orchitis is often associated with a urinary infection and it may occur in gonorrhoea. Mumps is a common cause. It may be difficult to distinguish from torsion of the testicle, which usually occurs in school boys about the age of puberty and is caused by twisting of the testis around its blood supply which is thus obstructed. If this is neglected and not corrected by surgery, the testis loses its normal function and viability.

Treatment of orchitis due to bacterial infection (urinary infection, gonorrhoea) is with an appropriate antibiotic. There is no specific treatment for mumps orchitis because it is a virus infection, but if the pain is severe, pethidine may be required for 24–48 hours to relieve it.

Medical advice should always be sought in those with suspected orchitis, both for help in relieving pain and nausea and because it can be very difficult to distinguish from torsion of the testicle.

Ornithosis
SEE PSITTACOSIS

Osteoarthritis

Due to 'wear and tear', and is most common in an ageing population. With increasing age, joint surfaces become irregular and this causes pain and restricted movement. The major weight-bearing joints, the hips and knees, are most commonly affected but the spine is often involved.

Treatment requires adequate pain relief and maintenance of good muscle tone, for if the muscles are allowed to weaken due to inactivity, mobility becomes more difficult. Simple analgesics such as paracetamol or aspirin are usually effective, and local warmth may help to relieve joint pain.

In severe osteoarthritis of the hips when the pain may be sufficiently severe to prevent any movement of the joint, great benefit may result from replacement with an artificial hip joint. Knee joints can also be replaced.

See also Arthritis.

Osteomyelitis

Infection of bone, which is now rare. The infection reaches the bone via the blood stream from a distant site (e.g. a boil or impetigo) and the bones most commonly affected are the tibia and femur in the leg. The condition causes severe pain in the affected bone, aggravated by movement and associated with a high temperature of 39–40°C (102.2–104°F). Treatment always requires high-dose antibiotic therapy and may involve an operation to drill a hole in the bone to release the pus.

Since the advent of antibiotics, osteomyelitis can usually be cured completely if detected sufficiently early, though diagnosis can be extremely difficult even for experienced specialists.

Osteopathy

Osteopathic treatments are based on the theory that disease is caused by disarrangement of bones and particularly the vertebral bones of the spine. Hence, by manipulating and realigning the bones it is hoped to restore normal health.

Whilst it is ridiculous to apply the theory to all disease, the cause of backache is often obscure and many derive benefit from spinal manipulation. Osteopathy is not formally recognized by the medical profession because few osteopaths have any formal training, either medical or non-medical, and cannot therefore determine whether manipulation is the

treatment required for any one patient with the obvious potential damage.

Manipulation (page 149) remains an extremely valuable form of treatment especially for bad backs and sciatica in patients carefully selected by experienced medical practitioners.

Osteoporosis

Loss of bone density. It is a natural process which occurs with increasing age, and as a result bones become brittle and liable to fracture. In old age simple falls can cause major fractures. Osteoporosis is one cause of backache in the old, when the vertebral bones may collapse resulting in pain, loss of height and a misshapen spine.

In women, osteoporosis usually occurs at the time of the menopause. There is evidence that this is hormonally related, as hormone replacement therapy may delay the onset of bone thinning. Osteoporosis also occurs in people receiving long-term oral steroid treatment in high dosage, in sufferers from rheumatoid arthritis and in people who are immobilized by illness for long periods.

Diets rich in calcium and vitamin D are often prescribed in an attempt to prevent its progression.

Otitis
(GREEK: *OUS*, EAR; *ITIS*, INFLAMMATION)

Otitis externa
Inflammation or infection of the skin lining the outer ear canal which leads into the ear down to the eardrum (*see* Ear).

Otitis media
Infection of the middle ear, the cavity of the ear lying on the inner side of the eardrum (*see* diagram, page 89). It may be associated with pain, discharge of pus and a raised temperature. (*See also* Ear infection.)

Otosclerosis
SEE UNDER DEAFNESS: IN ADULTS

Ovary

The female sex gland which forms the eggs (ova) from which the future offspring will grow after fertilization by a sperm (spermatozoon). There are two ovaries—one on each side of the pelvis, at the mouths of the Fallopian tubes which transmit the ova to the womb (uterus). (*See* diagram, page 263.)

The ovary also produces oestrogens, the female sex hormones which control the secondary sexual characteristics, including type and distribution of hair, body shape (including breast formation) and some features of personality and behaviour. They are also involved with primary sexual characteristics directly affecting reproduction, including regulation of the menstrual periods (page 169).

Inflammation of the ovary is called oöphoritis (Greek: *oophoros*, egg-bearing; *itis*, inflammation), and may cause sterility.

Overweight
(OBESITY)

Defined as 20 per cent above expected weight derived from life insurance studies and based on normal levels related to height, frame size and age (*see* Ideal weights, page 292). Obesity is synonymous with overweight.

Obesity is associated with an increased mortality rate. Disorders of the gall bladder, heart and weight-bearing joints are more common in the obese, and varicose veins and hernias are more trouble-some. Life insurance statistics show that death from diabetes mellitus is almost four times more common among the obese than in the general population.

Obesity is almost invariably caused by consumption of calories above the requirement for that individual. There is some evidence that thin people use up their food more efficiently whereas an obese person stores it as fat. Nevertheless, eating more than is required results in obesity.

Alteration of the diet is the only certain method of losing weight (*see* Reducing diets, page 292). The vast number of different slimming diets available suggest that there is no miracle cure but the safest method is to reduce the amount of food consumed in a balanced diet and the only necessary ingredient for success is perseverance. On any diet, weight falls rapidly over the first 2 weeks due to loss of body water but weight loss subsequently is much slower as the stored fat is used for energy. One way to maintain weight loss is to join a slimming or Weight Watchers club, as in this way peer pressure aids self-determination.

Slimming tablets are frequently prescribed. Amphetamines were used to aid slimming by reducing appetite but they have been withdrawn for routine use because of their addictive properties.

Unfortunately, there is little evidence to support the use of slimming tablets as few without the will to lose weight are helped by them, and many who are helped to reduce weight will regain it on stopping the drugs.

If weight gain is progressive, and associated with mental slowing, thickening of the skin, recent dislike of the cold, a gruff voice or loss of hair, medical advice should be sought to ensure that the thyroid gland is not under-active.

Ovulation

The time when an egg (ovum) is released from an ovary. It normally occurs every month and is controlled by hormones from the pituitary gland (*see* Periods). Ovulation usually occurs 2 weeks prior to the onset of the next period. When the menstrual cycle is regular, occurring every 28 days, ovulation takes place on day 14 of the cycle.

Ovulation starts at the menarche (the age when periods first begin) and ceases at the time of the menopause.

Ovulation may fail because of defective ovaries or during pregnancy, and is inhibited by the combined oral contraceptive pill.

Oxytocin

A hormone produced by the pituitary gland. It is produced in increased quantity during labour and stimulates the uterus to contract.

A drug similar to oxytocin is produced synthetically and is sometimes given to stimulate labour prior to childbirth.

P

Pacemaker

An electrical device used to regulate the heart rate. In the normal heart there is an area of muscle which acts as a natural pacemaker, known as the sino-atrial (SA) node. The SA node sends out regular electrical waves which are conducted to the rest of the heart muscle, causing contraction and hence a heart beat. The SA node's excitability is regulated by nervous and hormonal factors. Occasionally these impulses

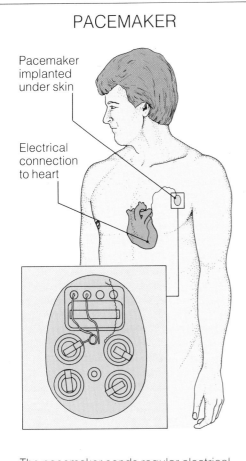

PACEMAKER

Pacemaker implanted under skin

Electrical connection to heart

The pacemaker sends regular electrical impulses to the heart at a rate of about 70 per minute.

ventricle of the heart. An energy source is then attached to produce intermittent electrical impulses at a controllable rate. Occasionally a permanent artificial pulse is required and a small pacemaker not much larger than a match box is placed under the skin in front of the right shoulder. It is regularly checked electrically without breaking the skin. They generally need replacing every 2-5 years. Batteries have a restricted life, so radioactive power packs are now used as a reliable long-term energy source.

Paget's disease

A bone disease of the elderly which causes thickening of bones, generally of the limbs, spine and skull.

Only one bone is usually affected and causes no disability or discomfort. Occasionally pain may occur in the spine and responds well to calcitonin, a hormone normally produced by the parathyroid gland. Very rarely, Paget's disease is sufficiently severe to cause bowing and enlargement of the tibial bones in the leg, and enlargement and deformity of the skull.

Pain

★ Medical advice should be sought for any unexpected acute or severe pain in any part of the body. (For further information, *see* specific entries such as Abdominal pain *and* Earache.)

Pain relief
SEE ANALGESIA

Palate

The roof of the mouth, and is formed by the hard palate in front and the soft palate behind with the uvula attached dangling down (*see* diagram, page 265). In the embryo it develops from two sides which meet and fuse in the middle. Occasionally, fusion is incomplete and results in a cleft palate.

Pallor
(PALENESS)

Reflects the amount of blood flowing through the small blood vessels (capillaries) in the skin. When the skin is warm, the fine capillaries open, allowing more blood to flow and this results in a healthy pink

are not conducted to the rest of the heart muscle. The ventricular heart muscle then loses its nervous and hormonal control and contracts at its natural rate, which is about half the normal resting rate. Also the heart rate cannot increase in response to exercise. This is known as complete heart block, and can be a serious handicap causing repeated fainting attacks because the slow heart rate results in a reduced cardiac output and reduced blood flow to the brain.

The problem is overcome by inserting an artificial pacemaker. For temporary pacemaking a wire is inserted along a blood vessel leading to the heart so that the tip can be placed on the muscle of the

complexion. Conversely, in cold conditions, the skin capillaries close to conserve heat loss from the body and the skin pales.

Pallor is seen commonly during faints, when there is transient circulatory failure—the lack of blood to the brain results in loss of consciousness and the diminished flow of blood in the skin causes pallor.

Palpitations

Describes an awareness of the heart beat, often noticed in the quiet of the night. It may just be an awareness of a normal heart beat sometimes with an occasional extra beat, and palpitation also occurs when the heart rate is rapid or irregular. A rapid heart rate is usually a reflection of underlying anxiety. None of these is necessarily due to an abnormality of the heart.

Palpitations which are recurrent or render the heart inefficient as a pump require treatment from a doctor. A well known example of the drugs used is digoxin (digitalis), which is most useful when the heart rate is persistently rapid and completely irregular (atrial fibrillation). Digoxin slows the heart rate and makes the heart pump more efficiently.

Pancreas

A gland which sits on the inside of the posterior wall of the abdomen, nestled within the curve of the upper intestine (see diagram, page 265).

Pancreatic juices are secreted into the duodenum and contain trypsin, amylase and lipase which break down ingested protein, carbohydrate and fat, respectively. Within the substance of the pancreas are small nests of cells which secrete insulin—which metabolizes the sugar (glucose) in the blood.

Acute inflammation of the pancreas causes severe abdominal pain (page 8) and peritonitis (page 172). Chronic pancreatitis destroys the glandular tissue and diminishes the secretion of digestive enzymes, leading to malabsorption and chronic severe diarrhoea. If insufficient insulin is present, diabetes (page 78) results.

Paracetamol

A commonly used pain-killing (analgesic) drug, obtainable without prescription in the UK. It has the same efficacy as aspirin although it does not exert an anti-inflammatory action. It is used in treating painful inflammatory conditions such as rheumatoid arthri-tis. Paracetamol and aspirin both have an anti-pyretic effect (i.e. they lower a raised temperature), of value in treating childhood infections, and essential when there is a previous history of febrile convulsion.

Paracetamol has no side-effects at the recommended dose, whereas aspirin often causes gastric irritation. When the normal dose is exceeded, severe and even fatal liver and kidney damage may occur. The normal adult dose is two (500 milligram) tablets 4-hourly but not exceeding eight tablets in 24 hours.

★ Paralysis

Weakness of muscles which may be partial or total. It results from damage to muscles or to the nerves supplying and controlling the muscles, including those parts of the brain which control the nerves.

A common cause of paralysis is a stroke. This is due to interruption of the blood supply to part of the brain and it usually results in paralysis or partial paralysis of one side of the body (hemiplegia).

Severe damage to the spinal cord results in paralysis on both sides of the body, and damage occurring high up in the spinal cord can cause paralysis of the arms as well as the legs (tetraplegia). Damage lower down the spine causes paralysis of the lower limbs (paraplegia). These traumatic injuries often occur during road traffic accidents.

Poliomyelitis, a virus infection, can produce paralysis. This may be sufficiently extensive to involve the muscles of respiration.

Damage may occur to single nerves; e.g. the nerve to the facial muscles is occasionally damaged at birth and may follow the use of forceps—fortunately, it usually recovers completely. Bell's palsy affects the same nerve in adults and also usually recovers spontaneously and completely.

Paranoia

A psychiatric disorder characterized by delusions of persecution. These are false reality judgements which would not be acceptable to other people of the same race, religion, sex and age.

Paranoid delusions are common in the elderly person suffering from dementia (intellectual impairment) especially when associated with depression. They are usually mild in the elderly and helped by carefully listening to their problems and helping them to understand.

Severe paranoia occurs with other psychiatric illnesses such as schizophrenia.

Many people get paranoid feelings to a minor degree on occasion but this invariably settles after a few days. If paranoia persists and interferes with a normal existence, medical advice should be obtained.

Paraplegia

Paralysis of the lower limbs. The causes include acute spinal injury, infections and tumours of the spine, blockage of the blood supply to the spinal cord, spina bifida and multiple sclerosis.

Paraplegia is a great handicap, with psychological problems in addition to the obvious physical ones. The prevention of pressure sores is of utmost importance, for their presence may force the most independent of paraplegics from a wheelchair to a bed. Pressure sores are especially likely to occur over bony prominences, such as the heels and ankles in addition to the more likely sites around the buttocks, base of spine and hips. Sores develop rapidly and may become deep and infected. They can be prevented by frequent posture changes.

Additional problems occur with loss of bladder and anal sensation. If bladder sensation is lost, the bladder usually remains full and there is difficulty in voiding urine. Catheterization (passage of a small flexible tube into the bladder) may be necessary. Likewise, constipation may be severe, and suppositories and enemas are required. Sexual feelings persist, and with guidance some experience can still be enjoyed.

Physiotherapy is extremely helpful in the early stages of rehabilitation, especially when the paraplegia has been caused by injury. Some people may learn to walk again; others, not so fortunate, may nevertheless achieve great independence in a wheelchair. The achievements of competitors in the paraplegic Olympic games is truly remarkable and a tribute to their tenacity and courage.

Parathyroids

Four small glands situated behind the thyroid gland. They secrete parathyroid hormone which regulates calcium absorption from the intestine, and loss from the kidneys. This hormone controls the manufacture and breakdown of bone in which calcium is stored.

Paratyphoid

A bacterial infection caused by *Salmonella paratyphi* A, B and C, resulting from the ingestion of infected food or water. Paratyphoid is a similar but less severe infection than typhoid. The illness is characterized by a protracted fever, diarrhoea, abdominal pain, and a rash appearing mainly on the trunk.

Treatment is by ensuring adequate fluid intake, which may have to be given intravenously. Appropriate antibiotics may be given if the blood stream is infected. The disease is best prevented by ensuring good hygiene and sanitation with a pure water supply, and high standards are required for people handling food. Two doses of TAB vaccine at 4- to 6-week intervals, one a year later and boosters at 3-yearly intervals provide protection against typhoid and paratyphoid A and B, and are given to travellers to the tropics.

Parkinson's disease

Named after James Parkinson who first described 'paralysis agitans' in 1817, it is characterized by poverty of emotional and voluntary movements, tremor and muscular rigidity. Parkinsonism usually occurs in the elderly and runs a steadily deteriorating course. It may, rarely, occur in the younger age groups following infections of the brain (encephalitis). It is also seen occasionally as a side-effect of certain drugs used as tranquillizers. The symptoms disappear with withdrawal of the drug.

The symptoms can be disabling. The tremor is marked in the hands, worse at rest and improved with purposive movement. The rigidity and poor movement may give difficulty in initiating walking. The gait is unusual, with no swinging of the arms and small shuffling steps. Sometimes the shuffling steps appear to be hurried in order to prevent falling over. There is a lack of facial expression, increasing difficulty with speaking, depression and occasionally intellectual impairment. (*See* chart, page 168.)

Treatment is aimed at reducing the symptoms. Social support and understanding, physiotherapy and occupational therapy may help to preserve mobility, and maintain morale. Drug therapy reduces tremor and muscular rigidity. The drugs commonly used are levodopa (in Madopar and Sinemet) and benztropine (Cogentin).

People with Parkinson's disease lose the power of emotional expression but frequently retain emotional feelings and intellectual ability. The loss of facial expression makes them appear slow witted but this is not necessarily the case and they understandably become very depressed—strong emotional support and understanding from their family and close friends is essential to overcome this.

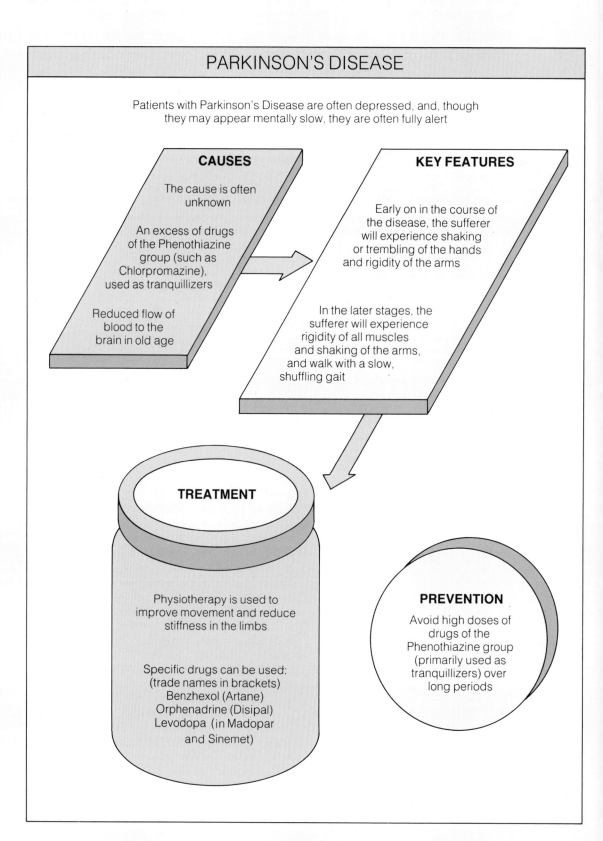

PARKINSON'S DISEASE

Patients with Parkinson's Disease are often depressed, and, though they may appear mentally slow, they are often fully alert

CAUSES

The cause is often unknown

An excess of drugs of the Phenothiazine group (such as Chlorpromazine), used as tranquillizers

Reduced flow of blood to the brain in old age

KEY FEATURES

Early on in the course of the disease, the sufferer will experience shaking or trembling of the hands and rigidity of the arms

In the later stages, the sufferer will experience rigidity of all muscles and shaking of the arms, and walk with a slow, shuffling gait

TREATMENT

Physiotherapy is used to improve movement and reduce stiffness in the limbs

Specific drugs can be used: (trade names in brackets)
Benzhexol (Artane)
Orphenadrine (Disipal)
Levodopa (in Madopar and Sinemet)

PREVENTION

Avoid high doses of drugs of the Phenothiazine group (primarily used as tranquillizers) over long periods

Paronychia
SEE WHITLOW

Parotid glands
(GREEK: *PARA*, BESIDE; *OTOS*, THE EAR)

Situated one each side just in front of the ears, and which secrete saliva via a small duct which opens into the mouth just opposite the pre-molar back teeth of the upper jaw. The parotid glands are most commonly inflamed and enlarged in mumps.

Parotitis

Inflammation of one or both the parotid glands. The parotid is a salivary gland situated behind the angle of the jaw below the ear. It is commonly inflamed in mumps and is responsible for the characteristic swelling (*see also* Mumps).

Swelling and pain in one parotid gland with meals suggests there may be a stone in the draining duct.

Patella

The small bone in front of the knee joint (page 143). It is held in place by the muscles and ligaments around the joint, and may slip if these are weak or damaged.

Pediculosis

An infestation with lice or nits (page 159).

Penicillin

The discovery of penicillin was a major medical advance; it was the first specific anti-bacterial agent to be discovered after sulphonamides.

The first clinical trials on penicillin were conducted in Britain in 1941. It had been known for a long time that the fungus *Penicillium* could suppress bacterial growth. In 1928 Fleming noted this effect and used the term 'penicillin' to describe the active substance produced by the fungus. Attempts to isolate penicillin were not pursued at that time, but in 1939 Chain and Florey, searching for antibiotics, first isolated penicillin. Following the first successful trials, arrangements were made for the production of penicillin in USA, and good supplies of penicillin were available by the end of World War II.

Penicillin rapidly replaced the sulphonamides because it is effective in a wide range of infections and much less toxic. Also penicillin is bactericidal (i.e. it kills the invading bacteria), whereas sulphonamides are bacteriostatic (i.e. they prevent the bacteria reproducing).

Penicillin is widely used for various infections, including streptococcal sore throat, bacterial meningitis, lobar pneumonia, gonorrhea and syphilis. In 1957 it became possible chemically to alter the structure of penicillin, and many different penicillins have been made. The semi-synthetic penicillins include ampicillin, amoxycillin, carbenicillin, cloxacillin and methicillin. The penicillins are well tolerated and relatively free of serious side-effects. Allergy to penicillin produces an itchy rash; the drug should be discontinued and future use of any of the penicillins avoided.

Penis
(LATIN: *PENIS*, TAIL)

The external male sex organ (*see* Genital tract: male).

Peptic ulcer

A term used to describe both stomach and duodenal ulcers. These are discussed under Stomach ulcer.

Perforated eardrum
SEE UNDER EARACHE

Pericarditis

Inflammation of the pericardium, the fibrous bag which encloses the heart. The inflammation may result from infection which often starts in the chest. Mild pericarditis is common after a heart attack.

It is usually painful, the pain being felt in the centre of the chest. It is often tight and worse with breathing and lying flat. It may be improved by sitting up and leaning forwards. Pericarditis is treated with pain-killing drugs (analgesics) at the same time as treating any underlying condition.

Periods
(MENSTRUATION)

Normally occur at regular intervals of 24–34 days (average 28 days) and last between 3 and 8 days (average 5 days). The normal age for the onset of periods (the menarche) is at puberty, between 10 and 16 years. Menstruation usually ceases during the fifth decade (the menopause).

Disorders of the menstrual cycle are common, and knowledge of the changes which occur during the cycle help in understanding these disorders. During each normal cycle an egg (ovum) is produced and released from the ovary. The lining of the womb (uterus) is thickened in preparation for receiving a fertilized egg. If fertilization does not occur, the lining of the uterus is shed, resulting in a period and the cycle is then repeated. All of the events are controlled by increasing and decreasing concentrations of hormones in the blood stream.

At the beginning of the cycle, part of the brain (the hypothalamus) releases two chemicals: (1) follicle-stimulating hormone-releasing factor (FSH-releasing factor), and (2) a smaller quantity of

luteinizing hormone-releasing factor (LH-releasing factor). These two substances stimulate the pituitary gland (situated beneath the brain) to release the appropriate hormones, i.e. follicle-stimulating hormone (FSH) and a smaller amount of luteinizing hormone (LH). The FSH passes in the blood stream to the ovary and stimulates the ripening of an ovum in the ovary as well as the production of another hormone, oestrogen, from the cells surrounding the ovum. The oestrogen in turn initiates the thickening of the lining of the uterus. As the level of oestrogen rises in the blood stream, it inhibits further FSH production reducing the amount of FSH-releasing factor. As the production of FSH-releasing factor diminishes there is a compensatory sharp increase in LH-releasing factor. The amount of LH in the blood stream rises and is the trigger for ovulation. The ovum bursts out of the ovary and enters the Fallopian tube on its way to the uterus.

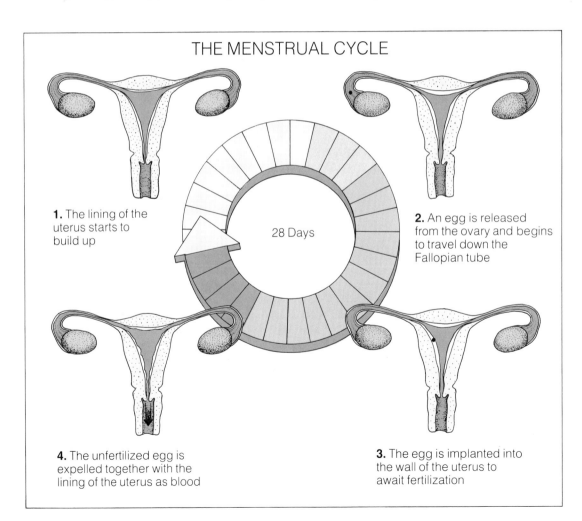

THE MENSTRUAL CYCLE

1. The lining of the uterus starts to build up

28 Days

2. An egg is released from the ovary and begins to travel down the Fallopian tube

4. The unfertilized egg is expelled together with the lining of the uterus as blood

3. The egg is implanted into the wall of the uterus to await fertilization

The cells which surround the egg in the ovary grow, to form a small gland called the corpus luteum. This gland produces progesterone, a hormone which continues to stimulate the lining of the uterus to make conditions ideal for receiving a fertilized ovum. If fertilization does not occur within 7 days of ovulation, the corpus luteum degenerates and ceases to function. The levels of oestrogen and progesterone fall rapidly, resulting in the shedding of the uterine lining and this usually occurs 14 days after ovulation. The low levels of oestrogen stimulate production of more FSH-releasing factor and the cycle is repeated.

Absent periods (amenorrhoea)

Considered abnormal, in the absence of pregnancy, in women of child-bearing age who have not had a period for 6 months or more. It implies that ovulation is not occurring. Commonly the function of the hypothalamus is altered due to factors such as weight loss and psychological upsets. Continued weight loss and absent periods are important features of anorexia nervosa, and restoration of weight is usually followed by return of the periods. Amenorrhoea is rarely due to failure of hormone production, from the hypothalamus, pituitary gland or ovary.

Amenorrhoea may follow stopping the oral contraceptive pill. In these circumstances the absent periods are probably not due to a side-effect of the pill. The pill has no over-all effect on future fertility although conception may be slightly delayed following cessation of the pill.

Amenorrhoea requires medical investigation to exclude pregnancy and to determine whether there is any underlying disease, whether the situation is reversible and whether conception is possible.

Heavy periods (menorrhagia)

Periods with excessive bleeding which are regular but sometimes prolonged. Fibroids and emotionally induced hypothalamic disturbance are two common causes and an intra-uterine contraceptive device (the coil) may make heavy periods worse. If the bleeding is disabling or produces anaemia (due to loss of iron), hormone treatment or the oral contraceptive pill may control the symptoms. In older women with fibroids a hysterectomy (removal of the uterus) may be necessary.

Irregular periods

Periods occurring irregularly with varying and often prolonged bleeding may indicate an abnormality of the uterus. Irregular periods are normal in early adolescence. This is due to the delay in establishing regular ovulation. In older women it needs further investigation, including a 'D and C'. A 'D and C' (dilatation and curettage) is an investigation performed under general anaesthetic. The cervix at the neck of the uterus is gently dilated to allow the passage of a small instrument to scrape the lining of the womb, and the scrapings are examined microscopically to detect any abnormalities.

A prolonged menstrual cycle of 6–10 weeks' duration followed by a heavy period may suggest that ovulation is not occurring. As a result, the lining of the womb continues to build up until it is shed with a much heavier bleed. The scrapings taken at operation will identify the thickening of the uterine lining.

Periods occurring infrequently

Periods only occurring at intervals of 6 weeks or longer are considered abnormal. The causes are similar to those for amenorrhoea (see above).

Periods occurring too frequently (polymenorrhoea)

The periods are heavy and regular but the overall cycle is much shorter than the usual 4 weeks and a period may occur every 2–3 weeks. Polymenorrhoea may follow pelvic inflammation due to infection of the Fallopian tubes, but, as with other menstrual disorders, may reflect underlying psychological problems.

Painful periods (dysmenorrhoea)

Typically occur in teenage girls. The pain occurs just before or with menstruation. It is only present in the ovulating woman and tends to improve with age. It is probably due to spasm of the uterus caused by prostaglandin, a chemical which is a constituent of the menstrual fluid. If there is no evidence of underlying uterine disease, pain-killing drugs which also have an anti-prostaglandin effect are given. Aspirin is the most common example. If it is ineffective, other drugs may exert a more pronounced anti-prostaglandin effect (e.g. indomethacin) and should be taken regularly 7 days prior to a period.

Another way to improve the pain is to stop ovulation, as dysmenorrhoea occurs only with irregular ovulation. This is achieved with the contraceptive pill.

Dysmenorrhoea also occurs in slightly older women. The causes include the intra-uterine contraceptive device (the coil), fibroids, pelvic inflammation and infection or endometriosis. Treatment obviously depends on the cause. A troublesome coil should be removed, and fibroids may need surgical removal. Pelvic inflammatory disease results from infection around the uterus, Fallopian tubes and ovaries, and may follow pregnancy, miscarriage, abortion, salpingitis and gonorrhoea—treatment is with antibiotics or surgery. Endometriosis is a condition in which the cells which line the womb (the endometrial cells) are present outside the womb (e.g. lying on the ovaries or the Fallopian tubes). These are sensitive to hormone change occurring during the menstrual cycle and go through the monthly changes of thickening, shedding and bleeding—which causes pain wherever the cells are found.

Investigation of dysmenorrhoea may require a D and C with laparoscopy: a flexible telescope with a fibre-optic system providing vision and light is introduced into the abdominal cavity under a general anaesthetic to observe the uterus, Fallopian tubes and ovaries. If necessary, a small piece of diseased tissue can be removed under direct vision for microscopic examination.

Most women experience variation in their periods during an otherwise healthy life, and some never have regular periods. These variations are rarely serious and usually settle after one or two further periods. If the changes persist, or if the periods are painful or associated with fever or discharge, medical advice should be obtained.

Peritonitis

A serious infection of the peritoneal cavity, which is that part of the body in which the intra-abdominal organs lie. These are all enclosed within a fine membrane—the peritoneum—which has pain receptors in its wall. The infection is usually caused by perforation of the gut, allowing bowel contents to escape into the peritoneal cavity. The most common cause is an acutely inflamed appendix.

The symptoms of peritonitis initially reflect those of the underlying cause (e.g. appendicitis). As peritonitis becomes established, there is severe abdominal pain which is typically made worse by movement, including coughing and breathing deeply. The pain may also be referred to the shoulder tip. The abdominal wall muscles are held rigid and the pulse rate and temperature rise. Vomiting is common. Similar features follow acute inflammation of the pancreas.

Treatment of peritonitis involves treatment of the underlying cause; e.g. removal of the appendix or closure of a perforated stomach ulcer, with appropriate antibiotics to counter the infection. The bowel usually ceases to function in peritonitis and for this reason oral fluids are avoided and replaced by intravenous fluids until bowel function returns as the infection subsides.

Peritonsillar abscess
(QUINSY)

A complication of acute tonsillitis, but is rare since the introduction of antibiotics. An abscess forms above the tonsils and the symptoms already present due to acute tonsillitis worsen. There is a high temperature, with difficulty in swallowing and opening the mouth, and earache. If a high dose of penicillin is given soon after diagnosis, the formation of the abscess may be prevented. Once the abscess has formed, unless it drains pus spontaneously, it may have to be drained surgically.

The development of a peritonsillar abscess is an indication for subsequent removal of the tonsils.

Pernicious anaemia

Results from a deficiency of vitamin B_{12}, which is essential for the production of blood cells. Dietary deficiency of B_{12} occurs in strict vegetarians (vegans) whose diet excludes animal meats and animal products, but pernicious anaemia usually occurs because of an inability to absorb vitamin B_{12} from the gut rather than a dietary deficiency. Normal B_{12} absorption requires a stomach acid to free it from food, and a glycoprotein (intrinsic factor) secreted by the stomach to combine with the freed B_{12}. It is only in this form that B_{12} can be absorbed into the blood stream from the ileum (the last part of the small intestine). In pernicious anaemia both acid and intrinsic factor are reduced or absent.

Treatment is by regular injection of 1000 micrograms of hydroxocobalamin, a more stable form of cyanocobalamin (vitamin B_{12}), given at 2- to 3-monthly intervals for life. If detected early and correctly treated, the outlook is excellent and the blood returns completely to normal unless the injections are stopped. If left untreated, some nerve tissues can be damaged, resulting in weakness and numbness in the legs. Further damage is prevented if vitamin B_{12} is given.

Perniosis
SEE CHILBLAINS

Perspiration
SEE SWEATING

Pertussis
SEE WHOOPING COUGH

Pessary

A *ring pessary* is a plastic flexible ring which is inserted into the vagina to support a prolapse. A vaginal prolapse results from weakness of the vaginal wall, causing protrusion of the wall into the vaginal cavity. This may cause discomfort and a feeling of fullness and sometimes disturbance of micturition. A vaginal prolapse may be minor and not warrant treatment, but if treatment is indicated and an operation is not advised the prolapse may be controlled with a ring pessary. The correct size of pessary provides maximum support but does not cause discomfort. A pessary should be changed approximately every 6 months.

The term *pessary* is also applied to drug formulations used to treat vaginal infections. The drug, usually an anti-fungal agent, is included in the pessary which is inserted into the vagina, where it dissolves.

Pethidine

A powerful pain-killing (analgesic) preparation. Although structurally dissimilar to morphine, it has a similar mode of action but is not as potent. Like morphine, continued use leads to dependence, and as a result its use is restricted within legal constraints under the Misuse of Drugs Act 1971.

Pethidine may be given in tablet or injection form. It is commonly used for pain relief following surgical operations, and is still used occasionally for pain relief during labour.

Petit mal

A form of epilepsy seen usually in children. The 'attack' is just a brief loss of awareness, usually for a few seconds. It is so brief that the 'absence' can be missed by an observer. There is no associated muscular spasm or jerking although it may be accompanied by eye blinking. There is no fit or fall.

Drug therapy is effective in producing a significant reduction or complete abolition of petit mal attacks in about three-quarters of those affected. The drug most commonly used is sodium valproate (Epilim).

Petit mal tends to improve with age, although rarely it heralds other forms of epilepsy in adult life. (*See also* Epilepsy.)

Pharyngitis

The pharynx is situated at the back of the mouth, and infection produces symptoms identical to those of acute tonsillitis. There is soreness of the throat, difficulty and pain on swallowing, a raised temperature, and enlarged glands in the neck. The infection is usually viral and antibiotics have little place in treatment. The infection is self-limiting but aspirin or paracetamol tablets taken regularly may give relief and reduce fever. Antiseptic lozenges, gargles and mouth washes do not reduce the length of the illness but can usually reduce symptoms.

Pharynx

The region behind the back of the nose, tongue and larynx (*see* diagram, page 265). The base of the skull is above and the cervical spine behind. The pharynx leads straight into the gullet (oesophagus).

Phenacetin

A compound incorporated in pain-killing tablets. There is good evidence that long-term use may lead to severe kidney damage, and phenacetin has therefore been withdrawn from the market. It is effective as a mild analgesic which, when absorbed into the body, is converted into paracetamol (page 166), probably the effective agent.

Phenobarbitone

A barbiturate drug used in epilepsy for its anticonvulsant properties. It was introduced in 1912 and until recently was the drug of first choice for treating many forms of epilepsy. The side-effects are drowsiness, and, rarely, irritability and hyperactivity in children.

Phenobarbitone is still occasionally prescribed as a sleeping tablet but safer drugs are now readily available and the use of phenobarbitone for sleeplessness has fallen dramatically over the past 10 years. (*See also* Barbiturates.)

Phenylketonuria
(PKU)

An inherited metabolic disorder which affects approximately 1 in 10,000–20,000 children. It is due to a deficiency of an enzyme (phenylalanine hydroxylase) which converts the amino acid phenylalanine to tyrosine. This deficiency results in an increased phenylalanine level which is toxic and damaging to the brain, causing mental deficiency. Raised levels also stunt growth and may cause eczema and convulsions.

Early detection is important. All newborn babies are tested for phenylketonuria by the Guthrie test, which is performed using a few drops of blood. Treatment is by dietary control to prevent high phenylalanine levels, though there is controversy about how long dieting is necessary. If dietary restriction is strict, neurological complications do not occur.

Phimosis

Narrowing of the foreskin, which causes difficulty in passing urine. It may result from recurrent infection of the foreskin, but may also be caused by forcibly retracting the foreskin in infants. The foreskin is often non-retractile in babies and infants, and only becomes retractile by the fourth year of life.

When phimosis is severe enough to cause ballooning of the foreskin and a poor stream on attempting to pass urine, it should be relieved by circumcision.

Phlebitis

Inflammation of one or more veins, and often occurs as a complication of varicose veins. The vein becomes painful, tender and red, and there is sometimes local swelling of the leg. Treatment is by supportive bandaging combined with rest and elevation of the leg. Anti-inflammatory and pain-killing (analgesic) tablets such as aspirin may be used to help ease the discomfort and reduce the inflammation.

Phlebitis also occurs as a complication of intravenous fluid therapy given in hospital. The fluid passes into a vein via a small plastic cannula inserted through the skin and the cannula may irritate the vein. The resulting phlebitis may be painful but is fortunately not serious and resolves spontaneously over 7–14 days.

Phlegm
SEE SPUTUM

Phobia

A pathological fear—e.g. claustrophobia, a fear of closed spaces; agoraphobia, a fear of open spaces.

School phobia
Dislike or fear of school to the extent that the child refuses to go. The term 'school phobia' is misleading, as often the fear is not of school itself but of separation from home and parents. Usually the child is well liked by school teachers and may be near the top of the class. Refusal may not be obvious but the child may develop recurrent headaches, abdominal pain or acute panic attacks at school time.

There may be an obvious precipitating cause; e.g. bereavement, maternal ill health, moving house or changing school. When this happens the parents are usually understanding and the prospects for an early return to school are good. There may, however, be no immediate precipitating cause. Often there are parental problems and marital disharmony, and it is difficult for the parents to have the same degree of insight and understanding—they may blame the school or other pupils. Return to school is not easy and psychiatric help may be required.

School phobia is very common particularly when sensitive and usually clever children change schools, and is rarely of serious importance. Many parents find that the combination of strong emotional support and small inducements are sufficient until the child has had time to make new friends. If school phobia persists for more than 3–4 months, advice should be obtained from teachers and the family physician.

Physiotherapy

The practice of aiding healing and recovery following illness by reconditioning the affected part to its previous function. Physiotherapy is highly skilled and requires many years' training usually at a specialized school attached to a medical school. Physiotherapists require detailed knowledge of anatomy and physiology, and comprehensive understanding of normal function. Physiotherapists are actively involved in treatment of acute lung infections, joint and muscle strains, and in rehabilitation following strokes, heart attacks, head injuries and bone fractures.

Pica

The term generally used to describe dirt eating, usually in children although it can apply to eating anything abnormal. Pica is common in children who are mentally subnormal. In older children, when not associated with subnormality, it may be to seek attention and underlying family discontent or anxieties may be present.

A normal child between the age of 5 and 12 months will take everything possible to the mouth. Most babies cannot distinguish dirt from anything else but grow out of eating everything after about 12 months. If the habit persists beyond 12 months, medical advice should be obtained to ensure that there is no underlying disease. It usually transpires that the baby is a little late in this respect, much as some crawl or sit up later than others.

Pigeon fancier's lung

A rare form of chronic pneumonia which causes progressive lung damage and breathlessness. It is caused by inhaling the secretions in pigeon droppings, to which the lungs of a few breeders are sensitive.

Piles
(HAEMORRHOIDS)

Swollen veins in the anus, which may enlarge to a sufficient extent to protrude. Piles are believed to arise as a result of the highly refined low-fibre Western diet, which produces more solid motions and constipation (page 64). This in turn leads to increased straining at defecation and increased pressure within the haemorrhoidal veins.

Piles may be painful or sore, and may irritate and bleed, causing anaemia. Bleeding from piles appears as bright red splashes around the lavatory pan or as streaks of blood on the stools or the toilet paper. A clot forming within them (thrombosed pile) can be extremely painful.

There are a number of methods of treatment, according to the severity of the symptoms and the size of the piles. If they are small, the piles can be sclerosed or clotted by injection of the enlarged veins; but if larger or protruding they may have to be removed surgically. The operation (haemorrhoidectomy) is straight-forward in expert hands and the results are excellent. (*See* chart, page 176.)

Pill
(CONTRACEPTIVE)

The oral contraceptive pill is the most reliable form of contraception. It is usually taken as a combined preparation containing two hormones—oestrogen and progestogen.

At commencement the first pill should be taken on the fifth day after the menstrual period has begun. It is taken daily for 21 days and then stopped, and restarted after 7 days. The cycle is then repeated and the pill restarted on the same day of the week each month, whether or not a period occurs during the week off the pill. Additional contraceptive methods should be used during the first month on the pill.

The combined pill contains oestrogen (usually ethinyloestradiol) and a progestogen. The concentration of the oestrogen determines whether or not the pill is a high or low strength. The common strength now used for ethinyloestradiol is 30 micrograms.

The combined pill works by suppressing ovulation. The artificial high level of oestrogen suppresses production of follicle-stimulating hormone (FSH). FSH is normally produced by the pituitary gland in response to low oestrogen levels and stimulates the ripening of an egg (ovum) in the ovary. As the ovum ripens, the cells surrounding it produce oestrogen in increasing quantities. This causes a fall in FSH production, which in turn produces a sudden compensatory rise in another pituitary hormone (luteinizing hormone, LH), which causes ovulation.

The combined pill is a very reliable form of contraception. The pregnancy rate is approximately 0.1–0.5 pregnancies per 100 fertile women per year. This compares with 2 pregnancies for a coil and 4–15 pregnancies with a sheath.

Pregnancies may occur because of failure to take the pill daily. The efficiency of the pill may also be altered by coincidental drug therapy, and in severe gastro-enteritis with diarrhoea and vomiting the pill may not be absorbed into the blood stream.

Unfortunately, the pill is not devoid of serious side-effects, which are more likely in older women and in those who have been on the pill for more than 10 years. The current recommendation is that women over the age of 35 years should not be taking the combined pill because of a greater chance of serious side-effects as a result of taking the pill than of being pregnant at this age. The most serious effects of the pill are heart attacks, strokes or thrombosis of the deep veins in the leg which may dislodge a blood clot to the lungs (pulmonary embolism). Complications are more likely to occur in heavy cigarette smokers, and a 40-year-old non-smoker on the pill may be at less risk than a 30-year-old smoker on the pill.

Other side-effects of the combined pill include nausea, weight increase and raised blood pressure. Nausea is common for the first month and usually wears off but occasionally an alternative preparation

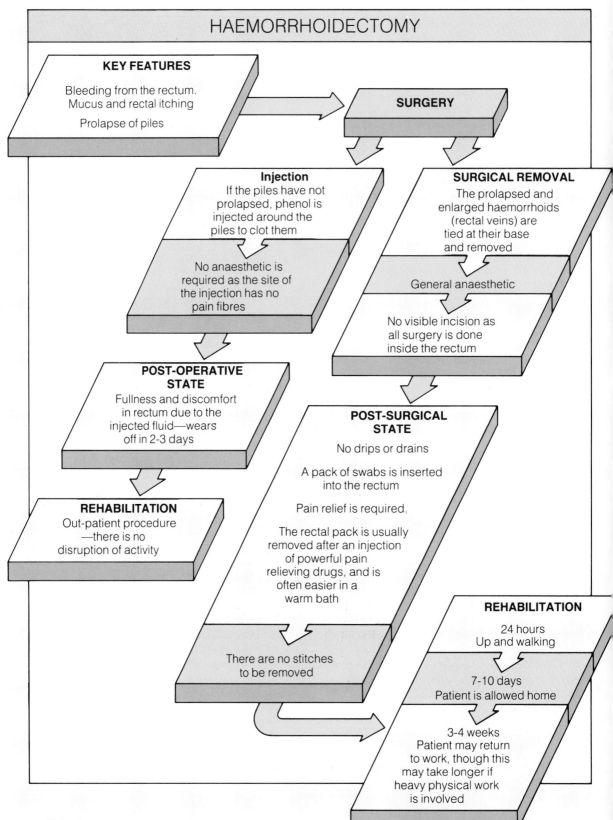

is required. Weight increase is a common problem and not restricted to pill users. Raised blood pressure developing in women on the pill is usually an indication to discontinue the pill and choose an alternative form of contraception.

There is no recognized association between the development of common cancers and taking the pill. The pill may even protect against the development of benign breast lumps. The pill is also used to improve painful and heavy periods.

The combined pill should not be used in liver disease, heart disease, previous history of deep vein thrombosis, pulmonary embolism or breast cancer. Expert supervision is required if the pill is used when there is pre-existing raised blood pressure, diabetes, migraine (if a migraine develops for the first time whilst taking the pill it should be immediately discontinued), severe varicose veins or multiple sclerosis.

Most of the evidence implicates the oestrogen component of the pill as the cause of these side-effects, and women over 35 years who wish to continue oral contraception are given a progestogen-only (mini) pill. Although this pill is not as effective in preventing conception as the combined preparation used in younger women, it is about as effective as a coil and becomes increasingly effective with increasing age. The progestogen-only pill has to be taken every day without a break; it alters the periods, which often become irregular and sometimes stop. It is also used by breast-feeding mothers, as progestogen does not suppress milk production.

Pimple

Any raised spot or blemish on the skin. 'Pimple' has no specific medical connotation (*see* Acne; Melanoma; *and* Moles).

Pins and needles

Pins and needles, and numbness, often occur in the fingers or toes when pressure has been exerted on a nerve. Common examples are when the legs have been crossed for any length of time or when the ulnar nerve is knocked at the elbow ('funny bone').

Pins and needles in the hands and arms may be due to cervical spondylosis or carpal tunnel syndrome. In *cervical spondylosis* there is a roughening of the vertebrae of the neck, which causes pressure on the nerves passing to the arms. The symptoms are often worse at night and may be

associated with pain. Severe symptoms may only be relieved if the neck is immobilized with a cervical (neck) collar. Others obtain benefit from physiotherapy. (*See also* Spondylosis.) *Carpal tunnel syndrome* (page 52) may produce similar symptoms. It is due to compression of the median nerve at the wrist as it passes underneath a fibrous band, the flexor retinaculum.

Pins and needles occur in nearly everyone at some time and only very rarely signify an underlying serious or chronic disorder of the nerves. If they persist, medical guidance should be sought.

Pituitary gland

One of the endocrine glands, which sits on the base of the skull, below the brain. The pituitary secretes a number of hormones, including:

Thyroid-stimulating hormone (TSH), which controls secretion from the thyroid gland.
Adrenocorticotrophic hormone (ACTH), which controls secretion of steroids from the adrenal gland.
Follicle-stimulating hormone (FSH) and luteinizing hormone (LH), which control the function of the ovary.
Growth hormone (GH), essential for normal growth and development.

An excess of ACTH causes Cushing's disease (*see* Adrenal glands), and excess GH causes acromegaly (page 12) in which the bones enlarge, resulting in increased stature, a large skull and jaw, and large hands and feet.

Placenta
(AFTERBIRTH)

Supplies blood, oxygen and nutrition from the mother to the fetus. It forms on the inner lining of the womb (uterus) where it embeds into the uterine wall and is thus in close approximation to the maternal blood in the uterus. Within the placenta there are blood vessels which are connected directly to the fetal circulation by the umbilical cord. Oxygen and nutrients such as protein and vitamins pass from the maternal blood stream to the fetal blood vessels in the placenta, and waste products pass the other way. Unfortunately, many drugs also pass across the placenta and they are best avoided during pregnancy.

The placenta produces specialized hormones which pass into the maternal blood stream. One of these, human chorionic gonadotrophin (HCG), is the basis of the pregnancy test; the hormone HCG passes into the urine, where its presence can be determined by immunological tests. Another hormone produced by the placenta causes enlargement of the breasts in preparation for breast feeding. Pregnenalone, a placental hormone, passes into the maternal circulation where it is converted to oestriol which is excreted in the urine. The quantities excreted over a 24-hour period reflect the health of the fetus and the adequacy of placental function. A fall in the level of pregnenalone in the blood may be the first indication that the pregnancy is not proceeding normally and that supportive intervention is required.

Plague
(BUBONIC PLAGUE; 'THE BLACK DEATH')

An infectious disease caused by a bacterium (*Yersinia pestis*), and now rare even in the developing world. It spreads to man via infected rats, and multiplies within the blood stream, producing fever, muscle aches and pains, headache and extreme exhaustion, and spreads to enlarge the lymph glands (the bubos). Untreated it may resolve spontaneously, but there may be spread to the lungs with pneumonia, progressive illness and death.

The bacterium is sensitive to antibiotics. The best protection is prevention and the disease has disappeared where there are good standards of sanitation.

Plantar wart
(VERRUCA) *SEE UNDER* WARTS *AND* CHIROPODY

Plasma

The liquid part of the blood which constitutes 50 per cent of the whole—the rest is cells—and contains proteins, and clotting factors which prevent excess bleeding after cuts and bruising.

Plasma can be given by transfusion after severe blood loss if replacement is urgent and there is insufficient time to wait for blood of the correct group to be obtained—only blood of the patient's own group can be given, and tests to ensure that the blood that is available is of a compatible group may take 1–2 hours.

Plastic surgery

A widely based specialty and not, as commonly believed, restricted to refashioning noses, breasts and face lifts. Plastic surgery is also required for the treatment of burns, congenital deformities, traumatic injuries and tumours. Following burns, surgery is required to reconstruct scarred and contracted skin. Bat ears are one of the commonest congenital abnormalities treated by plastic surgeons. Hare lips and cleft palates require much skill and perseverance, and a series of constructive operations may be continued through to adult life. Certain skin tumours are best dealt with by surgical removal, as wide skin clearance is required; expert plastic surgical techniques are employed to replace the area of lost skin.

Cosmetic operations are designed to improve the appearance of normal features. This may include removal of redundant skin around the eyelids, face and neck, or the alteration of the contours of prominent noses, receding chins or large breasts. These operations receive low priority under the National Health Service, although great psychological benefit may be attained by improvement of a feature which has caused social isolation, and this must be carefully balanced against the small operative and post-operative risks (e.g. wound infection) of a non-essential procedure.

Pleurisy

Inflammation of the pleural membranes which surround the lungs. It usually follows pneumonia. These membranes are in contact with the infected lungs and become inflamed, and this causes a sharp knife-like pain which is worse when a deep breath is taken or during coughing.

Pleurisy may result from a virus infection or, less commonly, from a non-infective cause such as pulmonary embolism, when a small clot arising in a deep vein in the legs (deep vein thrombosis) breaks off and travels to the lungs. This produces blockage of the blood supply to part of the lungs and the overlying pleural membranes become inflamed and hence painful. Rarely, pleurisy may be caused by a lung tumour invading the pleural membranes.

Pleurisy settles with successful treatment of the cause. The pain varies from mild to severe, and local warmth with pain-killing drugs (analgesics) may be required. Strapping the chest to relieve pain may well result in pneumonia and should be avoided.

Pneumoconiosis

An occupational lung disease caused by the inhalation of inorganic mineral dust, and is common in coal miners. Substances capable of causing pneumoconiosis include carbon, tin, coal, graphite, iron, silica, asbestos and beryllium.

Coal dust accumulates in the small air spaces in the lungs, and stimulates the production of multiple small scars (fibrosis). This is more likely to occur with coal with a high quartz content. If exposure is prolonged over 15–25 years, severe emphysema may develop. These changes are more likely in cigarette smokers. Diagnosis is based on x-rays of the chest, which show widespread scarring and large air spaces and cysts, but these changes may be quite marked before shortness of breath develops.

Pneumoconiosis due to silica (silicosis) or asbestos (asbestosis, page 28) tends to be more progressive than coal dust disease. Coal dust pneumoconiosis may remain mild and non-progressive, especially if further exposure is prevented. Occasionally, however, progressive and massive fibrosis occurs. This causes worsening lung function with increasing shortness of breath and eventually heart failure. Silicosis and asbestosis produce a similar clinical picture, but in addition asbestosis predisposes to the development of cancer of the lung and the pleura (the membrane surrounding the lungs).

Prevention is most important and can be effected by wearing masks, by damping the dust and by efficient ventilation systems. Pneumoconiosis is irreversible. Once it has developed, further exposure must be stopped. Smoking cigarettes should be prohibited as it increases the additional risk of chronic bronchitis.

Pneumonia

Infection of the lung tissues. When one lobe of the lung is involved it is termed lobar pneumonia, and more generalized infection is termed bronchopneumonia. Bronchopneumonia affecting both right and left lungs is sometimes referred to as 'double pneumonia'. Bronchopneumonia is commonest in children and the elderly, and it may occur with other infections (e.g. measles, whooping cough and chronic bronchitis).

Both lobar and bronchopneumonia are characterized by the production of infected green or yellow sputum sometimes containing blood, a high fever and shivering attacks (rigors). Pleurisy may complicate pneumonia and cause pleuritic chest pain later in the illness—the pain is localized, sharp and worse on inspiration and coughing. Lobar pneumonia is caused by a bacterium (*Streptococcus pneumoniae*) and responds well to treatment with penicillin. Bronchopneumonia caused by bacteria responds well to antibiotics, but it may also be caused by viruses which do not respond to them. Tuberculosis used to cause much lung disease, including pneumonia, but is now less common. Rare causes of pneumonia include psittacosis (page 188) and legionnaire's disease (page 145).

Pneumonia is a potentially serious infection which is best treated in hospital where oxygen, physiotherapy and constant nursing and medical supervision are available. With modern antibiotics the outlook is excellent unless the patient is very frail from another disorder or in extreme old age. Bronchopneumonia has been called the 'old man's friend' because it draws so many lives to a quiet, painless and dignified end.

Pneumothorax

A rare condition in which there is air in the chest between the lung and the inner chest wall. This occurs when the lung surface ruptures and air escapes from the lung and fills the potential space between the lungs and inside of the chest wall. A pneumothorax may occur spontaneously in a healthy person and is usually due to the rupture of a thin-walled cyst on the lung surface. It may occur in a chronic bronchitic who, as a result of the illness, has several large cysts within the lungs. Another (rare) cause is a penetrating injury—e.g. stabbing.

A pneumothorax causes a sudden sharp severe chest pain which is worse on breathing and may be made worse by movement. There is often shortness of breath. Young healthy people are the commonest group to develop a pneumothorax; usually the amount of air between the lung and chest wall is small, and disappears without specific treatment over 2–4 weeks.

If the pneumothorax is sufficiently large to compress the lung and embarrass breathing, the air is allowed to escape by inserting a narrow tube through the chest wall, and connecting it to an underwater seal drain. Air passes from the chest cavity and goes through the water valve and allows the lung to expand. Once the lung has been expanded for 24–48 hours, the hole in the lung usually seals spontaneously. When this does not occur, surgery becomes necessary to stitch the hole in the lung and to prevent continued leakage of air.

Poisoning

Intentional self-poisoning is becoming much more common and now accounts for up to 10 per cent of emergency hospital admissions from home.

In children, iron tablets or aspirin may be eaten as sweets. Both are extremely dangerous and may result in death. This is particularly tragic because it is easily preventable. Household chemicals are also of potential danger to children.

The common poisons, their clinical features and an outline of emergency treatment are given in First aid, page 276. *See also* Fungus poisoning; Gas poisoning; *and* Deadly nightshade.

Poliomyelitis
(POLIO)

A virus infection of the spinal cord and brain, and may take different forms. The least severe causes no symptoms but leaves the individual immune to further infection. Infection by the virus may also cause mild symptoms indistinguishable from a simple cold or a mild attack of gastro-enteritis with a brief period of diarrhoea. Polio virus can cause meningitis, which may resolve or progress to the most severe form of the disease—paralytic poliomyelitis. Paralysis may involve muscles in the legs or be more widespread. There may be a progressive ascending paralysis starting in the legs, which may ultimately lead to paralysis of the muscles of breathing. Recovery in most muscles occurs about a week after the onset of paralysis but the muscles which remain paralysed become wasted, leading to imbalance between opposing muscle groups and, hence, contractures with deformity and limited movement.

Polio is prevented by immunization (*see* Vaccination). Previous epidemics have affected mainly children and young adults, and prevention requires a continual and maximally used vaccination programme, concentrating on these age groups. Ideally, all children should be immunized starting at 3–6 months of age.

Polyp

An abnormal finger-like excrescence arising from a normally smooth surface. They occur at various sites and are usually not malignant growths.

Bowel polyps
Polyps may occur at various sites along the bowel, but are commonly seen in the large bowel and rectum. The polyps may be single or multiple. Early detection is important because some polyps predispose to cancer; when the polyps are small and single, they can be removed through a colonoscope (a flexible fibre-optic telescope) introduced via the rectum. If the polyp is large, surgical removal is required, including a short segment of intestine on either side of the polyp.

Nasal polyps
Occur with nasal allergy (hay fever), which causes persistent inflammation and thickening of the lining cells of the nose and leads to polyp formation. The presence of polyps may perpetuate symptoms with nasal discharge, a blocked nose and sneezing. When the polyps are very troublesome they can be removed. This is a simple operation but there is a high chance of recurrence.

Polyps in the uterus and cervix
These may cause bleeding between periods, blood spotting following intercourse, or a persistent (brown) vaginal discharge. These polyps may be seen on examination, protruding through the cervix. Whilst usually benign, a uterine polyp may represent a cancer of the uterus and careful removal is necessary. If the polyp is innocent it can be removed easily, but when a cancer is present a hysterectomy should be performed.

Posseting

Regurgitation of small amounts of food in babies. It is very common and usually occurs shortly after or during a feed, part of which is brought up with wind. Posseting is of no consequence other than producing a larger volume of washing, and all babies grow out of it. (*See also* Regurgitation.)

Medical advice should be obtained if the quantity of food or milk is large, if a baby is constantly miserable or fails to gain weight, or if it is acutely ill with fever, abdominal pain or diarrhoea.

Post-natal depression
SEE UNDER DEPRESSION

'Pot'
SEE CANNABIS

Prednisolone

A steroid drug, very similar to prednisone (next entry).

Prednisone

A steroid drug, usually prepared in tablet form. Prednisone, like other steroids, has a potent anti-inflammatory and anti-allergic effect; it is used in ulcerative colitis, rheumatoid arthritis, and in the treatment of life-threatening conditions such as leukaemia when it is combined with other drugs to induce and maintain remission. Prednisone is also of great value in an acute severe asthmatic attack. The drug is given initially in high doses, reducing rapidly and discontinuing after a few days. Intermittent short sharp courses are effective and avoid the unwanted long-term effects. (*See also* Steroids.)

Pregnancy

Pregnancy is suspected when a period is missed, particularly if they have been previously regular. Early pregnancy may cause nausea and vomiting characteristically in the morning, increased frequency of passing urine, and enlargement and discomfort of the breasts. Although these features suggest pregnancy, they do not confirm it. Pregnancy tests measure the level of hormones excreted in the urine. These rise soon after pregnancy starts and are measured in early-morning samples of urine and it is possible to obtain an answer within 2 hours. It is best to wait at least 2 weeks after the first missed period because too early a test may give a false result and fail to diagnose an existing pregnancy. If the periods do not begin again within a further 2 or 3 weeks of a negative result, the pregnancy test should be repeated and if there is still any doubt, medical advice sought.

Pregnancy is usually dated from the first day of the last menstrual period and the expected date of delivery is 40 weeks after that.

Complications
★ *Bleeding in early pregnancy*
Any vaginal bleeding during pregnancy is abnormal, but not necessarily serious. Bleeding in early pregnancy may be the first sign of a miscarriage (spontaneous abortion). Sometimes, when there has been scanty spotting of blood associated with mild pain and subsequently the bleeding has stopped, the pregnancy can continue normally. The episode of bleeding is termed a threatened miscarriage (abortion). In other cases, especially when the bleeding is heavy, a miscarriage may occur. When this has happened a small operation, under a general anaesthetic, may be performed to check that the womb (uterus) is completely empty. This helps to prevent complications. Spontaneous miscarriages (abortions) typically occur at between 6 and 12 weeks of pregnancy—in about one in every ten pregnancies. One cause is serious malformation of the fetus.

Other causes of bleeding in early pregnancy include infections and ectopic pregnancy. For example, candidiasis (thrush) can cause bleeding if the inflammation is severe. An ectopic pregnancy is a more serious but fortunately less common cause of bleeding. It occurs when the fertilized ovum implants outside the main uterine cavity in the Fallopian tube. As the pregnancy progresses there is little room for fetal growth and this results in severe pain and bleeding. (*See also* Ectopic pregnancy.) In some patients no cause for bleeding can be found.

★ *Bleeding in late pregnancy*
Vaginal bleeding after 28 weeks of pregnancy is called an ante–partum haemorrhage (APH). The commonest cause of APH is placenta praevia. This occurs when the placenta (afterbirth) lies too low in the uterus so that part of it lies near, or over, the opening of the birth canal.

Bleeding may occur as the opening of the birth canal begins to dilate. If the placenta completely covers the birth canal then a normal vaginal delivery of the baby will not be possible and a Caesarean section (page 51) will have to be performed. If the placenta just reaches the edge of the birth canal, a normal labour is possible.

Bleeding in late pregnancy often has serious consequences. Immediate medical advice is essential and immediate hospital referral is usual.

Toxaemia
A condition which occurs in late pregnancy. The name is confusing as it implies the presence of toxic substances in the maternal bloodstream. This was so termed because it used to be thought that fetal waste products were absorbed into the blood stream, causing the condition. Although the precise reason is still not known, it is not thought that this happens. Toxaemia is usually called pre-eclampsia or pre-eclamptic toxaemia (PET).

Pre-eclampsia is characterized by a rise in blood pressure associated with the loss of protein in the urine and sometimes with water retention causing swelling of the legs, arms and face. Pre-eclampsia affects the fetus as well. The afterbirth (placenta) does not work as efficiently and thus growth of the fetus may be retarded. Prematurity is more likely.

The severity of pre-eclampsia varies from individual to individual. In the mildest of cases, bed rest and perhaps sedation are all that are required. In the more severe cases, labour may need to be induced or the baby delivered by Caesarean section. This is for both maternal and fetal reasons. As the name implies, eclampsia follows pre-eclampsia and is manifest by convulsions. During these convulsions fetal loss is high and there is an associated maternal mortality. By delivering the baby in time this situation may be avoided. Eclampsia occurs only during pregnancy or shortly after delivery. Pre-eclampsia occurs in 4–7 per cent of ante-natal patients. It is more common in a first pregnancy and in multiple pregnancy.

★ *Vomiting*

Common in early pregnancy, it usually occurs at about the time of the first missed period (4 weeks), is at its worst at about 8–10 weeks and has usually disappeared by 12–14 weeks. The vomiting is typically early morning, although it can occur at other times. It is more common in first pregnancies, but is not present in everyone.

The vomiting may be reduced by taking more rest. If it is early morning, then a 'lie in' should be recommended. In some cases anti-sickness (anti-emetic) tablets may be used. Tablets have to be used with caution in early pregnancy in case the developing baby is affected. However, the ones used regularly for sickness in pregnancy appear devoid of side-effects.

Rarely, vomiting in pregnancy becomes so continuous that dehydration occurs (the condition is called hyperemesis gravidarum). This usually necessitates hospital admission and rehydration with intravenous fluids. The normal vomiting in pregnancy is partly due to a rise in hormone levels and occasionally to psychological factors.

Labour

The *first stage* of labour starts when regular uncomfortable contractions begin and cause the neck of the womb (the cervix) to dilate and the baby's head to descend further into the pelvis. During this phase, which may last several hours, the contractions become more frequent and stronger. The onset of labour may be suggested by a 'show' which is a plug of bloody mucus released by the cervix as it begins to thin and dilate. This may immediately precede contractions or may occur a day or so before.

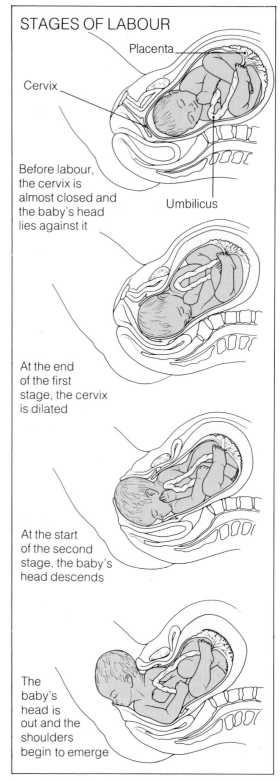

STAGES OF LABOUR

Placenta

Cervix

Umbilicus

Before labour, the cervix is almost closed and the baby's head lies against it

At the end of the first stage, the cervix is dilated

At the start of the second stage, the baby's head descends

The baby's head is out and the shoulders begin to emerge

The waters (amniotic fluid) may break before or during labour. They usually break as the contractions start. However, if the waters break and labour does not start, induction (*see below*) may be necessary to prevent infection entering the womb.

The *second stage* of labour is the expulsive phase of labour during which the baby is forced through the birth canal. It starts when the cervix is fully dilated and lasts until the baby is born. Both first and second stages of labour last longer in the first pregnancy than in the subsequent ones. The second stage of labour should not be allowed to exceed 1½ hours.

The *third stage* of labour is the delivery of the afterbirth (placenta). At the time of birth it is usual practice to give the mother an injection of ergometrine (or a related substance). This causes the womb (uterus) to contract, which prevents excessive blood loss and causes early separation of the placenta from the uterus. The placenta is delivered by gentle steady traction on the umbilical cord.

Induction of labour

Induction is the artificial stimulation of labour. It is used when prolongation of pregnancy is considered detrimental to the mother or fetus, or both. Induction is usually performed by artificial rupture of the membranes and by using intravenous drugs (oxytocin or prostaglandins) to stimulate and maintain uterine contractions. Two common indications for induction are post-term pregnancies and raised blood pressure.

Post-term pregnancies are eventually at risk from placental ageing and failure, which is of course detrimental to the fetus. It is usual practice to induce labour before the 42nd week of pregnancy. This emphasizes the need for good early ante-natal care when it is easiest to determine the likely length of the pregnancy. By physical examination, the gestation can be most accurately determined between 8 and 12 weeks. When ultrasound scanning is used to date pregnancies, it is also more accurate in early pregnancy. Both these methods become increasingly inaccurate with advancing pregnancy. It may be inaccurate—especially when conception occurs shortly after stopping the oral contraceptive pill—to estimate the expected date of delivery from the first day of the last menstrual period alone. Accurate dating of a pregnancy is important to help decide whether the pregnancy is post-term or not and thus to avoid unnecessary induction.

Raised blood pressure during pregnancy may be detrimental to both mother and fetus. A rise of blood pressure in late pregnancy may be associated with pre-eclamptic toxaemia. This condition can cause alteration of the kidney function in the mother and a deterioration in the placental function to the detriment of the fetus. Pre-eclampsia may lead to maternal convulsions (eclampsia). Eclampsia is associated with a high fetal mortality and a lesser but significant maternal mortality. Pre-eclampsia is a condition peculiar to pregnancy and thus induction and early delivery of the baby may be indicated. Pre-eclampsia may be detected by regular ante-natal care in which blood pressure is checked, and routine urine samples are tested to detect the presence of protein which may indicate an alteration in kidney function.

Some other indications for induction include ante-partum haemorrhage (discussed above, under Bleeding in late pregnancy), Rhesus incompatibility (page 195), maternal disease such as diabetes, or difficulties in previous labours.

Waters broken

This is usually the sign that labour is well under way. As the uterine contractions start, the baby's head is forced down and the pressure within the amniotic fluid surrounding the baby builds up. The membranes or 'bag' surrounding the amniotic fluid breaks under the pressure, allowing the fluid to flow out.

Sometimes the waters break before labour has begun. The reason for this occurrence is often not known. If this occurs, medical advice should be sought. Often when this happens labour contractions will start shortly afterwards. However, if labour does not start spontaneously it may need to be induced. The reason for this is that the baby loses its protective environment of amniotic fluid and is more susceptible to infection.

When labour is to be induced the waters are often broken artificially. One method is by carefully introducing a small plastic hook internally until the membranes are felt. The hook makes a small hole in the membranes, allowing the amniotic fluid to escape. Although this procedure sounds unpleasant it should not be painful, and is quite safe. One reason for doing this is that rupture of the membranes causes the body to release hormones which stimulate uterine contractions.

Another situation where the waters are broken artificially is when labour contractions have begun but the waters have not broken spontaneously and the labour is not progressing as quickly as it should. This is termed 'augmented' or 'accelerated labour'.

Pain relief in labour

Preparation for coping with labour pain usually begins during ante-natal care. The removal of fear of the unknown is an important aspect. The pregnant woman may be helped by an understanding of the normal course of labour. If the delivery is to take place in hospital then a guided tour around the delivery suite earlier in pregnancy may alleviate some fears of a strange and clinical environment. The involvement and education of husbands is encouraged so they may play a supportive role during labour. In addition, ante-natal classes teach different levels of breathing, and relaxation techniques which may help during and after contractions. These methods may be extended to include hypnosis.

The two most commonly administered pain relievers (analgesics) during pregnancy are pethidine and Entonox. Pethidine is a synthetic morphine-like drug which is given intramuscularly. Its drawbacks include drowsiness and nausea, and, sometimes, a dissociated feeling. The nausea is counteracted by giving a mild anti-emetic at the same time. The drowsiness is an important side-effect because the drug can cross the placenta and make the baby drowsy, too, by entering the fetal circulation. For this reason pethidine should not be given too close to the estimated time of delivery. Entonox is an equal mixture of oxygen and nitrous oxide. It is self-administered with a special mask, under professional supervision. Its two main advantages lie in its safety for the fetus and the woman's ability to use only as much as she feels she requires.

Epidural anaesthesia is another important form of pain relief during labour. Local anaesthetic is introduced into a space alongside nerves leaving the spinal cord. This numbs the nerves and hence the areas which are supplied to the nerves, which is usually from the waist downwards. It is a skilled procedure, usually performed by an anaesthetist. In some obstetric centres it is offered as a routine method of pain relief. In others it is used only in certain specific situations such as with raised blood pressure and in twin pregnancies.

Breech presentation

Occurs in 3–4 per cent of all deliveries: instead of arriving into the world head first, the baby comes out bottom first. It occurs more commonly in premature labours, where there is excessive amniotic fluid (hydramnios) and in multiple pregnancies. During the pregnancy there is considerable fetal movement and the fetus may be a breech presentation at certain times in middle pregnancy, returning spontaneously to head presentation later. After about 34 weeks there is less room for the baby to turn around and the fetal position remains fixed.

If a breech presentation is diagnosed, some obstetricians try to turn the fetus round by external manipulation. This procedure is not entirely without risks and is contra-indicated in certain situations. The main concern with breech presentation is at the time of delivery because the largest and hardest part of the baby comes last and it is too late to assess whether it can pass through the maternal pelvis or not. This presents problems chiefly in a first pregnancy when the size of the pelvis has not previously been shown to permit the passage of a baby during normal labour. Various measurements can be taken from a pelvic x-ray in late pregnancy to assess the possibility of a vaginal delivery.

When, in breech presentation, there is any doubt about the safe delivery of the baby, especially in a first pregnancy, it is usual to perform an elective Caesarean section. Vaginal delivery requires a skilled obstetrician. Once the body of the baby has been delivered, the baby's blood supply is cut off and it is essential that no delay should occur in delivering the head. In normal pregnancies, when the baby comes out head first, the head is often moulded and shaped to fit the pelvis because of its slow progress through the birth canal. However, no moulding occurs in breech delivery and the head is likely to be subjected suddenly to pressure within the birth canal. In order to protect the head from sudden changes in pressure and to effect a quick delivery the head is often delivered by forceps.

Forceps delivery

Forceps may be used to assist delivery of the baby when the second stage of labour is prolonged. The forceps blades, which are curved suitably for a baby's head, are positioned either side of the baby's face. Gentle traction is applied with each contraction to aid the delivery of the head. Forceps delivery can be an uncomfortable procedure and extra pain-relieving measures are required. This may be by the use of pudendal nerve block—a local anaesthetic injected with a special needle through the vaginal wall to block the sensory pain nerves supplying the lower part of the birth canal. If an epidural anaesthetic is used, there is no need for further anaesthesia.

Forceps delivery may be used in other situations; for instance, when the baby shows signs of distress and quick delivery is important, and maternal effort is not sufficient. Fetal distress may be detected by constantly observing the fetal heart rate during labour, particularly with attention to variation in the rate at each contraction. Fetal distress usually indicates that the fetus is suffering from oxygen starvation (hypoxia).

Forceps are commonly used in breech presentation to deliver the after-coming head.

Most forceps deliveries involve a safe straight-forward lift out of the baby's head. In some situations, however, the baby may be stuck in a horizontal position higher up in the pelvis. The fetus usually enters the pelvis with its head facing sideways. As the fetus is forced further into the pelvis, rotation of the head usually occurs so that the face is looking towards the mother's back. In some cases this rotation of the head does not occur, and further descent of the head is not possible because of the relative shapes of the fetal head and the maternal pelvis. The obstetrician then has to decide whether to deliver the baby by Caesarean section or with the use of special forceps (Kiellands) which first rotate the head and then pull the baby out. This type of forceps delivery is a highly skilled procedure and is performed only by a skilled obstetrician.

Termination
There are approximately 100,000 terminations performed each year in Britain. About half of these are performed in the National Health Service.

The Abortion Act 1967 requires the medical practitioners to recommend an abortion for one or more of the following reasons:
1   The continuance of the pregnancy would involve risk to the life of the woman greater than if the pregnancy were terminated.
2   The continuance of the pregnancy would involve risk of injury to the physical or mental health of the pregnant woman greater than if the pregnancy were terminated.
3   The continuance of the pregnancy would involve risk of injury to the physical or mental health of the existing child(ren) of the family of the pregnant woman greater than if the pregnancy were terminated.
4   There is substantial risk that if the child were born it would suffer from such physical or mental defects as to be seriously handicapped.

Methods for termination vary according to the duration of the pregnancy. Most abortions are performed on 12-week or less pregnancies (the 'weeks' are based from the first day of the last menstrual period). The method used in these pregnancies is a vaginal termination of pregnancy. It usually requires a general anaesthetic. The neck of the womb (cervix) is dilated to permit the introduction of a suction tube. The contents of the womb are sucked out, and then the lining is gently scraped to ensure that there are no remaining products of conception. This method is relatively free from side-effects. Occasionally the blood loss is excessive, requiring a transfusion. The uterus (womb) may be perforated, but surprisingly this complication rarely causes problems when performed under aseptic conditions and when protected by appropriate antibiotics. If the cervix is damaged due to forceful dilation, problems may ensue in subsequent pregnancies.

The problems of a damaged cervix may be twofold. First, the cervix which normally remains closed during the pregnancy may open early in pregnancy, often in the second trimester, causing spontaneous miscarriage (abortion). Secondly, the cervix may dilate at a later stage, causing a premature labour.

Other methods for termination are rarely used. Once a pregnancy has passed 14 weeks, the above method of termination is no longer safe. One method is by operation (hysterotomy). The fetus is removed in a similar way to the method used in Caesarean section. The main problem of this method is the womb has to be cut open and is left with a permanent scar. Unfortunately, the scar cannot be in the optimum position as in a Caesarean section because of the size of the uterus. This factor can cause problems in subsequent pregnancies, as the scar is likely to weaken during labour, making a normal delivery less likely.

Alternative methods for later abortions use hormones to stimulate uterine contractions and expel the fetus vaginally. The hormones used are prostaglandins and oxytocin. They may be given intravenously or introduced locally into the cervix or injected into the uterus. Whilst this method produces no uterine scar it is not devoid of side-effects. The discomfort of labour contractions is felt, and these can be very forceful. If the contractions are too forceful, the cervix may be damaged.

Fortunately, most abortions are performed early with the simplest method. There are times, however, when abortions have to be performed later. For example, amniocentesis, which can detect certain abnormalities, can only be performed at about 14–16 weeks, and some of the investigations following amniocentesis take 2 or more weeks to perform. Thus if major abnormality is present, termination is obviously going to occur late. The upper limit for abortion is 28 weeks' gestation. This limit is based on the legal definition of fetal viability independent of its mother under the Infant Life (Preservation) Act 1929. Nevertheless, with modern neonatal paediatric methods, viability has been achieved from 26 weeks. This fact and the fact that the occasional baby (out of 100,000) is born apparently alive has brought much pressure to lower the upper limit for abortion.

Premenstrual syndrome

A variety of changes experienced by many healthy women prior to menstruation. These range from a mild disturbance to irritability with depression. Some women also gain weight due to fluid retention, causing breast discomfort and a sensation of abdominal fullness. Even when fluid retention does not occur, symptoms may arise due to redistribution of fluid in the body. Headaches are common.

The cause of premenstrual tension is not understood. It is partly due to a hormone imbalance, and progesterone deficiency is present in about a third of sufferers.

Various treatments have been tried, including intermittent courses of diuretics (drugs which increase fluid excretion from the body via the kidneys), progesterone supplements in the form of dydrogesterone, and pyridoxine (one of the vitamin B group), and are often successful. Premenstrual tension in previously fit women usually settles without treatment after three or four periods, but if it persists, medical advice should be sought.

Prepuce
SEE FORESKIN

Proctitis

Inflammation of the rectum and anus. Fungus infection with thrush (page 223) is common, as is pain from piles (page 175) and fissures (page 19).

Progesterone

One of the sex hormones produced by the ovary during the menstrual cycle (*see* Periods). It prepares the lining of the uterus to receive a fertilized egg (ovum), and its continued secretion is necessary for successful embedding of the ovum and for the preservation of early pregnancy. Progesterone is also produced by the adrenal gland in both male and female and is converted there to other hormones, corticosteroids, androgens and oestrogens.

Progesterone deficiency has been implicated in repeated spontaneous abortion (miscarriage), premenstrual syndrome and puerperal depression. The evidence is controversial but treatment with progesterone derivative supplements is sometimes beneficial.

Progesterone is inactive when given in tablet form but synthetic compounds have been produced (progestogens) which overcome this. Progestogens are a component in the combined contraceptive pill, and do not cause the long-term unwanted effects generally attributed to the oestrogen component of the pill. Progestogens may be used alone as an oral contraceptive pill (mini pill) but are less efficient than the combined pill and may induce irregular periods.

Prognosis
(GREEK: *PRO*, FORE; *GNOSIS*, KNOWLEDGE)

The predicted outcome of an illness. The prediction is based on the particular illness or injury and its statistically known outcome according to previous medical experience, and the clinical state of the patient at the time. Accurate prognostication requires considerable skill, experience and knowledge and offers only the likely outcome for any one patient.

Prolapse

To slip forward or down out of place, as in prolapsed intervertebral disc of cartilage (slipped disc)—the cause of sciatica (*see* Backache)—or in prolapse of the vaginal wall into the vaginal cavity.

Vaginal prolapse is due to weakening of the vaginal walls, allowing them to protrude into the vaginal lumen. If the weakness is in the front wall, the bladder also protrudes into the vagina (cystocele). This may cause urinary symptoms with frequency of micturition and incontinence. A weak vaginal wall may allow the rectum to push forwards (rectocele). A rare genital prolapse, often associated with a cystocele or rectocele, results from weakness of the ligaments holding the uterus in place and allows the uterus to descend into the vagina. Occasionally, the descent is so marked that the uterus protrudes outside the vagina (procidentia). Prolapse is usually caused by a combination of muscle weakness following childbirth, and muscle thinning which occurs at the menopause as a result of low levels of circulating female hormones (i.e. oestrogen).

A prolapse can be held in place with a pessary (page 173) or cured by surgery. Pessaries are used when surgery is not advisable or delayed. They are made of flexible rings of inert polyethylene or polyvinyl which when correctly fitted lie behind the pubic bone and extend the length of the vagina giving support in place of the weakened muscles.

PROSTATIC ENLARGEMENT

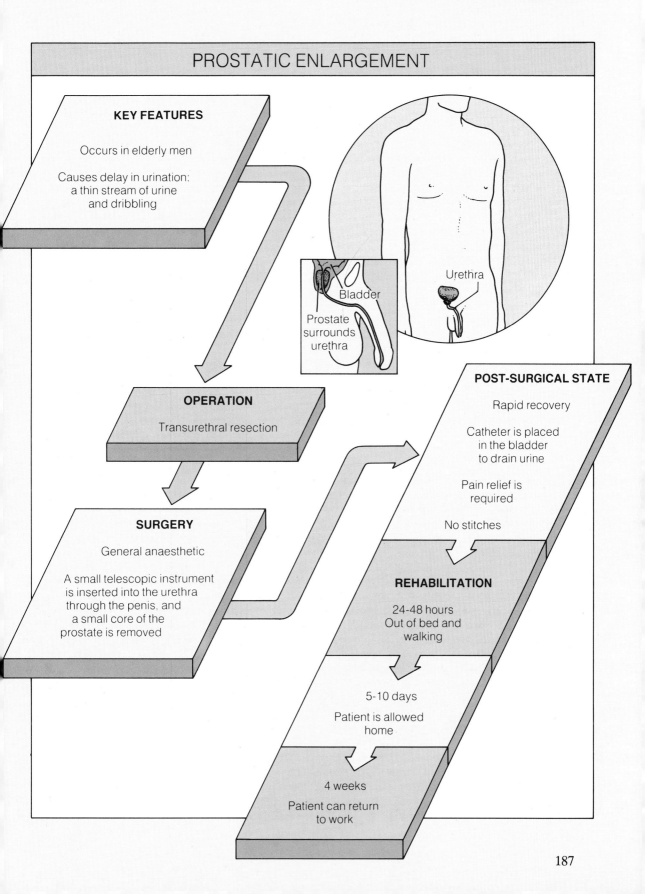

KEY FEATURES

Occurs in elderly men

Causes delay in urination:
a thin stream of urine
and dribbling

Urethra

Bladder

Prostate
surrounds
urethra

OPERATION

Transurethral resection

POST-SURGICAL STATE

Rapid recovery

Catheter is placed
in the bladder
to drain urine

Pain relief is
required

No stitches

SURGERY

General anaesthetic

A small telescopic instrument
is inserted into the urethra
through the penis, and
a small core of the
prostate is removed

REHABILITATION

24-48 hours
Out of bed and
walking

5-10 days

Patient is allowed
home

4 weeks

Patient can return
to work

Prophylaxis

This refers to treatment aimed at preventing disease rather than curing it. The commonest examples are immunization by injection against diphtheria, whooping cough, tetanus, hepatitis and yellow fever. Malaria is world-wide and any individual can prevent infection in himself by taking anti-malarial tablets during and for a period just after visiting a malarial zone.

Prostate

The prostate gland is present only in males, and lies immediately below the bladder, encircling the urethra which carries urine from the bladder to the penis. The gland produces a fluid which is excreted in seminal fluid at the time of ejaculation.

From middle age onwards the prostate gland enlarges. If the enlargement is sufficient, obstruction to the outflow of urine occurs. Initially the symptoms include frequency of passing urine, often at night, sometimes with discomfort, poor urinary stream with delay in starting, dribbling at the finish and the sensation of incomplete bladder emptying. This may progress to complete obstruction of urine flow, and if this occurs a flexible urinary catheter must be introduced to drain the bladder.

Treatment of an enlarged prostate is by surgically removing the gland. This may be achieved by entering the abdomen just above the pubic bone to expose the bladder, after which the prostate gland can be reached below the bladder and shelled out. Alternatively, a telescopic instrument (a cystoscope) is introduced via the penile urethra and small segments of the prostate are carefully removed with an electrically operated knife (transurethral resection, TUR). (*See* chart, page 187.)

Infection in the prostate gland (prostatitis) causes a generalized illness with fever as well as frequency and discomfort on passing urine. Treatment is with antibiotics; these may need to be continued for prolonged periods, as infection is slow to clear.

Psittacosis
(ORNITHOSIS)

A rare form of pneumonia (page 179), caused by the organism *Chlamydia psittaci*, and caught from infected birds—especially parrots. The infection responds rapidly to antibiotics if detected and treated early.

Psoriasis

A common non-infectious skin disorder present in about 1–2 per cent of the general population. In some cases it seems to run in families. The rash consists of red patches of skin with well demarcated edges sometimes slightly raised and with a roughened surface containing superficial silvery scales which are more obvious if the skin is rubbed. The rash is most marked on the elbows or knees, although any part of the body may be affected. Some of the patches may cover a large area, in contrast with psoriasis in children where patches are small and evenly distributed over the body. Psoriasis may also affect the scalp and the finger nails which are pitted, resembling a thimble. (*See* illustration, page 236.)

Psoriasis runs a chronic relapsing course and rarely completely disappears. Psoriasis in childhood usually resolves spontaneously within a few months but there remains an increased chance of developing chronic psoriasis in later life. Adult psoriasis may be precipitated by psychological stress and is often worse at puberty and the menopause but may improve with pregnancy. It results from over-activity of the skin, which consists of layers of cells. New cells are made by the basal layer and are gradually pushed to the surface as more cells are produced beneath. This cycle normally takes about 28 days to complete but in psoriasis the cycle is speeded up and more cells are produced and shed.

Psoriasis may be improved by a variety of ointments and pastes, and the most commonly used contain coal tar in various strengths. If the strongest coal preparation fails to help, dithranol can be tried. Steroid creams are not used routinely because of their long-term side-effects (*see* Steroids), but in severe disease are very effective, though the psoriasis often becomes worse on stopping them.

Other therapies which are used in severe psoriasis include ultraviolet light and methotrexate. Methotrexate is a cytotoxic drug (i.e. toxic to cells), which reduces the increased cell turnover in the skin. Unfortunately, it is also toxic to normal cells and should only be used under expert supervision.

Psychiatric illnesses

Occur with or without recognized and detectable brain damage. It is also likely that many of the non-physical 'diseases of the mind' may turn out to have a metabolic or biochemical basis. It follows that any attempt to label mental disorders as psychiatric or physical is often arbitrary and unhelpful.

With this proviso, most patients with psychiatric illnesses fall into one of the following groups, though there is often overlap between them.

1　Mental deficiency (page 152).

2　Organic or physical disturbance of brain function—the confusion of patients with meningitis (page 151), high fever, and alcohol or drug intoxication.

3　Psychotic illnesses (e.g. manic depression or schizophrenia, pages 149, 200), in which the patients appear to have bizarre behaviour and little or no insight.

4　Neurotic illnesses (neuroses)—e.g. anxiety (page 23), depression, (page 75), hysteria (page 130), and phobia (page 174)—in which the illnesses are almost an extension of normal responses; insight is usually retained.

5　Personality disorder in which behaviour is commonly regarded as abnormal (e.g. sexual deviants, drug addicts and psychopaths).

Many diseases contain a large element of stress and these are referred to as psychosomatic illnesses (page 190); e.g. asthma, ulcerative colitis and peptic ulceration.

Psychiatric treatment

Psychotherapy

May be used with an individual or a group. The therapist guides, rather than directs, the patient who is allowed to interpret as much as possible as he explores problems, feelings and previous experiences.He tries to crystallize his problems and then explain them, so relieving his anxiety. The therapy proceeds by suggestion, analysis and re-education.

Psychoanalysis

Performed on an individual basis using the technique of free association and interpretation. Free association is the consecutive ideas that come to mind following a word stimulus, the ideas being spoken out aloud to the analyst who gradually explores the unresolved needs and conflicts dating back to childhood. During analytical sessions various feelings, thoughts and fantasies may be developed by the patient toward the analyst which often reflect relationships which the patient may have had with other people in the past. This phenomenon is known as transference and is essential to the analytical procedure. The over-all object is to give the patient some insight into his unconscious make-up so that unresolved childhood conflicts may be resolved in a rational adult manner.

Behaviour therapy and behaviour modification

A commonly used form of treatment. Techniques such as systemic desensitization, deconditioning, flooding and relaxing are used by clinical psychologists, and are of benefit in a wide range of disorders, including phobias and compulsive disorders.

Unlike psychotherapy (discussed above), insight is not required. Unwanted feelings are unlearnt using principles which started with Pavlov and his dogs.

The best known example of 'conditioning' is the use of a bell which rings when a child wets a special pad in his bed with urine (see Bed wetting). The child gradually learns to associate distension of the bladder with wakefulness.

People with a distressing reaction to the sight of, for instance, spiders or snakes, can be 'desensitized' by learning to relax when shown a small non-frightening animal and to continue to relax when confronted with progressively larger specimens. If taken slowly and skilfully, treatment can result in a tolerance for creatures previously frightening.

'Aversion' therapy can be used to modify or stop an undesired kind of behaviour such as sexual deviation or alcoholism. An unpleasant experience such as a mild electrical shock is given at the same time as some feature of the unwanted behaviour. This form of treatment should obviously be used only when it is the patient who wishes to change behaviour, for otherwise it becomes more like 'brain-washing' used by corrupt governments in secret prisons.

Physical treatment

Involves the use of drugs and electro-convulsive therapy (ECT). ECT is used less frequently than in the past, and mainly in very severe depression (see also Shock therapy and Depression).

The drugs used are termed psychotropic agents, and are employed to effect changes in mood. The most commonly used are hypnotics (sleeping tablets), tranquillizers and antidepressants. In the past, barbiturates were commonly used as hypnotics and tranquillizers but they are drugs of dependence and have been superseded by another group of drugs—the benzodiazepines (e.g. nitrazepam, Mogadon; diazepam, Valium), which are used to control mild anxiety states. More potent tranquillizers such as chlorpromazine are required for severe agitation and acute schizophrenic excitement. A rare but well recognized side-effect of chlorpromazine in high dosage is irregular spontaneous movement of the limbs and tongue (see Parkinson's disease).

Antidepressants are commonly prescribed. Tricyclic drugs (e.g. imipramine and amitriptyline) are commonly used, and their antidepressant effect usually takes about 2 weeks to develop. Overdose may cause serious, even fatal, abnormalities of heart rhythm. Tetracyclic drugs such as mianserin are a new group of antidepressants which probably do not have such serious effects if an overdose is taken, either deliberately or accidentally.

The mono-amine oxidase inhibitors are another major group of antidepressants (e.g. phenelzine, Nardil) which are now rarely used because of the risk of producing a serious rise in blood pressure. This is most likely to occur on interaction with other drugs or tyramine-containing foods (cheese, chicken liver, pickled herring, Marmite, Bovril, Oxo and Chianti).

Lithium carbonate is used to treat manic depression, but strict dosage control by measuring blood lithium levels is necessary to avoid toxic effects. Features of toxicity include loss of appetite, nausea, abdominal pain, diarrhoea, vomiting, tremor, unsteadiness, weakness, thirst and drowsiness. Despite these many side-effects, lithium may be the only effective remedy for severe manic states which might otherwise prove dangerous or fatal.

Psychopath

People with psychopathic personalities characteristically exhibit superficial charm and good intelligence, and may show no remorse or shame for their poorly motivated antisocial and sometimes violent behaviour. They are unreliable, untruthful and insincere, have poor judgement and fail to learn from experience. Interpersonal relationships are shallow, with egocentricity and incapacity for love.

Psychopaths do not usually respond to treatment; those seriously affected often become criminals and end up in prison.

Psychosomatic disorders

An 'illness of the mind'. This concept tends to separate illness as being either a result of disorder of the mind or of the body, but the two are inseparable, as emotional disturbance may cause physical disorders and physical disturbance often induces emotional stress.

Certain illnesses have previously been considered psychosomatic—e.g. asthma, ulcerative colitis and psoriasis. A more likely explanation is that an individual is genetically predisposed to developing one of these illnesses and psychological events may be one of the stress factors required to trigger an attack. (*See also* Anxiety; Depression; *and* Psychiatric illnesses.)

Puberty

This is the age at which the ability to have children begins. It corresponds with increased sexual awareness and certain physical changes. In girls periods start and breasts develop. In boys facial hair starts to grow and the penis and testicles enlarge.

It is often a time of great emotional uncertainty about relationships with the outside world. Many children become irritable and difficult, particularly with their parents (with whom they are the most secure emotionally). Tolerance, great patience and understanding are required to help the adolescent through this difficult phase.

Puerperal depression
SEE DEPRESSION: POST-NATAL DEPRESSION

Puerperal fever
(LATIN: *PUERPERUS*, RELATING TO CHILD-BIRTH)

Fever following childbirth, which may be due to infection within the uterine cavity or vagina. This is potentially serious, as infection may spread to the blood stream. If detected early, it responds rapidly to antibiotics. Any woman who develops a fever for whatever apparent cause soon after delivery must seek expert medical advice immediately.

Pulmonary embolus

A blood clot in the lungs. It usually arises from a clot in a deep vein of the leg (*see* Thrombosis), part of which breaks off (the embolus) and flows along the vein, passing through the heart until it lodges in the lungs. This causes obstruction to the blood supply of part of the lung, and as a result that part no longer functions and degenerates.

The symptoms of a pulmonary embolus are a sudden sharp chest pain which is made worse by deep breathing or coughing, and shortness of breath.

Treatment is aimed at preventing further clots from forming. Heparin, an anti-clotting agent (anticoagulant), is given by intravenous infusion, and at the same time a slower acting anticoagulant (warfarin) is given by mouth. As soon as the warfarin starts to act, the heparin is discontinued, and warfarin is continued for 3–6 months in a daily dose which is carefully monitored to attain optimal and safe anticoagulation. A very severe pulmonary embolism which obstructs a major blood vessel to the lung may be removed surgically.

Thrombosis in the veins of the legs is more likely to occur after long periods of immobility and after operations. It is more common in the overweight and the elderly, and there is an increased risk of developing thrombosis whilst taking the combined oral contraceptive pill. Fortunately, very few thromboses in the veins cause pulmonary emboli.

Purgative

Also known as laxatives, aperients, cathartics and evacuants, purgatives are used to promote bowel action in constipation. They work by increasing faecal bulk (bran, Fybogel, Normacol), by stimulating intestinal contraction (senna, cascara) or by softening the faecal content (enemas, dioctyl).

Pyelitis

Infection in the kidney. It causes fever, shivering attacks (rigors) and loin pain, sometimes associated with frequency of micturition and burning on passing urine. A urine specimen examined in a laboratory usually reveals the infecting bacteria, which can then be treated with an appropriate antibiotic. It is much less common than cystitis (page 71), and after recovery from the acute illness, further investigation of the kidney should be performed.

Pyloric stenosis

Narrowing of the pylorus, the outlet from the stomach to the intestine (see Stomach). It occurs as a congenital abnormality within the first months of life, or may be acquired as a result of a long-standing peptic ulcer.

Congenital pyloric stenosis affects firstborn male babies, and there is often a family history of other children being affected. Symptoms start after 3 or 4 weeks, with frequent vomiting, which is often forceful and projectile. The appetite remains good but there is failure to gain weight. The treatment of choice is surgery, and Ramstedt's operation is performed to cut the thickened muscle causing the obstruction. This is a relatively minor operation with excellent results.

Pyloric stenosis occurring later in life results from ulcer scarring (see Stomach ulcer). The scars contract, causing obstruction at the stomach outlet, and this produces the symptoms of vomiting superimposed on pre-existing ulcer pain. Very large quantities are vomited, and food eaten 24–48 hours previously may be returned. Treatment once again is surgical, and the scarred pylorus can be either removed or bypassed.

Pyrexia

A fever, or temperature above 37°C or 98.4°F. It is usually a sign of infection, although it can occur in other illnesses (e.g. a low-grade fever for 1–2 days is often present following a heart attack).

The body temperature is recorded with a mercury thermometer, which in adults should be placed under the tongue. In children and infants it is placed under the arm or partially introduced into the rectum. The most accurate body temperature is obtained from the rectum, and least accurate from under the arm.

See also Fever.

Pyridoxine
(VITAMIN B$_6$) *SEE UNDER* VITAMINS

Quarantine

Strict isolation—originally of 40 days, imposed upon ships and travellers arriving at ports of entry and if likely to be incubating an infectious disease.

The length of time children with infectious diseases should stay away from school is listed on page 290.

Quinsy

An abscess which forms within and around an infected tonsil (see Tonsillitis *and* Peritonsillar abscess).

R

Rabies

A virus disease transmitted by the bite or licks of an infected animal. Rabies virus is spreading northwards within the wild animal population of Europe, though not yet as far as the United Kingdom, and occurs in most other parts of the world. The emergence of rabies in the animal population of the UK has been prevented by rigid animal quarantine and the Channel.

The infection develops 2–6 weeks after being bitten by an infected animal and causes headache, sickness, excitability, fear of drinking water, and finally convulsions, coma and death. Once rabies develops in a human it is almost always fatal.

New vaccines have been introduced to protect individuals against rabies, and are given to those at risk (e.g. animal handlers working in quarantine quarters) and to those bitten by a wild animal, usually a dog, whilst out of the UK. There is no risk to those bitten whilst in the UK because there is no rabies in the animals. However, this will only be true for as long as the rigid quarantine laws are successfully enforced.

Dogs kept as pets in the tropics and wherever rabies is prevalent should be vaccinated against the disease and, if necessary, be muzzled when away from their own environment.

In Europe the fox is a common carrier, but cats, skunks and vampire bats also may transmit infection.

Radiation sickness

Radiation hazards are a major risk of nuclear warfare, and of accidents in nuclear reactors and to those accidentally exposed to large doses of radioactive materials.

All cells are destroyed by excess radioactivity, and the cells exposed are destroyed and rapidly disintegrate. Later the bone marrow is destroyed and with it the formation of all blood cells stops.

The initial features are nausea and vomiting, followed later by prolonged weakness, loss of hair as the cells of the skin die, ulcers within the mouth and diarrhoea following the destruction of the fine lining cells of the mouth and intestine. As the bone marrow becomes involved, the blood cells are no longer formed causing anaemia from loss of red cells,

infection secondary to loss of white cells, and generalized bleeding into all tissues due to deficiency of platelets.

If the radiation dose is high the outlook is hopeless but the body can recover from smaller doses. Expert treatment is required and aims at preventing and treating infections which arise, maintaining normal fluid and salt intake, treating the anaemia and the prevention of bleeding.

There is an increased incidence of leukaemia developing in the survivors.

Repeated small doses of radiation may lead, after a latent period of many years, to cancer and leukaemia.

Radiotherapy

The use of x-rays and other forms of radiation employed to treat tumours. Small doses of x-rays are safe when used to take pictures of the body. However, in larger dose and strength they will destroy living tissue. Certain tumours are very radiosensitive—i.e. much more easily killed than normal tissue—and radiotherapy is the recommended treatment; e.g. some skin cancers and Hodgkin's disease may be completely cured by radiotherapy. Radiotherapy may also be used to prevent regrowth after a tumour is removed, or if it cannot be completely removed surgically.

Early experience with radiotherapy was disappointing but recent advances in accurate pinpointing (localization) of the cancers has allowed highly concentrated radiation to be focused on the tumours with excellent results and a minimum of side-effects for the patient.

Radius

The hand is attached to this, the smaller of the two bones of the forearm (the other is the ulna). It is connected to the ulna by muscles and a thin, strong, fibrous membrane. The upper end of the radius forms a modified ball-and-socket joint with the lower end of the humerus (see diagram, page 267), and this allows the forearm to rotate when twisting the hand. The lower end tends to fracture in falls onto the outstretched hand (Colles' fracture).

Rash
(LATIN: *RASUS*, TO SCRATCH)

Any skin lesion occurring in spots or patches. The most common group of diseases which produce rashes are the childhood virus infections; e.g. measles (page 149), German measles (page 111), chickenpox (page 56) and dermatological conditions such as eczema (page 92) and psoriasis (page 188). (*See also* Skin disorders, pages 235–238.)

Chemical irritation is a common cause of rashes, and is seen in the nappy rash of infants (page 157), the dermatitis caused in a few adults by washing-up liquids and powders, and with a few drugs.

The rashes of virus infections disappear as the infection subsides, and the chemical rashes settle when the irritant is removed or no longer used. Rashes which persist require further investigation and specialized treatment, often by an experienced dermatologist.

Raynaud's disease

A condition affecting the hands in cold weather. The small arteries supplying blood to the hands go into spasm when the hand is cold. This causes the fingers to go white and then blue, and pins and needles or numbness may be felt in the finger tips. As the blood suddenly returns to the fingers, they become red and very painful.

In mild cases, avoiding cold water and wearing woollen socks and gloves in the winter may be sufficient to reduce the symptoms to acceptable levels. However, Raynaud's disease may be very severe, and should then be managed by clinicians with special experience of the disease.

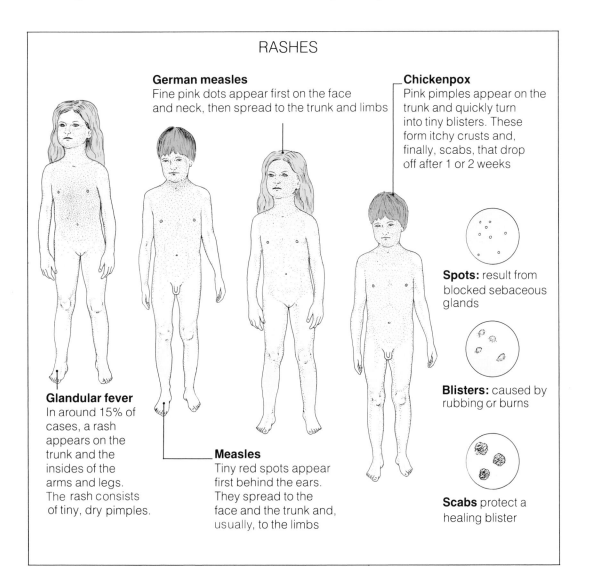

RASHES

German measles
Fine pink dots appear first on the face and neck, then spread to the trunk and limbs

Chickenpox
Pink pimples appear on the trunk and quickly turn into tiny blisters. These form itchy crusts and, finally, scabs, that drop off after 1 or 2 weeks

Spots: result from blocked sebaceous glands

Glandular fever
In around 15% of cases, a rash appears on the trunk and the insides of the arms and legs. The rash consists of tiny, dry pimples.

Measles
Tiny red spots appear first behind the ears. They spread to the face and the trunk and, usually, to the limbs

Blisters: caused by rubbing or burns

Scabs protect a healing blister

Occasionally, cutting the nerves which are responsible for causing the arterial spasm (sympathectomy) may be curative. Some drugs (e.g. propranolol, Inderal) occasionally cause similar symptoms, which cease when the drug is stopped.

Rectum
(LATIN: *RECTUS*; STRAIGHT)

The final, straight, part of the digestive tract, ending at the anus. The inner lining contains a large plexus of veins, which may enlarge and form haemorrhoids (piles). The rectum is very sensitive, hence the pain of haemorrhoids (page 175).

Reflux oesophagitis

The cause of heartburn (page 122). It is due to a defect in the valve between the stomach and the gullet (oesophagus), and this allows the acid secretions in the stomach to flow backwards (reflux) into the oesophagus. This causes inflammation of the fine inner lining of the oesophagus and gives pain. Sometimes reflux oesophagitis is associated with a hiatus hernia (page 126). The pain may be noticed on stooping or on lying flat in bed, because both postures encourage the acid to flow into the lower oesophagus.

Pain at night can be partially relieved by sleeping propped up, and during the day by removing tight

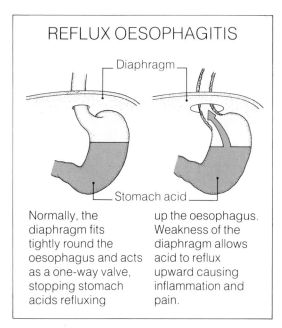

REFLUX OESOPHAGITIS

Diaphragm

Stomach acid

Normally, the diaphragm fits tightly round the oesophagus and acts as a one-way valve, stopping stomach acids refluxing up the oesophagus. Weakness of the diaphragm allows acid to reflux upward causing inflammation and pain.

clothes and corsets which increase the intra-abdominal pressure. Antacids (e.g. milk, Asilone, Rennie) are used to neutralize the acid secretions of the stomach, and recently discovered drugs—cimetidine (Tagamet) and ranitidine (Zantac)—may improve symptoms by reducing the amount of acid produced.

Regional ileitis
SEE CROHN'S DISEASE

Regurgitation

Babies
Regurgitation (posseting) in babies is very common, although some babies are more prone to it than others. Small amounts of food, often with wind, are brought up after every feed. Small amounts may be regurgitated between feeds. This understandably leads to parental anxiety, mainly the fear that baby is not getting enough feed. It is also distressing because the baby constantly smells, as do the carpet and furniture.

Provided that the baby continues to put on weight, appears to be developing normally and is otherwise healthy, persistent regurgitation is not serious. If, however, the regurgitation consists of large quantities or the baby is unwell, then medical advice should be sought.

Most babies with regurgitation grow out of it by about 1 year, or when they begin to walk. Until that time, regurgitation may be minimized by ensuring that the baby is not over-fed, that winding is carefully performed, and that the baby is propped up for a short time after feeding. Thickening the feeds with Carobel or Nestargel may partially resolve it.

Adults
Regurgitation of food in adults is rare and often associated with difficulty in swallowing. Food sticks in the gullet (oesophagus) and is almost immediately regurgitated. This is a potentially serious disorder, and requires careful clinical assessment and investigation. (*See also* Swallowing difficulty.)

Reiter's disease

A venereal disease (page 241) which produces a urethral discharge, soon followed by fever, and severe destructive joint disease usually of the ankle, knee and spine. It occasionally follows dysentery. It usually responds to antibiotics but the outcome is variable and joint damage may be permanent.

Renal disease
SEE CYSTITIS; KIDNEY FAILURE; KIDNEY STONES; *AND* PYELITIS

Respiratory distress syndrome

This is confined to newborn babies—usually those born early (premature, or pre-term, babies), of whom about 5 per cent will develop respiratory distress. As the name implies, the babies have great difficulty in breathing, because their lungs are immature and unable to expand fully. This results in a reduced amount of oxygen reaching the blood stream, and there is a compensatory increase in respiratory effort, with rapid shallow breathing. Modern management has greatly improved the outlook, particularly if the babies are looked after in Special Care Baby Units. In severe cases, artificial respiration with a ventilator may be required until the infection subsides.

Retina

The light-sensitive layer on the inner wall of the back of the eye (*see* Eye). The retina may become detached after blows to the eye and can be successfully stuck back by expert ophthalmic surgery using laser beams. Damage to the retina may seriously impair vision in poorly controlled diabetes (page 78) and high blood pressure (page 41). (*See also* illustrations, pages 69–70.)

Rhesus disease in the newborn

Rhesus incompatibility occurs in infants born to mothers with Rhesus-negative blood. If a Rhesus-negative mother has a Rhesus-positive baby, she may develop a reaction to the baby's blood. During the first pregnancy small amounts of the baby's blood mix with the mother's across the placenta. In this situation the baby's blood is incompatible with the mother's and she develops antibodies which destroy the baby's blood cells which have entered her blood circulation. In itself this causes no problems, but once these antibodies have been made they remain, and if stimulated again by Rhesus-positive cells they produce a more rapid and sustained response. Thus in the first pregnancy there is rarely any problem because the reaction is small. However, if in a subsequent pregnancy the new baby is also Rhesus positive, the antibody reaction may be massive and the mother's antibodies pass across the placenta, enter the fetal circulation and destroy the baby's red blood cells, causing anaemia and jaundice.

During ante-natal care, blood is taken for blood grouping to ascertain whether the mother is Rhesus positive or negative. If she is Rhesus negative, a further blood sample is taken at birth from the baby's umbilical cord to determine the baby's blood group. If the baby is Rhesus positive, antibodies are likely to develop in the mother's blood, and she can be vaccinated to prevent their formation. If the baby is Rhesus negative, no reaction will occur and there is no need for vaccination.

Rheumatic fever

Now very uncommon (as a consequence of improved living standards and nutrition), it is a rare complication of throat infection caused by the bacterium *Streptococcus* and is characterized in its worst form by fever and severe joint pains. The pains flit from one joint to another and the joints are excruciatingly tender. A rash on the legs also may occur. The most serious effect of rheumatic fever is damage to the heart valves.

Treatment includes rest for the inflamed joints and heart, aspirin to relieve pain and inflammation, and penicillin to destroy the bacterium.

Recurrent rheumatic fever may, after many years, result in narrowing or incompetence of the mitral and aortic valves of the left side of the heart (page 253), which may have to be replaced if the efficiency of the heart is seriously decreased.

Rheumatism
(FIBROSITIS)

'Rheumatism' and 'fibrositis' are terms applied to aches and pains in joints and muscles. They virtually never denote serious disease, but become more common with increasing age. These pains may respond to heat treatment, massage, physiotherapy, or simple pain-relieving drugs such as paracetamol and aspirin, but tend to recur.

'Rheumatic disease' is a more specific term describing diseases which affect joints. These disorders include rheumatoid arthritis (page 197), osteoarthritis (page 163), rheumatic fever (*see above*), and gout (page 114).

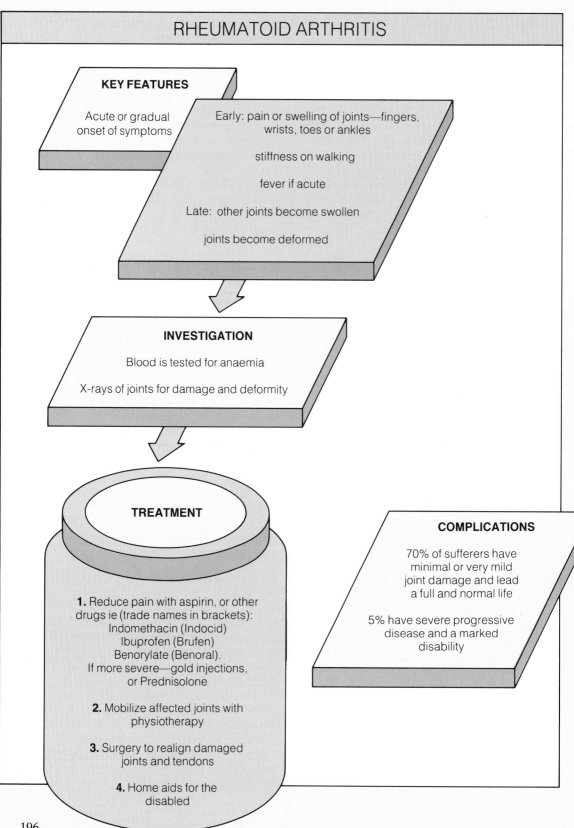

RHEUMATOID ARTHRITIS

KEY FEATURES

Acute or gradual onset of symptoms

Early: pain or swelling of joints—fingers, wrists, toes or ankles

stiffness on walking

fever if acute

Late: other joints become swollen

joints become deformed

INVESTIGATION

Blood is tested for anaemia

X-rays of joints for damage and deformity

TREATMENT

1. Reduce pain with aspirin, or other drugs ie (trade names in brackets):
Indomethacin (Indocid)
Ibuprofen (Brufen)
Benorylate (Benoral).
If more severe—gold injections, or Prednisolone

2. Mobilize affected joints with physiotherapy

3. Surgery to realign damaged joints and tendons

4. Home aids for the disabled

COMPLICATIONS

70% of sufferers have minimal or very mild joint damage and lead a full and normal life

5% have severe progressive disease and a marked disability

Rheumatoid arthritis
(SEE ALSO ARTHRITIS)

Approximately 3 per cent of the population in Britain suffer from rheumatoid arthritis and over two-thirds of these are young and middle aged women. It is characterized by pain and swelling in the joints, usually associated with stiffness in the morning. Several joints are involved though the small joints in the hands and fingers are commonly affected first. There may be later involvement of wrists, knees, shoulders, ankles, elbows and, rarely, the hips. The pain and swelling are caused by inflammation within and around the joint.

Rheumatoid arthritis may run any of a number of courses. Many cases are mild with minimal deformity, and about half develop little or no disability. At the other extreme, 10 per cent develop increasing disability and handicap. In between, the disease runs a remitting, relapsing course with variable disability.

Treatment requires the use of pain-killing (analgesic) and anti-inflammatory drugs. Many drugs combine both these capabilities. Aspirin is the best known and, if well tolerated, is very effective. Other drugs in common use are indomethacin (Indocid) and ibuprofen (Brufen). Steroids (e.g. prednisolone) are very powerful anti-inflammatory drugs but have serious unwanted effects (*see* Steroids) if taken for long periods in high doses. They are used only for severe rheumatoid arthritis which does not respond to other measures.

Gold and penicillamine are reserved for those with persistently active and progressive disease because side-effects are common and need careful expert supervision.

In addition to drug therapy, physiotherapy and occupational therapy are valuable lines of treatment. Special techniques for coping with disability may be learnt, and equipment and appliances can be modified to individual requirements for use in the home—particularly in the kitchen and bathroom—to allow even a severely disabled patient to maintain full activity and independence.

Rhinitis

Inflammation of the nose, usually caused by a virus infection (e.g. the common cold) or by allergy such as hay fever. The symptoms include nasal irritation and discharge which may be associated with sneezing. There is no specific treatment for the infections because they are due to viruses which do not respond to antibiotics. If the discharge is excessive, nasal decongestants such as pseudoephedrine (in Actifed) or xylometazoline (Otrivine) reduce the quantity of secretions and partially relieve the symptoms. Antihistamines are used to suppress allergy but produce drowsiness and may make driving unsafe.

Rhythm method
SEE UNDER FAMILY PLANNING

Riboflavine
(VITAMIN B_2)

Present in yeast, milk, liver, eggs and leafy vegetables. Gross deficiency of riboflavine causes soreness of the lips, mouth and tongue, and irritation in the eyes. Eventually the corners of the mouth crack and fissure, and the lips may ulcerate.

The recommended daily intake for an adult male is 1.8 milligrams. Dietary deficiency is very rare in the developed world, and is usually combined with generalized malnutrition and deficiency of other vitamins. (*See also* Vitamins.)

Rickets

Rickets is due to defective bone formation during growth. The features are 'beading of the ribs' (small swellings where each rib joins the breastbone, or sternum) swelling of the bones at the wrists and curvature of the long bones of the legs (bow legs or knock knees).

Rickets is caused by deficiency of vitamin D (calciferol). Vitamin D is present in milk, egg yolk and liver oils especially fish (halibut and cod), and is also manufactured in the skin on exposure to sunlight. Vitamin D is not present in breast milk and breast-fed babies are usually given supplements until the age of 6 months. Vitamin D is converted in the body to cholecalciferol, a chemical which is essential for the intestinal absorption of calcium, required for new bone formation. Dietary deficiency is rare in Britain although it may occur in the children of Asian immigrants.

Rarely, despite adequate vitamin D intake, rickets may be caused by kidney disease. Healthy kidneys chemically alter vitamin D to a more active compound which is responsible for controlling blood calcium levels and bone formation.

The recommended daily intake of vitamin D is 400 international units. The treatment of dietary-deficient rickets is vitamin D 500 international units daily by mouth. Rickets due to disease of the kidneys is more difficult to treat and requires higher doses of vitamin D. There is a small danger of overdosage with vitamin D, and treatment should be monitored by careful clinical assessment.

Rigor

The shaking or shivering which occurs with high fluctuant fevers. Rigors are a common feature in patients with malaria (page 148) who, at the height of the fever, develop drenching perspiration and shaking of the entire body with chattering of their teeth. Rigors indicate very high fevers irrespective of thermometer readings, and nearly always signify the need for urgent medical assessment.

Rigor mortis
(LATIN: *RIGOR*, STIFFNESS; *MORS*, DEATH)

The fixed nature of the body after death.

Ringworm

A fungal infection of the skin, usually the feet, groins, scalp and nails. (*See* illustrations, page 236.)

Infection of the feet—athlete's foot (page 32)—produces thickened, soggy, white skin between the toes, with some itching. The infection may spread to the legs, causing a red itching rash. Occasionally nails are infected and are irregularly thickened.

Ringworm in the groin (tinea cruris) is characterized by a red rash with a sharp edge between infected and normal skin often associated with intense itching. It is commoner in males.

Scalp ringworm occurs nearly always in children, and causes localized loss of hair over the infected area. Some cases are due to contact with animal ringworm, though many are spread from human to human.

Cattle ringworm may occur in farmers who have been in contact with infected cows, and may also be acquired from contact with farm gates or in the cattle market. This infection causes multiple, round, well demarcated areas of infected skin which commonly starts on the wrists and spreads to the rest of the body.

Treatment of ringworm is either by the use of an anti-fungal cream which is applied directly to the rash or by taking tablets of the anti-fungal drug griseofulvin. The tablets have to be taken for several months in severe ringworm infections.

Rodent ulcer

A small ulcer in the skin of the face, which slowly grows until treated. They can be cured completely if detected early and treated by radiotherapy or removed surgically. Surgery requires great expertise to ensure complete removal and a good cosmetic result. (*See* illustration, page 237.)

Rubella
SEE GERMAN MEASLES

Rupture

The lay term for a hernia. There are many types of hernia but 'rupture' usually refers to an inguinal hernia in the groin. It is due to a weakness in the groin muscles and results in a swelling in the groin which gets larger with coughing or standing up and goes away on lying down. It may or may not be painful. (*See also* Hernia.)

Safe period
SEE FAMILY PLANNING

Salicylates

A group of drugs used to ease pain and reduce inflammation and fever. Aspirin (acetylsalicylic acid, page 29) is the best known. The name is derived from the word salicin, which is an extract obtained from willow bark, used as a substitute for quinine in the eighteenth and nineteenth centuries. Aspirin is the commonly used modern preparation and is prepared synthetically.

Salivary glands

Several glands produce saliva . They are the parotid glands (situated just in front of the ears), the submandibular glands (just below the inner borders of the jawbone, or mandible) and the sublingual glands (underneath the tongue). These glands secrete saliva into the mouth by small ducts, which may become blocked by small stones. The gland involved swells up when production of saliva is stimulated—by eating or anticipating food. All of these glands can be inflamed in mumps, but the parotids are the most commonly involved.

Salmonella

The genus of bacteria which cause typhoid (page 231) and food poisoning (page 105).

Salpingitis

Infection of the Fallopian tubes, the tubes along which the eggs (ova) produced by the ovaries pass to reach the womb (uterus). The infection causes abdominal pain, fever, irregular periods and, sometimes, a vaginal discharge. Treatment is with an appropriate antibiotic and although the acute infection can be successfully treated, it may result in sterility. This is because the acute infection and inflammation heal with scarring and narrow the Fallopian tubes sufficiently to block the passage of the ova; this prevents fertilization.

Salpingitis frequently occurred following illegal abortion, because of poor attention to sterility. This has become rare since the alteration of the laws on therapeutic abortion and the consequent decline in illegal abortion. Gonorrhoea is now the commonest cause.

Scabies

An infestation of the skin, caused by a mite (*Sarcoptes scabiei*) which is spread from person to person by direct skin contact. The mites cause an allergic reaction in the skin with an intense itching red rash around the sites of skin penetration—commonly the webs of the fingers and the wrists and elbows, buttocks and armpits. The adult female burrows under the skin, laying eggs, which hatch after a few days. The young emerge from the burrows and develop into adults, when mating occurs and the cycle repeats itself. Once in a burrow, the female never emerges. Infection persists because the young re-infest the patient.

Treatment is extremely effective. The standard method is to bathe, dry the skin and apply benzyl benzoate lotion with a paint brush from the neck downwards, allowing it to dry on the skin. This is repeated on the second day. On the third day, after bathing and painting again, clean clothes should be worn. The itching usually disappears within a week. The dirty clothes which have been impregnated with the lotion can be washed normally.

Scan

CAT scan (computerized axial tomography)
Produces clear pictures of the internal organs with the use of x-rays. Its major present use is to study the internal brain structures when searching for bleeding and tumours. (*See* illustrations, pages 201–2.)

The CAT scan has revolutionized some aspects of radiology, particularly neuroradiology, and usually replaces the more invasive forms of examination which were much more unpleasant for the patient and often required a general anaesthetic. With the CAT scan, the patient lies with his head resting within the scanner, and this then moves round and takes x-ray pictures. The process is completely painless and no anaesthetic is required.

Ultrasound scanning
Employs high-frequency sound waves which are aimed at body structures. The waves rebound from the surfaces between two structures and are detected in the same way as radar.

Ultrasound scanning is valuable during pregnancy because the sound waves used are harmless. One of its uses is in determining the age of the fetus, to estimate the date of delivery. (Conventional methods of determining this date depend on the date of the last menstrual period and on the size of the womb (uterus) as felt on examination, both of which are unreliable.) Early scanning is more accurate in determining both the length of pregnancy and the growth rate of the baby.

Ultrasound scans are also employed for amniocentesis (page 16), a procedure whereby the amniotic fluid is withdrawn for examination to detect abnormalities in the fetus—particularly mongolism and spina bifida. The scan is used to define the best area for removal of fluid without endangering the placenta or the fetus.

Scarlet fever

An acute bacterial (streptococcal) infection which causes a high fever, severe sore throat and a generalized bright red rash over the entire body. The severe form of the disease has been disappearing progressively over the last 20 years and is now rarely seen. Prior to antibiotics, complications were common and affected the kidneys to produce varying degrees of kidney failure (page 141), the heart to cause damage to the valves (page 120), and the ears to cause deafness (otitis media, page 88).

Schistosomiasis
(BILHARZIA)

An endemic disease of the tropics, caused by blood flukes. After man is infected, the organism is shed in urine or faeces and the schistosomes then infect fresh-water snails which inhabit calm water. The parasite multiplies inside the snail liver and is shed back into the water in a form which is able to penetrate human skin. Hence the life cycle of the parasite is perpetuated. Multiplication of the organism depends upon the presence of certain species of snails, and schistosomiasis can exist only where they are found.

In the developed world, two forms of schistosomiasis are seen. *Schistosoma haematobium* is found in Africa, and particularly in the Nile valley, the east coast, the Congo and Nigeria. After infecting man, the flukes pass to the blood vessels in and around the bladder, to cause urinary bleeding with frequency of micturition. There may be additional features of fever and general exhaustion in the early stages soon after infection. The eggs (ova) of the fluke can be detected in the urine. *Schistosoma mansoni* also occurs in Africa and produces a similar initial illness, but with intestinal symptoms of diarrhoea which may be severe, with blood and mucus in the stools.

The best treatment is prevention, and travellers should not bathe or wash in, or drink from, ponds and rivers. Destruction of the intermediate snail hosts prevents spread. Infected patients respond to a number of drugs such as niridazole (Ambilhar) but it is important to confirm the diagnosis before starting treatment.

Schizophrenia

The term applied to a group of mental disorders with a wide range of symptoms typified by disorders of thinking, feeling and behaviour to other people and the external world. It usually develops in adolescence. The cause is unknown, though a schizophrenic-like illness may be induced by some drugs (e.g. mescaline, LSD, amphetamines), epilepsy or sleep deprivation.

The most significant symptoms include delusions, auditory hallucinations and passivity experience. A *delusion* is a false unshakeable belief which is out of keeping with the individual's educational, cultural and social background. A *hallucination* is the apparent perception of a sensation which is not actually present. Hallucinations relating to hearing are very common, and the schizophrenic may hear voices which are not there or his own thoughts spoken aloud, or voices commenting on his actions, or voices arguing with each other. Often the voices are critical and produce the feeling of paranoia (page 166). *Passivity experiences* are experiences which feel

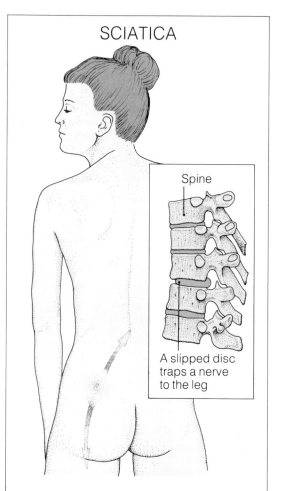

SCIATICA

Spine

A slipped disc traps a nerve to the leg

A vertebral disc which slips out of place may trap one of the nerves from the spinal cord to the leg. The resulting pain may be very severe, shooting down the back of the leg to the knee, or even the foot.

Scanning

Two techniques are commonly used–X-ray scanning and isotope scanning.

In both the patient lies resting on a bench and either the scanner moves over him or the bench moves beneath a fixed machine. With X-ray scanning films are taken of the tissues under examination and retained for later analysis. This is particularly useful for scanning the abdomen, for enlarged organs e.g. the liver and pancreas. It has therefore acquired the name of "cancer scanner" but has many other uses.

With isotope scans, a radioactive isotope is injected into a vein and is taken up preferentially by the tissues being examined. Pictures of these can then be taken for analysis. Isotope scans are of great value in detecting diseases of the liver, kidney, thyroid, brain and bones.

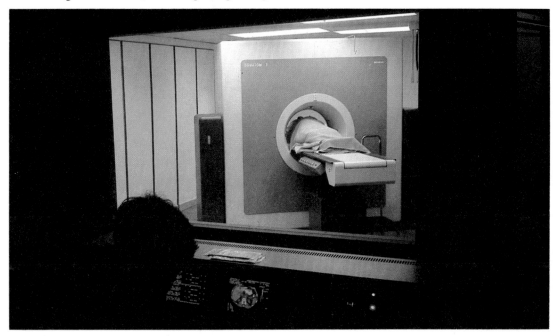

The patient lies on a bench as the scanner moves around him or her. A technician sitting in a control room monitors the scanner's progress on a T.V. screen.

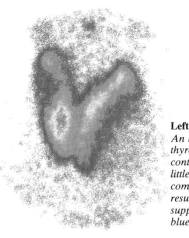

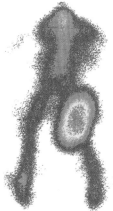

Left
An isotope scan of the thyroid gland. The gland contained many cysts with little blood supply. These compress the normal gland resulting in poor blood supply, which appear as blue areas.

Right
An isotope scan of the blood flow in a transplanted kidney. The red areas indicate good blood flow, while the blue areas indicate poor flow.

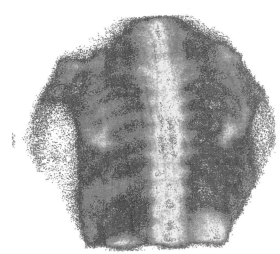

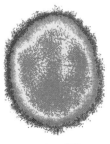

Right
An isotope scan of the liver showing the blood supply. The regions with good flow show hot (red) areas. The abscess in the upper part of the liver displaces normal cells and appears to have little blood flow and appears blue.

Left
An isotope scan of the vertebrae and ribs–the isotope being taken up by the bones. Areas of good blood supply show in red, poor supply in blue.

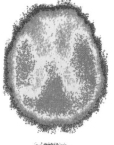

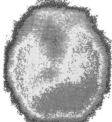

Several radio-iodine scans of a normal brain taken at different levels through the head. The regions of good blood supply show as hot (red) whereas areas with little supply show as cold (blue).

202

as though they are being made from outside the self. These include passivity of thought (e.g. experiences of thoughts being controlled), mood, emotion and volition.

Schizophrenia tends to run in families, although the incidence in the general population is very low (0.5 per cent).

A complete cure for schizophrenia is unusual. The outlook has improved with the introduction of tranquillizing drugs, occupational rehabilitation and social support which can prevent severe progression of the disease. Many chronic schizophrenics lead a relatively normal life integrated into their local community, though unfortunately a small number eventually need long-term institutional care because they can no longer cope alone.

Sciatica

Pain felt down the back of the leg, due to pressure on the roots of the sciatic nerve where they leave the spine. The pressure is usually caused by prolapse of an intervertebral disc (*see* Disc). The pain corresponds to the distribution of the nerve down the leg, and may be felt in the buttock, back of the thigh and calf, and sole of the foot. The severity varies from a dragging ache down the back of the leg to a sudden severe shooting pain which makes further walking or movement of the leg impossible.

Treatment depends on the severity of the pain. If sudden and severe, rest on a firm bed is recommended. The most comfortable position is usually flat on the back, until the acute pain subsides.

Once the acute period has passed, mobilization can be started with advice about sensible posture and care when bending, lifting and twisting, and physiotherapy to strengthen the back muscles. Analgesics to relax muscle spasm, traction to the spine and manipulation are sometimes very effective. Recovery is usually excellent, although it may take up to 6 weeks. Sciatica may recur, and regular exercise and care in lifting and twisting should be maintained.

Scoliosis

Curvature and twisting of the spine is universally present to a minor degree but rarely sufficient to damage health in any way. If severe, it may constrict the lungs, which become susceptible to bronchitis and pneumonia.

Scrotum

Swelling of the scrotum is caused by excess fluid (*see* Hydrocele), by enlargement of the testes (*see* Orchitis) or by hernias (page 124). It may be difficult to distinguish between them, and medical advice should be sought as testicular swellings may be malignant and are cured by removal if detected early.

Scurf
SEE DANDRUFF

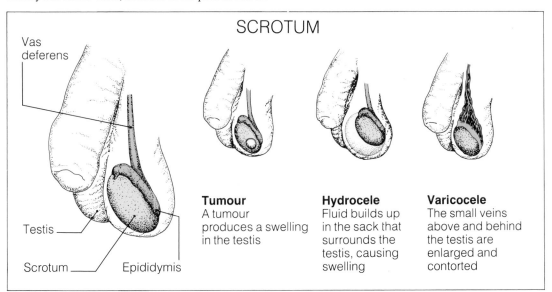

SCROTUM

Vas deferens

Testis

Scrotum — Epididymis

Tumour A tumour produces a swelling in the testis

Hydrocele Fluid builds up in the sack that surrounds the testis, causing swelling

Varicocele The small veins above and behind the testis are enlarged and contorted

203

Scurvy

An illness due to a deficiency of vitamin C (ascorbic acid) in the diet. It is a rare occurrence in the developed world, though it does occur in tramps who live rough and occasionally in the old if they live alone without support from friends or family and take an inadequate diet. Scurvy causes bruising of the skin, especially marked on the buttocks and back of the thighs. The bruising may occur spontaneously and is not related to previous injury. The gums also become swollen and bleed easily.

Scurvy responds rapidly to treatment with vitamin C tablets. Prevention requires a diet with adequate vitamin C, i.e. fresh fruits and vegetables.

The term 'Limeys' for British sailors comes from their habit of eating limes to prevent scurvy, a common disease among eighteenth century sailors. This is an interesting example of preventive medicine, occurring long before the chemical nature of the disease or the vitamin was known.

Sea sickness
SEE TRAVEL SICKNESS

Sedatives

Sedatives and hypnotics are amongst the most frequently prescribed drugs, and are used to relieve anxiety during the day (sedatives) or induce sleep at night (hypnotics).

Anxiety is often a feature of more deep-seated psychiatric trouble, and sedatives should be prescribed only after careful assessment of the patient's worries—often the anxiety diminishes after the problems and fears have been explained and understood (see Anxiety). The most widely prescribed sedative for anxiety is diazepam (Valium). Sleeping tablets in common use are discussed with sleep disturbance (page 208).

Senile dementia

Caused by a decrease in the number of functioning brain cells. To a certain extent, loss of brain cells is an unavoidable consequence of ageing, though most elderly people retain their full mental faculties.

The features of dementia develop slowly, with impairment of intellect and personality. There is usually memory loss for recent events whilst childhood can be clearly recalled. An early sign is emotional lability with rapid and sudden mood swings usually appearing as depression with weeping. As the process continues, neglect of personal care and hygiene occurs. Inappropriate behaviour due to impaired judgement and critical faculties is common, and in severe cases disorientation in time and place occurs. There is loss of identity and increasing dependence on help from others, whilst at the same time there is an inability to recognize the need for help. Rational conversation and communication eventually become impossible.

The process is progressive but the rate of progression varies enormously from individual to individual. There is no method of reversing or preventing senile dementia, but a number of well recognized diseases (e.g. hypothyroidism, page 224; brain tumour, page 45; multiple and minor strokes, page 217; and alcoholism, page 14) simulate it and should be excluded by careful medical examination and investigation.

Septic/septicaemic

Septic means infected and usually refers to a boil on the skin. *Septicaemia* denotes spread of infection to the blood.

Serum

The liquid part of the blood from which thrombin and prothrombin, the proteins which control clotting, have been removed.

Serum hepatitis

A virus infection of the liver usually caused by injection of infected serum and common in drug addicts. It is less commonly caused by tattooing with an infected instrument and by sexual intercourse. All blood used for transfusion is tested for the virus before use. (*See also* Hepatitis.)

Sexual problems

The common problems are impotence and premature ejaculation in men, and frigidity and pain on intercourse in women.

Impotence
The inability to obtain or sustain an erection, and

occurs on occasions to nearly every sexually active man. The reasons are often ill understood, and include inexperience, tiredness, anxiety, a phase of depression and fear of pregnancy or venereal disease. Alcohol will 'provoke the desire but take away the performance' (*Macbeth*). Only if impotence persists is there cause for concern. The cause is invariably psychological, though some diseases of the nervous system and a few drugs may produce impotence.

The management of persistent impotence requires the help of those with special interest and experience in the field. Considerable time and patience must be spent in attempting to get to the root of the problem, and this may be most upsetting to both partners, such as a hidden dislike of one partner for the other or buried homosexuality. If the couple have had a previously stable and happy relationship, there is a good chance that the problem will disappear with time, though it may take many months of understanding and affection from both the couple with or without psychiatric help.

Premature ejaculation and failure of ejaculation

These are ill understood. Again they have affected many healthy and sexually active men from time to time even in the most stable and contented relationships. The possible causes include inexperience, over-excitement and alcohol. Only if they persist is there need for concern, and expert advice should then be sought.

Frigidity

Features vary from total revulsion to failure to achieve orgasm. Failure of orgasm is common from time to time both in women and in men, and is rarely cause for concern unless it persists. Arousal is generally slower in women, and inexperience and hurry from the male partner is frequently the problem. Other factors include fear of pregnancy, venereal disease and pain on intercourse, particularly if earlier experiences have been unpleasant. If orgasm is never reached and is of concern, expert psychiatric advice should be sought, preferably by both partners; considerate and skilled guidance may be sufficient to overcome the problem.

The more severe forms of frigidity appear as total lack of sexual feelings or desires. There may be an obvious cause such as pain on intercourse, or a more deep-seated psychiatric problem. Frigidity is often ascribed to religious or family guilt related to an excessively puritanical upbringing. Whether this is true or not, those with serious degrees of frigidity with total lack of sexual feelings are well advised to seek psychiatric advice.

Pain on intercourse

May be caused by local ulcers or infection of the vulva, vagina or cervix. In the first instance, careful examination by a skilled gynaecologist is required to exclude or treat these disorders. If none exists, and the pain persists, counselling from an experienced psychiatrist or therapist may be invaluable.

Shingles

An infection caused by the varicella or *Herpes zoster* virus, which also causes chickenpox. It arises the following way: following chickenpox infection in childhood, the virus remains in the body (in the sensory nerves which lead from the skin to the spinal cord). It usually remains dormant within these nerves throughout life but occasionally, and usually in middle or old age, the virus can become active again and produce an attack of shingles. This often follows a minor infection such as a cold or an acute attack of bronchitis. These suppress the natural immunity against the shingles virus and allows it to break out.

Shingles starts with pain, numbness and pins and needles in the band of skin which is served by the sensory nerve. This is followed by a rash of small blisters which burst and crust (see illustration, page 235). Shingles remains infectious until the last blister has crusted. Unfortunately, there is no safe and effective treatment and the infection should be allowed to run its natural course. Calamine lotion in oil may ease local irritation, and analgesic agents to relieve pain and sleeping tablets may help during the acute phase. Following shingles the area of skin involved may remain painful for several months (post-herpetic neuralgia), and very occasionally is excruciating. If this persists and pain is not improved with powerful pain-killers (analgesics) such as pethidine, the nerve transmitting the pain can be destroyed with phenol injections or cut surgically.

Shock therapy
(ELECTRO-CONVULSIVE THERAPY, ECT)

Used in the treatment of severe depression. The patient is first rendered completely unconscious and relaxed under a short-acting anaesthetic. An electric current is then applied to the patient's head through electrodes on each temple. The occasional complications of this procedure are temporary memory loss and headache.

Shock therapy is of value in a small number of patients with extreme and severe depression who do not improve with antidepressant tablets. The mode of action of ECT is unknown. The late Dr Richard Asher, famed for his objective statements about medical practice, referred to ECT as 'a shuffle and redeal' of the brain cells. Medical opinion has swung strongly away from its use in the routine management of depression but there is no doubt that in a few patients with very severe depression with strong suicidal drives, ECT can miraculously reverse the depression, sometimes for only a short while.

Shortness of breath

Breathlessness is normally associated with vigorous exercise and is the body's response to replace oxygen used up during exercise. Certain illnesses are commonly associated with breathlessness.

Anxiety
Some people express anxiety by over-breathing. The unpleasant sensations produced by this serve only to increase the anxiety and a vicious spiral can result.

Asthma (page 31)
During an asthmatic attack there is marked breathlessness associated with wheezing. This is due to narrowing of the small breathing tubes (bronchi) which carry oxygen deep into the lungs. Narrowing of the airway is due mainly to contraction of the muscles of the walls, resulting in partial obstruction to air flow. There is a decrease in the oxygen reaching the blood and the brain and hence a sensation of breathlessness. Once the asthmatic attack has abated, lung function rapidly returns to normal, and breathlessness disappears.

Chronic bronchitis (page 48)
Usually occurs in cigarette smokers and is characterized by recurrent chest infections with cough, the production of sputum and wheezing. Lung function becomes worse during these infections, and never returns completely to normal. The small airways leading into the lungs and the fine lung tissues are permanently damaged, causing both obstruction to air flow and defective transfer of oxygen into the blood across the lungs (page 147).

Heart disease
Can cause shortness of breath, even if the lungs are normal. When the heart is pumping inefficiently, blood flow through the circulation is reduced and blood pools in the lungs, reducing the oxygen exchange to the blood stream. The characteristic features are breathlessness on exertion and paroxysmal attacks of breathlessness at night induced by lying flat. One of the commonest causes of heart pump failure is atheromatous narrowing of the coronary arteries which supply oxygen to the muscle of the heart (see Arterial disease and Heart).

Industrial lung disease (see also Industrial diseases)
Many industrial dusts can damage or destroy the tissues of the lung (e.g. carbon, tin, iron, coal, graphite, silica and asbestos). Coal-workers' pneumoconiosis results from the inhalation of coal dust particles, which remain in the lung to produce chemical damage. If exposure is heavy and prolonged, irreversible changes in the lung occur. Changes are more likely to be severe in cigarette smokers, who also develop chronic bronchitis, and they are much more likely to develop severe progressive breathlessness.

Infection
During a chest infection (e.g. acute bronchitis and pneumonia), oxygen is not efficiently absorbed into the blood stream. This results in a reduction of oxygen to the brain, which is perceived as breathlessness and followed by a compensatory increase in respiratory effort.

Breathlessness other than after exercise is abnormal and requires careful medical assessment. Acute breathlessness is a sign of serious illness and ★ medical advice should be sought urgently.

Shoulder joint

A modified ball-and-socket joint (see diagram, page 267). The head of the humerus is held by the surrounding muscles and ligaments against a shallow socket in the outer aspect of the shoulder blade (scapula). This allows the arm to move in virtually all directions at the shoulder, but, because the socket is very shallow, the joint is unstable and prone to dislocate easily (see Dislocation).

Siamese twins
SEE TWINS

Sickle cell disease

A hereditary disease occurring mainly in inhabitants of Africa, India and the Mediterranean. It results in the formation of an abnormal haemoglobin, the oxygen-binding protein of red blood cells, rapid destruction of these cells and anaemia (*see* Anaemia).

Sickness

The sensation of a need to vomit. (*See* Pregnancy: vomiting; Travel sickness; *and* Vomiting.)

Sight

SEE BLINDNESS; BLURRED VISION; CATARACT; COLOUR BLINDNESS; DOUBLE VISION; GLASSES; GLAUCOMA; *AND* SQUINT

Sigmoidoscopy

The insertion of a hollow metal tube into the rectum, which allows the inner lining of the lower bowel to be observed directly. The term is derived from the 'S' or sigmoid shape of the lower end of the colon.

Sinusitis

Inflammation of the nasal sinuses by viruses or bacteria; it is very common, particularly with a cold. The typical features are of fever, pain over the affected sinuses—usually the nasal sinuses, giving pain behind the cheeks and in the upper jaws and teeth—and a nasal discharge. Fluid produced in the largest sinuses drains via a small aperture high up in the nose (*see* diagram). This hole is small and easily blocked, resulting in a build-up of fluid in the sinuses which is static and hence easily infected.

Usually, sinusitis settles spontaneously within a few days. If bacterial infection supervenes, antibiotics may be required; should infection be sufficiently frequent and painful, it may be necessary to create an artificial hole in the septum to allow secretions to drain more easily. The operation is straight-forward in the hands of experienced otolaryngologists and is usually performed with a local anaesthetic.

Skeleton

The skull, vertebral column, rib cage, pelvis and

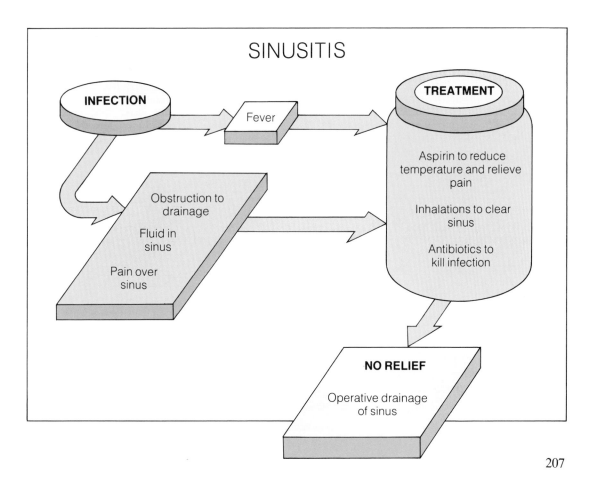

SINUSITIS

INFECTION

Fever

TREATMENT

Aspirin to reduce temperature and relieve pain

Inhalations to clear sinus

Antibiotics to kill infection

Obstruction to drainage

Fluid in sinus

Pain over sinus

NO RELIEF

Operative drainage of sinus

bones of the limbs are the framework which supports and protects the delicate organs of the body (e.g. the brain within the skull, and the heart and lungs within the rib cage) (*see* diagram, page 259). The muscles and tendons are fixed to the skeletal bones.

The bones also store calcium, which is essential for muscular contraction (including that of the heart).

Skin diseases
SEE PAGES 235–238

Skin tests

Used to determine allergy to foreign substances (allergens); e.g. a dilute solution of a grass pollen may be tested in a hay fever sufferer. The solution is dropped onto the forearm skin and the surface of the skin is gently and painlessly broken with a needle. A positive or allergic reaction develops within 10 minutes with redness and swelling around the puncture site and this denotes hypersensitivity or allergy. As well as allergy against various grass pollens, sensitivity to the house dust mite (*Dermatophagoides pteronyssimus*) may be implicated in non-seasonal hay fever and asthma.

Allergic individuals (and their families) with eczema, hay fever and asthma may have positive skin reactions to a variety of allergens which do not produce symptoms in them, and conversely some will be negative for those which do. Sufferers from hay fever or seasonal asthma who are sensitive to a single allergen (e.g. house dust mite) can be desensitized and this can produce considerable relief or cure.

Sleep disturbance

Loss of a night's sleep is common and is caused by short-term anxiety, excitement or caffeine (tea or coffee) at night.

Chronic loss of sleep is caused by emotional strain, fear (*see* Nightmares), anxiety (page 23) or depression (page 75), and returns to a normal pattern if the underlying problem is resolved. Sleep walking is rare and ill understood, and probably is caused by an underlying anxiety. It may be a hysterical response to an underlying and apparently insoluble problem (*see* Hysteria).

Hypnotic drugs taken at night induce a sleep state for a few hours. There are many available and drugs commonly used to induce sleep include flurazepam (Dalmane), temazepam (Normison, Euhypnos), nitrazepam (Remnos, Mogadon, Somnased), and dichloralphenazone (Welldorm).

Sleeping sickness
(TRYPANOSOMIASIS)

Infection is transmitted by the bite of the tsetse fly which inhabits the African continent. Man and large animals are the reservoirs of infection. The life cycle begins after ingestion of infected human or animal blood by the fly, in which the organisms multiply. They then pass to the salivary glands of the tsetse fly to be injected into its next victim.

The disease begins with a fever and general ill health which progresses slowly over 2–4 months. The body organs are all progressively involved, and after 6 months or so the infection in the brain causes headache, inability to concentrate, poor memory and apathy, leading finally to drowsiness and coma.

Slipped disc
SEE BACKACHE; DISC; SCIATICA; *AND* SPONDYLOSIS

Smallpox

A serious viral infection, caused by the variola major or the variola minor virus. The former is more severe and carries an over-all mortality of 40 per cent. Variola minor is a milder variant with a mortality of less than 1 per cent.

The spots are similar to those of chickenpox but the distribution is different. In smallpox the spots are mainly on the face and limbs, whereas in chickenpox they are mainly on the trunk.

A world-wide vaccination programme organized by the World Health Organization has just cleared the world of smallpox infection. However, close surveillance is continuing to ensure that it does not recur. Apart from the Birmingham laboratory accident in August 1978, the last reported case in the world was in Somalia in October 1977.

Smoking

A short history of smoking
Until the middle of the nineteenth century, tobacco was smoked only in pipes. It was also chewed and taken as snuff. Cigarette smoking was first introduced after the Crimean War and increased in popularity at the end of the nineteenth century when machinery for making large numbers of cigarettes was introduced. Since 1920, cigarettes have domin-

ated tobacco sales; of male smokers, only 5 per cent are now exclusively pipe or cigar smokers.

Women seldom smoked before World War II, but since 1950 there has been a steady upward trend in the number of women who smoke regularly, whilst smoking in men has remained unchanged.

After both World Wars consumption fell and the cost of smoking increased. There were also brief falls following the Royal College of Physicians' reports in 1960 and 1971, which emphasized the dangers of smoking.

The only group in the community in whom the consumption of cigarettes has fallen is the medical profession. This is of interest because they are also the only group in whom death rates from the two major killers associated with smoking—lung cancer and heart attacks—are declining.

Dangers of smoking

Smokers are prone to a number of diseases including:
1 Cancer of the lung
2 Heart attack
3 Arterial disease
4 Chronic bronchitis and emphysema
5 Some other cancers
6 Stomach and duodenal ulcers

The extra number of deaths per year in the United Kingdom as a result of smoking are as follows:

Cause	
Lung cancer	940 (19 per cent)
Chronic bronchitis and emphysema	470 (10 per cent)
Coronary heart disease (heart attacks and angina)	1,520 (31 per cent)
Other cardiovascular disease (including strokes)	1,000 (21 per cent)
Other diseases	920 (19 per cent)
	4,850 per 1 million smokers

Smoking and lung cancer

This accounts for over 35,000 deaths per year in the UK. In men under 65 the death rate is beginning to fall, but it is still rising in women. The risk of death from lung cancer is directly related to the number of cigarettes smoked and the age of starting. It is reduced by smoking filter-tipped cigarettes, and pipe and cigar smokers are less at risk—probably because they inhale less. Giving up smoking reduces the risk of death from lung cancer so that after 10 years'

abstinence the risk is little more than in those who have never smoked.

Lung cancer is a preventable disease and its incidence is already falling among doctors, of whom only 20 per cent smoke compared with 50 per cent 20 years ago. If the rest of the community were to cut down to the same extent, death from lung cancer would fall by 80 per cent over the next 20 years.

It must be stressed that one expects exceptions to the rule; e.g. the 90-year-old man who is hale and hearty despite having smoked regularly all his life (Churchill is the most frequently quoted example), and at the other end of the scale is the man who has never smoked in his life but still dies of cancer of the lung. Nevertheless smoking significantly increases the chances of dying from cancer of the lung.

Smoking and chronic bronchitis and emphysema

Over 27,000 people per year die from chronic bronchitis and emphysema in the UK, and smoking is the chief cause of bronchitis though atmospheric pollution and exposure to coal smoke also cause it.

Smokers of filter-tipped cigarettes, pipes and cigars are less affected. Stopping smoking halts further damage to the lungs, but most of the damage already sustained is probably permanent. Severe emphysema, which is the result of the bronchitis, is very uncommon in non-smokers.

Patients with bronchitis have a persistent cough and often find it difficult to 'get up' the phlegm. Cigarette smoke, by irritating the lungs and liquefying the phlegm, makes it easier at the time for the smoker to cough up his phlegm, but in the long term each cigarette increases the damage to the lungs.

Chronic bronchitis causes a slow but progressive deterioration in health with increasing shortness of breath over a period of years until exhaustion occurs with the slightest effort.

Smoking and arterial disease

About 40,000 people between the ages of 35 and 64 die each year from coronary heart disease (heart attacks) in the UK, and almost 10,000 of these deaths could be attributed to smoking. Under the age of 65, smokers are twice, and heavy smokers are three and a half times, as likely to die of a heart attack as non-smokers.

Death rates from coronary artery disease in the population as a whole continue to increase; in only one group—doctors—is the death rate from heart attack falling, as the result of the fall in their consumption of cigarettes.

Pipe smokers and cigar smokers are less at risk, probably because they inhale less. Cigarette smokers who switch and continue to inhale are probably failing to decrease the risk. Diseases of the arteries of the leg which may cause pain in the calf on walking, or even gangrene, are closely related to smoking. If gangrene occurs, amputation may be required. Amputation is rarely performed in non-smokers.

Smoking in pregnancy
The babies of mothers who smoke during pregnancy weigh less on average (0.2 kilogram, 0.5 pound) than those who do not, and babies weighing less than 2.5 kilograms (5.5 pounds) at birth are twice as common in mothers who smoke. This is particularly so when smoking takes place after the fourth month and is related not to reduction in the length of the pregnancy but to retarded growth.

Stillbirths and deaths in the first week of life occur nearly 30 per cent more often in the babies of mothers who smoke regularly after the fourth month of their pregnancy.

Smoking and children
The smoking habit begins early in life. Some children start to smoke when they are 5 and one-third of regular adult smokers began before they were 9 years of age; about 80 per cent of children who smoke regularly continue to do so when they grow up. The earlier one starts to smoke and the longer this continues, the greater the risk to health.

Children are very influenced by others, and if parents or teachers smoke they are more likely to do so. The babies of parents who smoke are more likely to develop pneumonia in the first year of life, which is probably related to the smoky atmosphere in the home.

Harmful contents of cigarettes
The three known harmful components are:
1 *Tar* These compounds produce cancer when applied to the skin and lungs of experimental animals.
2 *Nicotine* Some smokers become dependent on nicotine.
3 *Carbon monoxide* It is absorbed by the blood more readily than oxygen and the oxygen is displaced. It may be this which damages the unborn child and one of many factors causing coronary artery and other blood vessel diseases.

There are also a number of irritant substances in the smoke which narrow the air passages to the lung, and interfere with the normal mechanisms for removing secretions. These effects may predispose to chronic bronchitis and cancer of the lung.

Treatment
Many non-smokers and some doctors adopt a rather unsympathetic attitude to regular smokers because they do not understand that a cigarette smoker may be nearly as dependent on tobacco as a drug addict on his drug.

A regular smoker has only a 20 per cent chance of giving up. There is no more than a 30 per cent success rate at the best smoking withdrawal clinics, and tremendous will power is needed.

The main deterrents to taking up smoking are parental influence and fear of disease; anyone reaching the age of 20 without becoming a smoker is much less likely to smoke. The regular childhood or teenage smoker is very likely to become dependent on tobacco and find it impossible to give up. Determination is the major factor in success.

Some points which may help are:
1 It will not be easy during the first 2–4 weeks and you may feel physically unwell—be prepared for a difficult phase but remember that you will feel better later.
2 Choose a particular day after which you will stop smoking as quickly as you can and prepare yourself mentally for it. The night before D day get rid of all cigarettes.
3 Immediately after D day (especially in the first 2 weeks) avoid stressful or tempting situations, especially drinking alcohol with friends who smoke.
4 If you have occasional lapses, don't give up but do not think you can have the odd cigarette on a special occasion or you may revert.
5 Use the money you save to buy something else regularly; e.g. books, records or something expensive on hire purchase.
6 You must remain determined not to slip back for at least a year (not even a cigar).

Many smokers find it difficult to give up suddenly. For them, the MD4 cigarette holders may be helpful. The MD4 is a package of four cigarette holders, each of which filters the cigarette smoke just a little more than the last so that the smoker receives less and less nicotine. (The MD4 is available at most chemists.)

How to smoke more safely if you can't kick it—ten points to remember:
1 Smoke fewer cigarettes.
2 Switch to a low tar brand—these as a rule have less nicotine.
3 Always smoke filter-tipped cigarettes and preferably those with a 'ventilated' filter, which can be recognized by the ring of perforations around the

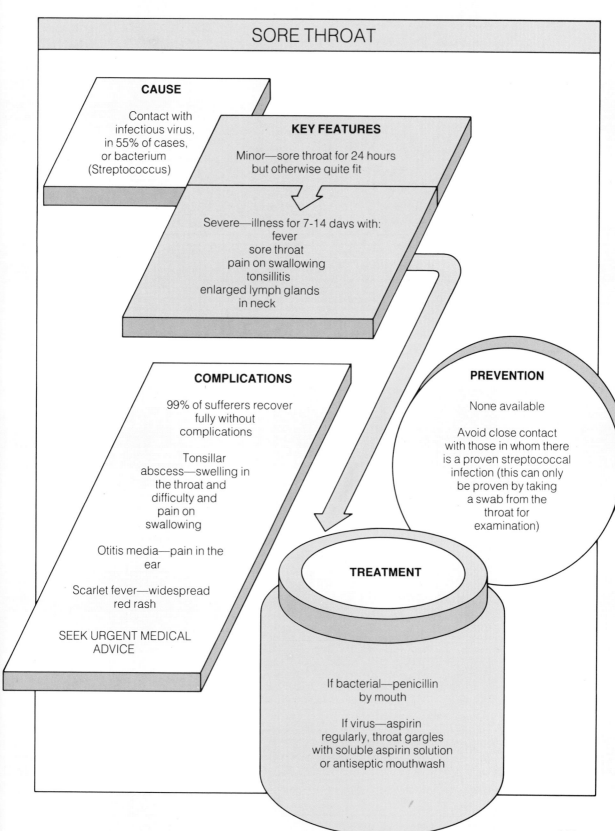

SORE THROAT

CAUSE

Contact with infectious virus, in 55% of cases, or bacterium (Streptococcus)

KEY FEATURES

Minor—sore throat for 24 hours but otherwise quite fit

Severe—illness for 7-14 days with:
fever
sore throat
pain on swallowing
tonsillitis
enlarged lymph glands in neck

COMPLICATIONS

99% of sufferers recover fully without complications

Tonsillar abscess—swelling in the throat and difficulty and pain on swallowing

Otitis media—pain in the ear

Scarlet fever—widespread red rash

SEEK URGENT MEDICAL ADVICE

PREVENTION

None available

Avoid close contact with those in whom there is a proven streptococcal infection (this can only be proven by taking a swab from the throat for examination)

TREATMENT

If bacterial—penicillin by mouth

If virus—aspirin regularly, throat gargles with soluble aspirin solution or antiseptic mouthwash

211

junction of the filter and the tobacco.
4 Do not inhale.
5 Take fewer puffs from each cigarette and leave a larger stub at the end. Most of the damaging tar and nicotine enters the lung during the last one-third of the cigarette.
6 Do not relight a half-finished cigarette.
7 Take the cigarette out of your mouth between puffs.
8 Try using cigarette holders (e.g. MD4, 'Tar Gard').
9 Try to switch to smoking a pipe or cigars (but remember that if you inhale you may not be any better off).
10 Remember, the only safe cigarette is one that is unsmoked.

The various diseases which smoking produces have been discussed and the cumulative effect of all this unnecessary disease is enormous. Apart from the individual suffering, it is estimated that smoking results in about 50 million working days lost in Britain per year. There is also a marked reduction in life expectancy among smokers; on average a smoker shortens his life expectancy by 5½ minutes for every cigarette he smokes, and a regular smoker is twice as likely to die before his 65th birthday.

Snoring

Results from vibration of the tongue against the palate whilst sleeping flat on the back. It never indicates serious illness but may be the cause of considerable disharmony. A gentle nudge will make the snorer roll over, which allows the tongue to drop away from the palate.

Sore throat

Extremely common at all ages, but particularly in the 5–15 year age group. Over 95 per cent are caused by viruses—the same ones which cause colds and influenza. (See chart, page 211.)

The pain may be associated with difficulty in swallowing solids but not liquids though this, too, may be painful. The throat is inflamed and red, and the glands in the neck may enlarge in response to the infection. Aspirin gargles three times daily and aspirin by mouth will reduce the inflammation, pain and fever within 24–48 hours. Further relief may be obtained with ice cream which numbs the throat, and anaesthetic lozenges which are best sucked before meals to decrease the pain of swallowing.

Rarely, sore throats occur with glandular fever (page 111)—when a white covering can be seen over the tonsils and there is gross enlargement of the neck glands—and are occasionally due to bacterial infection (streptococcal throat). It is not possible to distinguish viral sore throats from bacterial, although the vast majority are viral and improve rapidly within 24–36 hours with simple therapy. If not, and particularly in children in whom bacterial sore throats are more serious, medical advice should be obtained.

Earache is associated with sore throats; if it lasts more than 12 hours, particularly in children, the family physician should be consulted as this may be the first sign of middle ear infection (otitis media, page 88).

Spastic children

Spasticity means stiffness and is applied to children who have weak and stiff limbs, usually as the result of brain damage (i.e. cerebral palsy or paralysis). The term is often applied to children with cerebral palsy although not all children with cerebral palsy have spasticity of the muscles.

Cerebral palsy is permanent, non-progressive, brain damage resulting either from infections occurring in the womb (uterus) during development, or from birth injury with or without oxygen deprivation. Brain damage may occur in the first few weeks of life as a result of meningitis, encephalitis or trauma. Cerebral palsy may result in spasticity of the muscles of the arms and legs, which prevents normal movement and causes abnormal postures.

In addition, or alternatively, some children have involuntary movements and unsteadiness, with inco-ordination and poor balance. The involuntary (athetoid) actions are irregular, slow, writhing or rotating movements of the limbs, trunk and face.

Treatment for these children depends on the extent of involvement and whether there is associated mental handicap. The most severely affected require special schooling and residential care with expert physiotherapy, occupational therapy, teaching and nursing facilities. Those less severely handicapped and with normal intelligence should receive a normal education. The Spastics Society continues to give great support to children with all degrees of handicap and actively supports research into the underlying causes of the disorder and the best methods of overcoming it.

Spastic colon

This common condition, usually of young and

middle-aged women, causes a change of bowel habit with intermittent diarrhoea or loose motions and abdominal pain (which is sometimes colicky), usually in the lower left side of the abdomen. The pain may be relieved by defecation. Associated symptoms are common and may include headaches, dizziness, tiredness, loss of concentration, depression and anxiety.

The symptoms of spastic colon are caused by excess muscular activity in the bowel wall. The condition is painful but completely benign and does not progress to more serious disease, and the knowledge of this alone may be sufficient reassurance. Various drugs are used to improve the symptoms, including tranquillizers, anti-spasmodics (e.g. mebeverine, Colofac) and anti-diarrhoeals. Recently the use of regular cereal dietary fibre (e.g. bran) has been very successful in reducing excessive bowel activity.

If there is associated weight loss or if the symptoms persist unrelieved after careful explanation, bran or bulk diets and anti-spasmodics, it may be necessary to investigate in more detail with sigmoidoscopy (page 207) and a barium enema (page 36) in the unlikely event that there may be another bowel disorder present.

Spectacles
SEE GLASSES

Speech and voice disorders

Speech is initiated from the 'speech centre' of the brain, which controls the power of verbal expression. Accurate and clear speech depends upon the normal function of the cells within the brain which control the lungs and larynx, the nerves to the larynx and the muscles which move the vocal cords.

Expression is impaired by damage to the 'speech centre' and commonly follows a brain haemorrhage. Damage to the laryngeal nerves due to the pressure of a tumour within the chest (often a cancer of the lung) may make the voice gruff. Swelling of the vocal cords from a tumour, during acute infection with laryngitis, or in hypothyroidism will make the voice hoarse (*see* Hoarseness *and* Thyroid disease).

Slurred speech
The commonest cause is excess alcohol but strokes and barbiturate poisoning can produce the same effect.

Stutter and stammer
These are caused by poor co-ordination of the complex nerve and muscle interactions needed to produce clear speech. There is no detectable abnormality in the brain, controlling nerves or muscles of the lung or larynx. Stuttering and stammering are made worse by lack of confidence and can be greatly improved or completely overcome by constant practice and parental reassurance.

Sperm count

A test performed during investigation for infertility. The sperm are counted under a microscope, noting the percentage of normal shape and the percentage of sperm which are moving (motile). There is a very wide range of normality, but for chance of conception to be good the count should be: volume of more than 2 millilitres (0.08 fluid ounce) with more than 50 million sperm per millilitre, of which more than 40 per cent should be motile after 4 hours. A smaller number does not definitely mean infertility but it gives a general indication.

Seminal fluid is also collected after vasectomy to ensure that no sperm are present and the operation has been successfully performed.

Spermicidal

Spermicidal preparations are used for contraception. They are prepared as a cream, gel, foam or as vaginal pessaries, and inserted into the vagina prior to intercourse. If used as the only means of contraception the failure rate is high, and they are therefore normally used as an adjunct to barrier methods (i.e. with a sheath or diaphragm).

Spina bifida

A congenital abnormality occurring approximately once in 400 births, which results from failure during development of the vertebral (spine) bones to enclose completely the spinal cord.

In most cases the defect is so small that there is no nerve exposure or damage and the defect can only be detected on x-rays, which show the failure of one or two vertebral bones to completely encircle the spinal cord. These defects are of no consequence and require no treatment. In the most severe instances the nerves have no covering at all and are exposed on the back at the lower end of the spine. As a result, most of the nerves are damaged and there is partial or complete paralysis in the lower limbs, sometimes associated with absent sensation. The nerves to the bladder and rectum may also be damaged, causing loss of control. There is often an associated abnormality in the brain which causes obstruction to the fluid (cerebrospinal fluid) flowing around the brain. As a result, the pressure increases and enlarges the head (hydrocephalus).

Treatment of severe cases is complex and requires specialized neurosurgery. The first aim is to cover the exposed nerves in the back with skin to prevent further damage and infection. If hydrocephalus develops, the pressure is relieved by inserting a drainage tube into the head. Any deformities of the limbs or disorders of bladder function require specialist attention.

Spinal cord

The part of the central nervous system which carries impulses from the peripheral sensory nerves up to the brain, and from the brain down to the motor nerves which move the muscles. The cord is enclosed within a bony spinal column which consists of 24 separate vertebral bones held together by ligaments and the

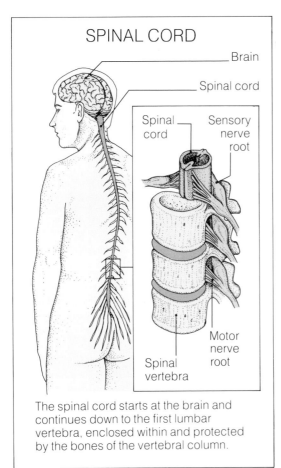

SPINAL CORD

The spinal cord starts at the brain and continues down to the first lumbar vertebra, enclosed within and protected by the bones of the vertebral column.

surrounding muscles. This arrangement gives excellent protection to the spinal cord and still allows the vertebral column to bend.

Spleen

The spleen and lymph glands act to destroy infectious material within the blood stream as it filters through, and are also the site of manufacture of antibodies against infectious organisms.

The spleen sits high up against the diaphragm on the left side of the abdomen, protected by the lower ribs. It enlarges in response to most common infections, and is frequently damaged in road accidents—after which it may have to be removed.

Loss of the spleen is of no consequence except in children who become especially prone to infection with the bacterium *Pneumococcus*. A vaccine is available to immunize children from whom the spleen has been removed.

Spondylosis
(SPONDYLITIS)

The changes which affect the bones of the vertebral column with increasing age. The spinal column carries the entire weight of the body above the pelvis and also allows a great range of movement. The bones and ligaments are protected against jarring and damage by two mechanisms: the spinal column is held in a springy S-shaped arm of strong muscles and between each vertebral body there is a shock absorber, the disc. An intervertebral disc consists of a very tough fibrous ring with a gelatinous substance packed inside. A 'slipped' disc occurs when the central gelatinous material breaks through a defect in the surrounding fibrous bag. After the age of about 20 years the gelatinous material begins to dry out slowly and the disc becomes brittle and inelastic. The vertebral bodies come closer together and this puts more strain on the vertebral bodies which become irregular and develop bony protrusions from their sides. This is spondylosis.

Usually spondylosis causes no symptoms, and the changes of spondylosis are only diagnosed on x-ray. In a few, spondylosis causes neck or back ache and slightly diminished spinal movement.

Occasionally, the bony excrescences press on passing nerves, which gives rise to pain along the nerve; e.g. spondylosis in the neck (cervical spondylosis) causes pain down the arms. Usually the acute pain resolves spontaneously in 2–6 weeks although the bony changes do not improve.

Ankylosing spondylitis

A rare disorder of young men in whom the joints of the pelvis and spine begin to fuse. Pain in the lower back may be severe and movements diminished by the fixed spinal vertebrae. If detected early, pain relief with suitable analgesic drugs and carefully guided physiotherapy will help to reduce the spinal fixation to a large degree and may even prevent any long-term complications.

Sprains

Occur at joints and are due to over-stretching or tearing of the surrounding ligaments and tissue. This produces severe pain, swelling and bruising around the joint. Immediate treatment with a cold compress and taking the weight off the joint will reduce the swelling. In severe sprains, immobilization of the joint with firm supporting bandages will ease the pain. An x-ray may be required to exclude the possibility of an underlying fracture. If a complete tear has occurred, the joint can be rested in a plaster cast, to allow the tear to heal spontaneously.

Rarely, a tear may leave a joint unstable and this may have to be corrected surgically.

Sputum

Phlegm coughed up from the lungs, and its presence means that the amount of secretion normally produced by the respiratory tract—the trachea and bronchi—is excessive.

Its consistency and colour vary according to the cause. Thick green and yellow sputum indicates an infection in the lungs (e.g. acute bronchitis). Thin clear frothy sputum may be coughed up if there is increased fluid in the lungs; this is often associated with shortness of breath, especially at night time when lying flat. It is due to fluid accumulation in the lung as a result of inefficient contraction of the heart, and treatment with water-losing (diuretic) tablets is usually effective.

Occasionally blood may be coughed up alone or mixed with sputum. Although the commonest cause of this is chronic bronchitis, coughing up blood is understandably very worrying, and medical advice should always be sought.

Squint

In children

The eyes look in different directions. Early detection is very important to prevent the development of a lazy eye. In children less than 8 years the image from a squinting eye will be suppressed by the brain and this can give rise to a lazy eye—i.e. the child will only see through the non-squinting eye (uni-ocular vision). When suppression continues beyond the age of 8, the area of the brain which receives sensory stimuli from the squinting eye will no longer function, and the squinting eye is effectively blind although the eye itself is normal.

Squints may be obvious during the first few months of life, but may be more difficult to detect as they appear intermittently and become apparent only during an acute infection such as measles.

The earlier treatment is started the better the outlook. Initially, the good eye is covered to make the squinting eye work harder. In many children, whose squint develops between the ages of 2 and 4 years, there is associated long sightedness and correction of this may reduce the squint. An operation may be necessary to realign the squinting eye, and also for cosmetic reasons to prevent the obvious embarrassment and ridicule of children growing up with a squint.

In adults

Squint or double vision in adults with previously normal vision usually indicates damage to one of the muscles controlling the eye, and should be reported to a doctor as a matter of urgency.

Stammer
SEE SPEECH AND VOICE DISORDERS

Starch

The major source of dietary carbohydrate, it is present in cereals, potatoes, legumes and other vegetables. Starch is a polysaccharide—i.e. it contains hundreds of smaller glucose molecules joined together; it is digested into separate glucose molecules by intestinal enzymes and the small glucose units can then be absorbed into the blood.

Sterilization

Female sterilization is achieved by occluding the Fallopian tubes. This prevents the passage of the egg (ovum) from the ovary to the womb (uterus). The operation is usually performed through a laparoscope (a flexible tube with fibre-optic light source through which slender instruments can be passed under direct vision). The laparoscope is inserted via a small incision below the umbilicus. Inert gas is inserted into the abdomen to allow more space and visibility; once the Fallopian tubes have been visualized, clips are applied. The procedure is usually performed under a general anaesthetic.

Male sterilization, or vasectomy (page 241), is a simpler procedure performed with either local or general anaesthetic. A small incision is made in each side at the top of the scrotum, and the tubes carrying sperm from the testes to the penis (the vasa deferentia) are cut and tied. Three specimens of seminal fluid are collected subsequently to ensure the absence of sperm.

Sterilization is a permanent procedure. It is usually without side-effects although it is not always possible to predict later psychological effects.

Steroids
(STRICTLY, CORTICOSTEROIDS)

A group of chemically related hormones secreted into the blood stream, principally by the adrenal glands. These hormones are essential for normal life, and regulate salt balance and blood pressure, and the utilization of glucose as a source of energy. Absence of these hormones causes muscular weakness and a reduced resistance to infection.

Steroids are now made synthetically for use in certain illnesses, and are given in the form of tablets (e.g. prednisolone, prednisone, cortisone, fludrocortisone), injection (hydrocortisone), inhaler (beclomethasone, Becotide) or cream (topical steroids) to be applied to the skin. Steroid treatment is used to control severe allergic reactions (e.g. asthma). They are also used to suppress inflammatory disorders such as rheumatoid arthritis and ulcerative colitis.

The long-term use of steroids, unless given in small doses as replacement therapy for Addison's disease (a rare disorder of adrenal insufficiency) may produce unwanted effects which must be balanced against the severity of the original illness. These effects can be partly avoided by using intermittent short courses of steroids. The unwanted effects are weight gain, diabetes mellitus, raised blood pressure, acne, muscle wasting, bruising, thinning of bones, and increased risk of stomach ulcers. Another potential danger is suppression of the normal production of steroids by the adrenals. Return of normal production may take some time, and for this reason steroids should never be stopped abruptly. A 'steroid card' should always be carried, indicating

dosage and duration of treatment because an increased dose is required with accidents, surgery, and other illnesses. They do not occur if the daily dose is small or with long-term inhaler therapy in asthma.

Topical steroids are used to treat eczema and dermatitis. There are many available preparations of varying potency, and they are prepared either as creams or ointments. Long-term topical treatment, especially with the more potent preparations, may cause thinning of the skin, increased visibility of underlying blood vessels which may be pronounced on the face, stretch marks, easy bruising and even adrenal gland suppression following absorption into the blood stream.

Steroids are used only for serious diseases and require expert monitoring throughout treatment. They should be used only with medical guidance.

Stings

Bees leave their sting in the skin. The sting should be removed, and because the sting is alkaline a weak acid such as vinegar may be applied. A local antihistamine cream may reduce the inflammation if used immediately.

Wasps generally do not leave their sting behind, although they do so later in the 'season'. The stings are acid and a weak alkali such as bicarbonate of soda can be applied.

Occasionally stings cause a severe allergic reaction with puffiness of face and neck and swelling of the throat. This constitutes a medical emergency and immediate help should be sought because the symptoms can be relieved by an injection of adrenaline, which all family physicians carry.

Stomach

Part of the digestive system (*see* diagram, page 265) in which swallowed food is mixed by the muscular contractions of the stomach wall and also partially digested by the pepsin and strong hydrochloric acid normally secreted by the cells lining its wall.

Stomach ache
SEE ABDOMINAL PAIN

Stomach ulcer
(GASTRIC ULCER; PEPTIC ULCER)

Ulcers commonly occur in the stomach or in the duodenum, and 1 in 5 men and 1 in 10 women will probably develop an ulcer during their lives. Smoking cigarettes and psychological stress probably do not cause ulcers although they may delay healing in an established one. Likewise, moderate alcohol intake does not predispose to ulcer development.

Stomach ulcers produce pain in the middle of the upper abdomen, and the site can often be localized by pointing. The pain is gnawing or burning in character and is relieved by milk, food and alkalis, and tends to come and go over 2–7 days with pain-free periods of 2 weeks to 2 months in between attacks. There may be associated vomiting. The severity of the pain does not relate to the size of the ulcer nor does it imply that it is about to burst.

Treatment involves avoiding spicy foods and alcohol during episodes of pain, stopping smoking, and taking antacids and specific drugs to heal the ulcers. Antacids are taken in the form of alkaline mixtures (aluminium hydroxide, magnesium trisilicate) and they act by neutralizing acid secretions in the stomach to relieve pain. More specific drugs include carbenoxolone (Biogastrone) which is related to liquorice and promotes ulcer healing. A newer drug, cimetidine (Tagamet), acts by preventing acid secretion from the stomach. This improves healing, but, as with carbenoxolone, relapse may occur after discontinuation of treatment. When medical treatment fails, or the symptoms are persistent, recurrent and disabling, surgical treatment should be carefully considered.

Stomatitis

Small shallow ulcers or sores in the mouth and on the tongue. Commonly viruses infect the delicate lining of the mouth which becomes ulcerated and very painful. The ulcers normally resolve spontaneously within about 10 days and the condition is harmless albeit extremely unpleasant. It is often recurrent. (*See* Mouth ulcers.)

Strangulated hernia

A hernia results from muscular weakness in the abdominal wall, allowing abdominal contents (i.e. bowel or intestines) to pass through the defect, giving rise to swelling under the skin. The most common site is in the groin (inguinal hernia). Occasionally when the defect is small the blood supply to the intestine within the hernia is occluded—or 'strangulated'—

leading to gangrene if left untreated. The earliest symptom of strangulated hernia is severe pain in the hernia. This eventually leads to generalized abdominal pain and tenderness. Surgery is essential to reduce the hernia and, if necessary, remove any gangrenous bowel.

Strawberry birthmark
SEE BIRTHMARK

★Stroke
(CEREBROVASCULAR ACCIDENT)

Caused either by obstruction to a blood vessel supplying part of the brain (cerebral thrombosis) or by bleeding into the brain (cerebral haemorrhage).

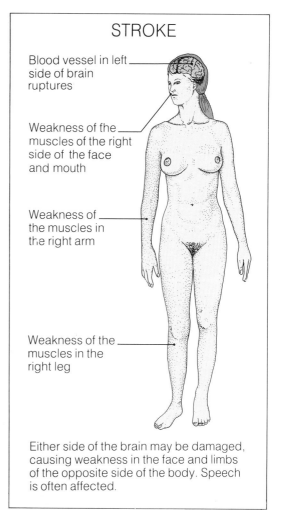

STROKE

Blood vessel in left side of brain ruptures

Weakness of the muscles of the right side of the face and mouth

Weakness of the muscles in the right arm

Weakness of the muscles in the right leg

Either side of the brain may be damaged, causing weakness in the face and limbs of the opposite side of the body. Speech is often affected.

The affected area of brain is destroyed and the functions controlled by that part of the brain cease. Commonly this results in paralysis or partial paralysis of an arm and leg on the other side of the body. This may be associated with loss of sensation as well as weakness, and the arm and leg feel numb.

Other functions which may be lost include speech and vision. Loss of speech is due to an inability of the brain to express thoughts in words; i.e. the patient knows what he wants to say but cannot do so despite a normal speaking apparatus. The inability to converse often gives the impression that understanding is lost. There may be loss of vision to the side of the paralysis but visual loss is fortunately not complete.

Recovery following strokes is variable. Return of function is most marked in the first few weeks, but improvement can occur up to 1 year later.

Skilled physiotherapy and occupational therapy will aid a return to physical independence by strengthening muscles to take over lost function and by teaching the use of physical aids in the home. Many patients who have suffered severe strokes are able to develop new skills and, despite some physical restriction, lead a very full life.

There is a definite correlation between raised blood pressure and an increased incidence of strokes, and earlier detection and control of blood pressure should reduce the number of strokes.

Stutter
SEE SPEECH AND VOICE DISORDERS

Stye

A small boil in the skin of the eyelid. This infection occurs at the base of the lash at the lid margin, causing local pain, redness and swelling. Styes usually settle spontaneously after a few days after discharging a small bead of pus. Bathing with warm water and mild pain-relieving drugs (paracetamol, aspirin) lessen the pain but do not speed healing.

Subnormality
(MENTAL HANDICAP)

Mental subnormality may be divided into two categories. The first includes those severely handicapped to such an extent that they are unable to lead an independent existence. Their intelligence quotient (IQ) is usually less than 50 and there are often physical handicaps. The second group, the

mildly subnormal, can be as independent as normal adults, and physical handicaps are uncommon.

A common cause is Down's syndrome (mongolism) which is due to a chromosome abnormality. Rubella (German measles) infection during early pregnancy may be associated with subnormality, which is also more likely to occur when there is a family history of mental handicap, if there is severe breathing difficulty at birth and if birth is premature. Severe infections (e.g. meningitis), and severe head injury soon after birth predispose to subnormality.

Warning signs are often present during the first year of life when the four main fields of development (posture and movement, vision and manipulation, hearing and speech, and social behaviour) are retarded. Lack of interest in the surroundings, poor responsiveness and poor concentration are important features, and posture and movement are least affected unless there is associated physical handicap.

The child who is subnormal may be perfectly contented. However, the difficulties for the parents both in emotional and financial terms may be very great, and the families need great understanding from the doctors and the social services.

Sudden infant death syndrome
SEE COT DEATH

Suicide

The third most common cause of death in the 15–45 year age group in England and Wales, and accounts for one-third of all deaths in students. There has been a decrease in successful suicides from 12 per 100,000 in 1960 to 8 per 100,000 in 1980, but there has been an increase in suicide attempts which approximate to 50,000 a year.

Death by suicide is more common in older males, particularly if they are physically ill, divorced, separated, widowed or living alone. There is often a previous history of mental illness (depression 70 per cent, and alcoholism 15 per cent). The method of suicide is often an active one, such as drowning or shooting. Over half of the successful suicides have spoken about it and most have visited their family doctors shortly beforehand.

Those who fail in their suicide attempts have different characteristics, and are more likely to be females in their twenties. The attempt often follows a precipitating event and the method used is usually a drug overdose.

Often, a suicide attempt in response to a recent

problem can be fairly easily managed by the patient and his/her medical and psychiatric advisers. However, any attempt must be taken seriously, and a careful assessment of the individual patient's mood, response and mental state must be made quickly—though not hurriedly—as longer term psychiatric support may be required.

Sunstroke

A rare but dangerous medical emergency. It usually occurs during physical activity in an unaccustomed hot climate. The normal body-temperature-control mechanisms are unable to cope, resulting in unconsciousness, rapid pulse, raised temperature—40°C (104°F) or higher—and hot flushed skin. This leads to shock and death unless vigorous treatment by cooling is begun.

More common and less severe is fainting after excessive exercise in the heat. The skin is cool, sweaty and pale, and recovery is rapid after removal from the heat and on lying down for a short time.

See also Heat stroke.

Suppository

A drug preparation which is inserted and allowed to dissolve in the rectum (or, less commonly, the vagina). Suppositories are commonly used to treat constipation, the pain of haemorrhoids or vaginal infections. Suppositories for the vagina are usually known as pessaries.

Swallowing difficulty

Swallowing is co-ordinated from a group of nerves in the mid-brain. Disorders of this area of the brain or the nerves which send information to the oesophageal muscles cause difficulty in swallowing. This may occur in multiple sclerosis, poliomyelitis or following a severe stroke.

Difficulty in swallowing is usually associated with the feeling of a lump in the throat and a choking sensation. This may be an expression of an underlying anxiety state, often due to the fear of cancer. Difficulty in swallowing from obstruction in the gullet (oesophagus) gives the sensation of food sticking in the chest behind the sternum and is associated with pain and regurgitation of food.

There are a number of causes of mechanical obstruction. Acid reflux (*see* Hiatus hernia) from the stomach may cause local scarring and narrowing. A

valve system normally operates at the junction of the oesophagus and stomach, and this prevents the acid stomach secretions flowing back into the oesophagus. When the valve is incompetent, the acid irritates the oesophagus, initially causing heartburn; persistent irritation leads to scarring and narrowing (strictures). Severe peptic strictures may be stretched (under general anaesthetic) with dilators of increasing size. Sometimes in the older age group difficulty in swallowing may be due to a tumour.

Oesophageal strictures may occur in children following the accidental ingestion of a corrosive agent (e.g. cleaning solution, Domestos). The fluid burns the lining of the oesophagus, and this is followed by scarring and narrowing.

The inability to swallow is most uncomfortable. In most people the cause is never found and it settles without any treatment. However, it is important to ensure that no serious underlying disease is present and medical advice should be obtained.

Sweating

There are two types of sweat gland found in man: the eccrine and the apocrine. The eccrine glands are widely distributed in the skin and respond to body heat, exercise, stress and anxiety. Heat is removed from the body by evaporation of the sweat, and this helps to reduce body temperature during acute infections and in hot climates. The apocrine glands are present in the groins and armpits, and produce a distinctive odour of considerable importance in lower animals. (Some odour is caused by chemicals called pheromones, which are believed to be important stimuli to sexual attraction.)

Occasionally, the apocrine glands in man produce excess secretion—and social embarrassment. There is no cure but frequent washing, and antiperspirant/deodorants usually control the unpleasant odour.

Syphilis

An infectious disease spread by sexual contact (venereal disease), which is increasing in frequency throughout the world. The infection is caused by the organism *Treponema pallidum*, which gains entry into the blood stream through a mucous membrane—usually the genital skin. After 2–6 weeks an ulcer or a sore develops at this site. In males the sore is usually on the penis, and in females on the external genital skin or cervix. The sore may be found at other sites on the body, such as the lips, throat, fingers and anus.

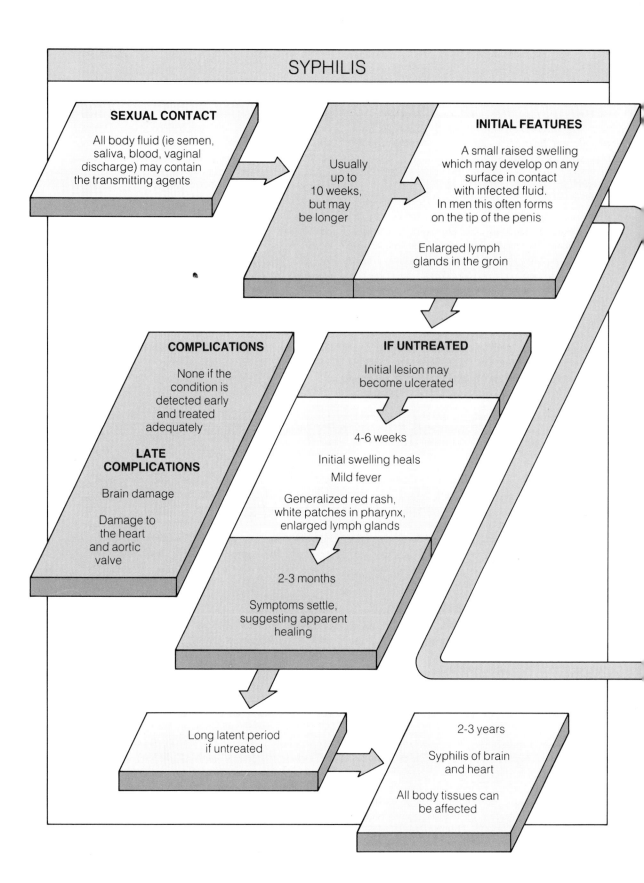

SYPHILIS

SEXUAL CONTACT

All body fluid (ie semen, saliva, blood, vaginal discharge) may contain the transmitting agents

Usually up to 10 weeks, but may be longer

INITIAL FEATURES

A small raised swelling which may develop on any surface in contact with infected fluid. In men this often forms on the tip of the penis

Enlarged lymph glands in the groin

COMPLICATIONS

None if the condition is detected early and treated adequately

LATE COMPLICATIONS

Brain damage

Damage to the heart and aortic valve

IF UNTREATED

Initial lesion may become ulcerated

4-6 weeks

Initial swelling heals

Mild fever

Generalized red rash, white patches in pharynx, enlarged lymph glands

2-3 months

Symptoms settle, suggesting apparent healing

Long latent period if untreated

2-3 years

Syphilis of brain and heart

All body tissues can be affected

T

The sore disappears without treatment, and a few weeks or months after the initial infection a generalized skin rash develops which covers the whole of the body, including the palms, soles and scalp. This also resolves spontaneously and without treatment but the parasites remain in the body and eventually produce the symptoms of late syphilis, with damage to the brain, heart and main blood vessels.

If a woman has syphilis while pregnant the baby will be infected during development, causing teeth deformities, deafness and sometimes brain damage.

Syphilis is treated with penicillin given by injection. The earlier treatment is started the better the chance of cure and the lower the likelihood of serious late complications. Contacts must be carefully examined and treated if infected.

TAB

The vaccine used to immunize travellers against typhoid and paratyphoid A and B (*see* Vaccination). It is advisable to be vaccinated well before leaving because TAB sometimes causes illness similar to mild influenza, lasting for 1–4 days.

Talipes
SEE CLUB FOOT

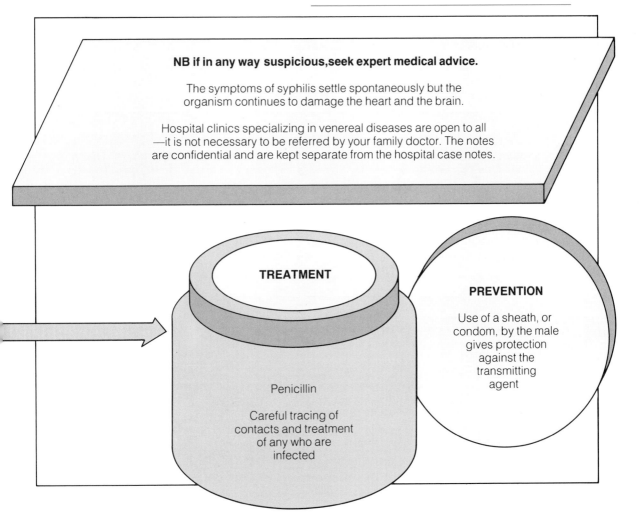

NB if in any way suspicious, seek expert medical advice.

The symptoms of syphilis settle spontaneously but the organism continues to damage the heart and the brain.

Hospital clinics specializing in venereal diseases are open to all —it is not necessary to be referred by your family doctor. The notes are confidential and are kept separate from the hospital case notes.

TREATMENT

Penicillin

Careful tracing of contacts and treatment of any who are infected

PREVENTION

Use of a sheath, or condom, by the male gives protection against the transmitting agent

Tantrum

Temper tantrums in children are very common and are experienced by most families at least once. Probably the best approach is to ignore the child during the tantrum and not to let him have his own way. It is difficult to leave a room with a child screaming and rolling about but it is the simplest way to deflate the situation. Tantrums usually reflect jealousy of a brother or sister or a feeling of unfair treatment. Less commonly they indicate underlying discontent or problems within the family unit. Whatever the cause, tantrums will continue if they attract too much attention or if the child succeeds in manipulating the situation to his advantage. (*See also* Breath-holding attacks.)

Teeth

SEE FLUORIDES; TEETH DEVELOPMENT IN CHILDREN (PAGE 290); *AND* TOOTHACHE

Tennis elbow

This painful condition of the elbow results from tears of the muscle attachment at the elbow. Typically there is an area of tenderness just below the bony prominence on the outer side of the elbow. With time the pain disappears, but if it persists it can be relieved by an injection of hydrocortisone and local anaesthetic into the painful spot. Although common in tennis players, any activity which puts strain on the muscle attachments will give the same symptoms.

Testes
(TESTICLES)

The male sex glands. They produce sperm (spermatozoa) which pass via the seminal tubules to the penile urethra and are ejaculated into the vagina at sexual intercourse.

The sperm have a tail which propels them through the central canal of the cervix into the womb (uterus) and on to the Fallopian tubes to fertilize the female egg (ovum). A normal man produces 2–5 millilitres of seminal fluid in each ejaculate containing about 50 million sperm per millilitre.

The testes also produce the hormone testosterone, which controls the development of the male characteristics of body structure, depth of voice and growth of beard.

See also Orchitis.

Tetanus

Caused by a bacterium (*Clostridium tetani*) which is present in soil. Most people are protected against tetanus by routine active immunization during childhood. Those at most risk work in outdoor occupations such as gardening, farming or outdoor sports and athletics, and they should keep their immunization up to date.

Tetanus develops in dirty wounds, especially when they have not been cleaned and dressed properly. The bacteria multiply in the wound and produce a poison (toxin) which spreads along nerves and in the blood to the rest of the body. The toxin causes muscular spasm typically starting in the jaw, which becomes fixed and clenched; i.e. lockjaw or risus sardonicus (sardonic smile). The muscular spasms spread to the rest of the body, interfering with breathing and other essential functions. Although the introduction of Intensive Care Units has greatly improved the outlook for patients with tetanus, the

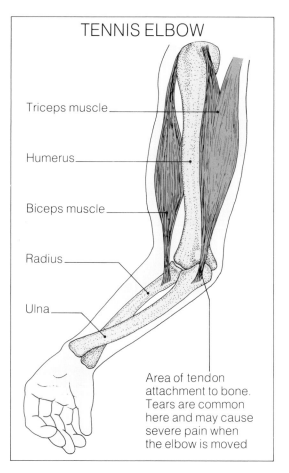

TENNIS ELBOW

Triceps muscle

Humerus

Biceps muscle

Radius

Ulna

Area of tendon attachment to bone. Tears are common here and may cause severe pain when the elbow is moved

illness is potentially fatal—especially in the elderly and very young. It is therefore important to ensure that all injuries sustained in the garden, at sport or on the road should be treated properly by careful washing with soap and water. Immunity to tetanus should always be kept up to date by booster injection and repeated every 5–10 years.

Thalassaemia

An inherited disorder which occurs in peoples originating from south-east Asia and around the Mediterranean. They make an abnormal haemoglobin, the oxygen-carrying protein within the red blood cells, which makes these cells less stable and causes anaemia (see Anaemia).

Thiamine
(VITAMIN B₁)   *SEE UNDER* VITAMINS

Thirst

Thirst due to dehydration is stimulated by dryness of the mouth and also from a specialized group of cells in the brain (the thirst centre) where hydration of the body is monitored. A deficit in body fluid activates the centre, creating the sensation of thirst. The greater intelligence and highly developed social behaviour of humans adds another dimension to the monitoring of hydration, and a regular beer drinker is able to consume many pints of beer in the absence of any thirst.

Persistent severe thirst (polydipsia), particularly if associated with an increase in urine output and weight loss, suggests the presence of diabetes (page 78). Sugar in the urine draws water out of the body via the kidneys, which causes the dehydration of diabetes.

Another but very rare cause for excessive fluid loss from the kidneys is deficiency of a pituitary hormone (the 'anti-diuretic hormone') which retains water filtered from the blood by the kidneys. This occasionally follows head injury, and spontaneous recovery can occur in the following months. It is treated by replacement therapy using lypressin.

In psychogenic polydipsia, excess thirst and drinking occurs for psychological reasons and not because of excess urine loss.

Persistent thirst may indicate diabetes or excess fluid loss from diseased kidneys, and these should be excluded by careful clinical investigation.

Thrombosis

The formation of a blood clot inside a blood vessel (artery or vein). Thromboses usually occur in three sites in the body: the heart (coronary thrombosis—see Heart attack), the brain (cerebral thrombosis—see Stroke) and the leg. The last occurs in one of the deep veins of the legs and hence is termed a deep vein thrombosis (DVT).

DVT is a common complication of immobilization in bed. It is commoner after a surgical operation in the elderly and the overweight. Women on the contraceptive pill may be at risk during surgery, and the surgeon should be informed so that special precautions can be taken. A clot forms in the vein and obstructs the return of blood to the heart. This results in swelling of the calf with pain and tenderness.

The leg is elevated to reduce the swelling, and sometimes supported by an elastic stocking. Anticoagulant tablets may be given to prevent the clot becoming larger. The dose must be very carefully controlled by frequent blood tests. A DVT is not itself serious but part of the clot may become free and pass upward in the blood stream to the heart and onwards into the lungs (pulmonary embolus, page 190). This produces central chest pain and sudden shortness of breath.

Weight reduction prior to surgery and early mobilization after an illness or operation are important preventive measures for patients at particular risk. A short course of injections of heparin (an anticoagulant) over the period of surgery is sometimes used to prevent a DVT. Once a DVT has occurred, it is an absolute contra-indication to taking the oral contraceptive pill, as this predisposes to further clot formation in susceptible women.

Thrush

A yeast infection known also as candidiasis or moniliasis. The yeast (*Candida albicans*) is present on the skin of normal people. Infection occurs when the organism starts to multiply, and this is most likely in individuals with a decreased resistance to infection such as babies and the elderly, the very ill and diabetics. Candidiasis may also occur in pregnant women and those taking the oral contraceptive pill, and in people taking steroid drugs or antibiotics.

Oral candidiasis appears as white spots on the tongue and inside of the cheeks, and, in babies, must not be confused with spots of milk left in the mouth after a feed. Occasionally a nappy rash is due to *Candida*. Medical advice should be sought when oral candidiasis is suspected. Candidiasis improves rapidly with anti-fungal agents (e.g. nystatin). When a nappy rash does not respond to the usual care with barrier creams and frequent nappy changes, or is severe, advice may be obtained at a Well Baby Clinic or from the family physician. If candidiasis is diagnosed, an anti-fungal cream will be prescribed.

A common site of infection in adults is the genital area. In women this causes an irritant vaginal discharge (*see* Vaginal discharge), and men may suffer from an irritant rash on the end of the penis. These respond to anti-fungal preparations.

In the elderly and obese, thrush may occur in damp skin folds where two skin surfaces are in contact, such as under pendulous breasts and between rolls of fat. Prolonged immersion of the hands in water predisposes to nail fold infections (*see* Whitlow). These infections are prevented by frequent washing and keeping the skin dry with talcum powders, and by using protective gloves.

Thumb sucking

A habit of nearly all normal children, who grow out of it—usually by the age of 3 or 4. It is harmless.

Thyroid disease

The thyroid gland is situated in front and either side of the wind pipe (the trachea) in the neck. It produces the thyroid hormones, including thyroxine, which regulate the metabolic rate of the body. An increase in the production of thyroid hormone increases the rate at which the body works. Thyroid disease occurs when the thyroid gland is either over-active or under-active.

Over-activity of the thyroid, when excess thyroxine is produced, is called thyrotoxicosis or hyperthyroidism. Like bellows to a fire, this makes the body burn energy faster. The patient's weight falls despite an increased appetite, the pulse speeds up, and there is a feeling of warmth at all times, restlessness and a tremor of the hands. Sometimes this is associated with protuberant staring eyes and a swelling of the gland. Treatment depends on the severity of the illness and the age of the patient. Anti-thyroid tablets (e.g. carbimazole) are frequently used to block the formation of excess thyroid. Alternatively, part of the gland can be removed surgically. In older patients a minute dose of radioactive iodine can be taken by mouth, and this, selectively taken up into the thyroid gland, suppresses the activity of the cells.

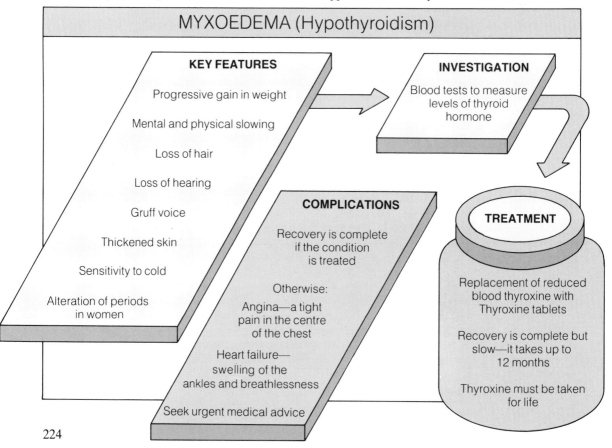

MYXOEDEMA (Hypothyroidism)

KEY FEATURES

Progressive gain in weight

Mental and physical slowing

Loss of hair

Loss of hearing

Gruff voice

Thickened skin

Sensitivity to cold

Alteration of periods in women

INVESTIGATION

Blood tests to measure levels of thyroid hormone

COMPLICATIONS

Recovery is complete if the condition is treated

Otherwise:

Angina—a tight pain in the centre of the chest

Heart failure—swelling of the ankles and breathlessness

Seek urgent medical advice

TREATMENT

Replacement of reduced blood thyroxine with Thyroxine tablets

Recovery is complete but slow—it takes up to 12 months

Thyroxine must be taken for life

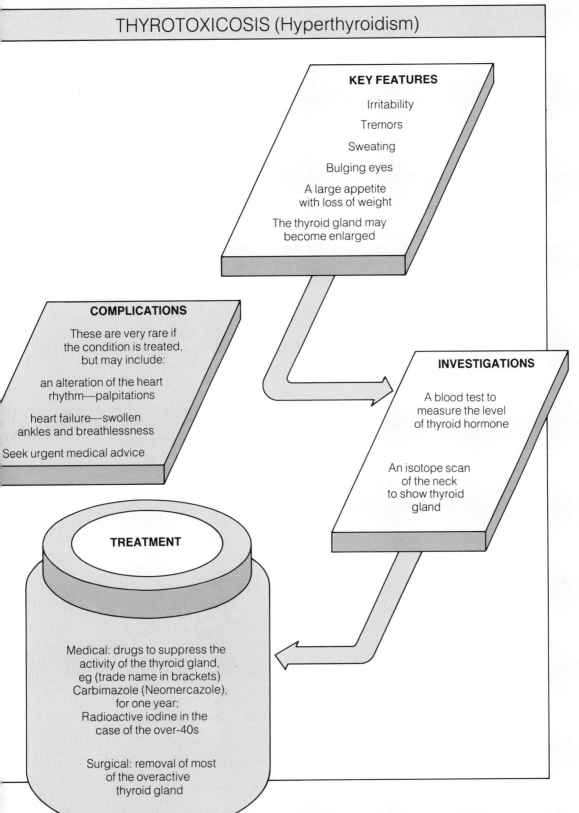

THYROTOXICOSIS (Hyperthyroidism)

KEY FEATURES

Irritability

Tremors

Sweating

Bulging eyes

A large appetite
with loss of weight

The thyroid gland may
become enlarged

COMPLICATIONS

These are very rare if
the condition is treated,
but may include:

an alteration of the heart
rhythm—palpitations

heart failure—swollen
ankles and breathlessness

Seek urgent medical advice

INVESTIGATIONS

A blood test to
measure the level
of thyroid hormone

An isotope scan
of the neck
to show thyroid
gland

TREATMENT

Medical: drugs to suppress the
activity of the thyroid gland,
eg (trade name in brackets)
Carbimazole (Neomercazole),
for one year;
Radioactive iodine in the
case of the over-40s

Surgical: removal of most
of the overactive
thyroid gland

Under-activity of the thyroid gland is called hypothyroidism or myxoedema. Insufficient thyroid hormone results in a general slowing down. Weight increases, the pulse slows, and there is intolerance to cold and mental slowing. The voice becomes gruff, the face filled out, yellow and pale, with straggling hair and the skin dry. As with thyrotoxicosis, a swelling or goitre may be present. Treatment is very simple with between one and three thyroxine tablets daily. The dose varies from individual to individual but must be continued for life. Because this is the natural body hormone, once the dose is correct, there are no side-effects or risks.

Swellings of the thyroid (goitres, page 114) occur with over- or under-activity of the gland. They may also slowly develop even when the thyroid is producing the correct amount of hormone. A goitre is not serious but may be unsightly; rarely, it may grow to a very large size and cause pressure on the trachea or oesophagus. For these reasons the gland may have to be removed surgically.

Some thyroid swellings may be due to cancer but this is very rare and very amenable to treatment. For this reason, early medical advice should be sought by anyone in whom a thyroid swelling develops, irrespective of whether or not they feel unwell.

Tibia

The shin bone (*see* diagram, page 259). It is the larger of the two bones between the knee and the ankle, and takes nearly all the weight. The smaller bone, the fibula, lying alongside, forms a part of the ankle joint but not part of the knee. The two bones are held together by a thin strong fibrous sheet and the surrounding muscles.

Tic

SEE TWITCHING EYELIDS

Tongue

The tongue is frequently examined but rarely gives useful clinical information. Most changes are due to eating and drinking different foods, and are of no consequence. These include whitening and furring of the tongue, 'geographical tongue' and darkening at the back of the tongue.

Whitening and furring of the tongue is due to thickened skin which results from soft milky diets and is also common in smokers.

Geographical tongue describes a tongue which looks like a map. This is due to shedding of irregular groups of cells, leaving 'islands' of thickened cells behind. The cause is not known, but it does not indicate general ill health nor is it really a 'disease'.

Darkening of the back of the tongue is due to brown colouring of the taste buds, or rarely to a fungal infection but this can only be confirmed by removing the fungus by scraping the tongue and examining the scrapings with a microscope.

The main value of inspecting the tongue is to assess dehydration, when the tongue quickly loses its glistening moist appearance.

A tongue which is sore and appears bright red and smooth may signal severe anaemia due to lack of iron or vitamins (*see* Anaemia).

Localized soreness is caused by ulcers. Small ulcers are common, and come and go causing few problems. Recurrent ulcers result from bad teeth when the tongue continually rubs against a roughened tooth or worn denture and becomes sore and ulcerated. When an ulcer persists for more than 2 weeks or increases in size, medical advice should be obtained.

Tonsillectomy

The tonsils and adenoids are lymph glands (page 147) which drain infection from the throat and pharynx. Removal of the tonsils (tonsillectomy) and adenoids is still one of the most commonly performed operations, for which the major indication is recurrent tonsillitis (*see below*).

Many ear, nose and throat (ENT) specialists now agree that tonsils have often been removed unnecessarily. Recurrent tonsillitis is a genuine problem in the young school child, but most children grow out of it by about 10 years of age. All children develop sore throats and may have large tonsils. Neither is a reason to remove the tonsils. Operation is very occasionally necessary if a child has recurrent sore throats with severe fever and illness.

The adenoids are usually removed at the same time as the tonsils, to prevent recurrent ear infections (otitis media, page 88). The adenoids are situated above the tonsils in the back of the nasal cavity and their enlargement blocks the 'drainage' from the ear, down the Eustachian tube to the nose, and predisposes to ear infection.

Tonsillitis

Infection of the tonsils, resulting in a sore throat. The tonsils appear red and inflamed.

The majority of infections are caused by the viruses which usually cause colds. A few are due to a

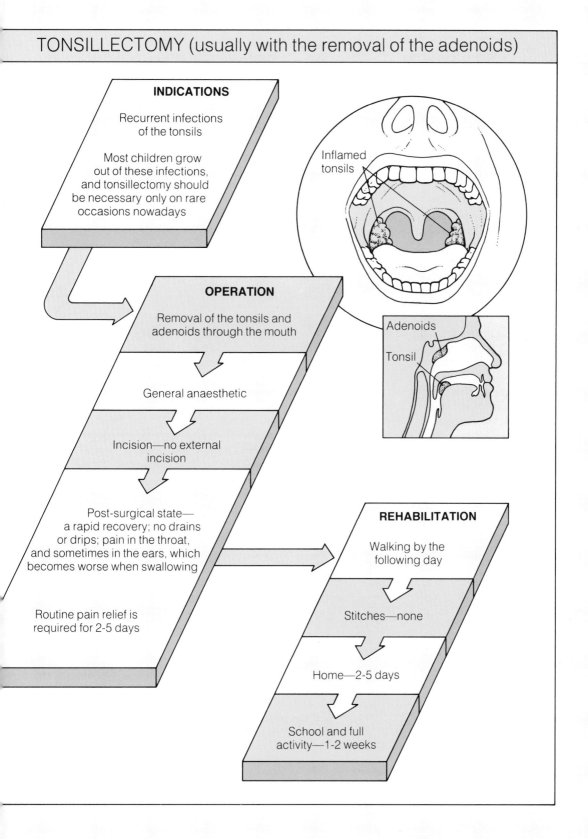

TONSILLECTOMY (usually with the removal of the adenoids)

INDICATIONS

Recurrent infections of the tonsils

Most children grow out of these infections, and tonsillectomy should be necessary only on rare occasions nowadays

Inflamed tonsils

Adenoids

Tonsil

OPERATION

Removal of the tonsils and adenoids through the mouth

General anaesthetic

Incision—no external incision

Post-surgical state— a rapid recovery; no drains or drips; pain in the throat, and sometimes in the ears, which becomes worse when swallowing

Routine pain relief is required for 2-5 days

REHABILITATION

Walking by the following day

Stitches—none

Home—2-5 days

School and full activity—1-2 weeks

bacterial infection, which responds to penicillin. Rarely, bacterial infection of the tonsil results in the formation of a large collection of pus. This peritonsillar abscess—also termed a 'quinsy'—may be sufficiently large in small children to obstruct swallowing or breathing. Quinsies usually respond to injected penicillin, but may have to be drained if they obstruct the posterior pharynx.

In the teenager, glandular fever ('kissing disease', page 111) is a possible cause of tonsillitis.

Toothache

The commonest cause is caries of the soft tooth pulp and irritation of the sensitive nerves in the pulp base. Careful dental examination to confirm the cause, removal of the damaged infected tissue and refilling of the cavity comprise the best way to relieve pain, unless the damage is so extensive that the tooth has to be removed.

If a dentist is not available, some relief may be obtained by placing a warm compress against the jaw in the region of the tooth and taking pain-killers (analgesics) such as aspirin or paracetamol. Local drops containing oil of cloves may also help. Failing this, a stiff alcoholic drink will help.

Dental abscesses at the root of the teeth are less common. They produce tender swellings which may appear to involve the entire jaw. Antibiotics are required, usually penicillin to which most mouth bacteria are sensitive, and the abscess may have to be drained. The diagnosis can be difficult for the inexperienced to confirm, and therapy should be planned by an experienced dentist.

Wisdom teeth are the back molars, which erupt late, but sometimes fail to do so, or press against and crowd the other nearby teeth. They can be left alone if they cause no trouble, but, if painful, can be removed. This requires a full anaesthetic and a hospital stay of 2–4 days if the wisdom teeth are impacted deeply within the jaw.

Toxaemia (pre-eclampsia)
SEE UNDER PREGNANCY: COMPLICATIONS

Trachea

The upper part of the airways, leading from the larynx to the large bronchi (see diagram page 255).

Tracheitis

Inflammation of the trachea. It is very common, and

usually results from a virus infection. The symptoms are cough with pain or soreness behind the upper chest on breathing in. Steam inhalations may relieve the pain, which settles in 2–3 days as the underlying infection subsides.

Trachoma

A tropical disease of hot, arid regions with poor hygiene, and the commonest cause of blindness world-wide. The eye is infected with a minute organism (Chlamydia trachomatis), inducing a severe reaction in the tissues of the cornea which swell and scar and eventually obscure sight. The infection usually responds to antibiotics but the result is unpredictable.

Tranquillizers

The term is often used synonymously with sedatives, which are used in the treatment of anxiety (page 23) and sleeplessness (page 208). Powerful tranquillizers such as the phenothiazines (e.g. chlorpromazine, Largactil) are used to treat severely disturbed or aggressive patients, and in psychiatric disorders such as schizophrenia (page 200) and manic depression (page 149).

Weaker tranquillizers include some of the benzodiazepines such as diazepam (Valium) and chlordiazepoxide (Librium). These are used for limited periods in patients whose life is adversely affected by excess stress.

Travel sickness

Sea, car and air sickness are forms of motion sickness. The sickness may be associated with vertigo (a spinning sensation).

Sea sickness results from unaccustomed stimuli affecting the balance receptors (the labyrinth) within the ear (page 88). The swelling motion of the sea continuously alters the position of the labyrinth and the nervous impulses stimulate the 'vomiting centre' in the brain.

Car sickness is caused by a similar mechanism but in addition there may be an accumulation of exhaust fumes from the traveller's or other cars, particularly in heavy traffic.

Air sickness may have a similar mechanism to sea sickness but fear of flying is often a major factor.

The most effective treatment, especially for short journeys, is hyoscine. It may, however, cause drowsiness, blurred vision and a dry mouth. For long journeys, antihistamines are more appropriate but less effective and they also cause drowsiness. There are many proprietary preparations available and all are equally effective and can be obtained without prescription (e.g. Avomine, Kwells, Sea-legs).

Tremor

Everyone has a tremor, which is best seen in the hands if the arms are outstretched, and this tends to increase with age. The normal tremor is so fine that it is usually unnoticeable. Certain situations such as anxiety, over-activity of the thyroid gland (*see* Thyroid disease) or an alcoholic binge cause an exaggeration of this normal phenomenon. In some cases an obvious tremor may be inherited and may be accentuated by stress, fatigue, exercise or cold. This tremor is an isolated feature of no serious medical consequence except for the nuisance and embarrassment it may cause, particularly as it is popularly associated with the tremor of alcoholics.

A coarse tremor occurs in patients suffering with Parkinson's disease (page 167). The tremor is worse at rest and with emotion, and improves on movement. Certain drugs may cause a similar tremor.

Very occasionally a tremor develops during active movement of the hand towards an object, and with no tremor at rest. This is due to inco-ordination and is a feature of diseases of the cerebellum (page 55), the part of the brain which controls smooth co-ordinated movements.

Trichomonas vaginalis

A parasite which infests the vagina (*see* Vaginal discharge).

Trigeminal neuralgia

Severe spasmodic pain which shoots along the fifth (the trigeminal) cranial nerve in the face (*see* Neuralgia).

Tropical diseases

Travellers to the tropics are exposed to certain

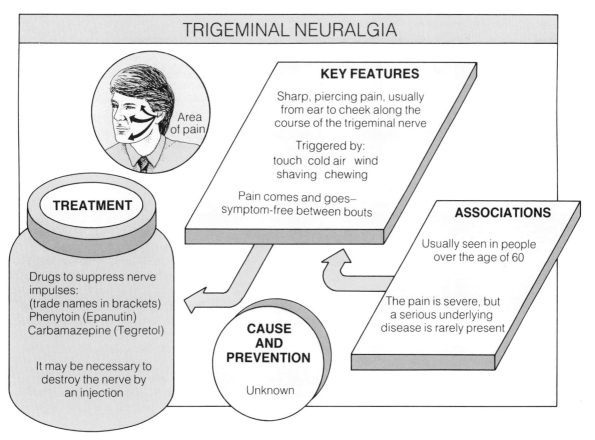

TRIGEMINAL NEURALGIA

KEY FEATURES

Sharp, piercing pain, usually from ear to cheek along the course of the trigeminal nerve

Triggered by:
touch cold air wind
shaving chewing

Pain comes and goes—symptom-free between bouts

Area of pain

TREATMENT

Drugs to suppress nerve impulses:
(trade names in brackets)
Phenytoin (Epanutin)
Carbamazepine (Tegretol)

It may be necessary to destroy the nerve by an injection

CAUSE AND PREVENTION

Unknown

ASSOCIATIONS

Usually seen in people over the age of 60

The pain is severe, but a serious underlying disease is rarely present

diseases which are less common or do not occur in the non-tropical world. Poliomyelitis (page 180) and diphtheria (page 83) are very common in parts of the tropics, and tetanus (page 222) more common in the developed countries.

Returning travellers bring back a number of tropical diseases, of which malaria (page 148) is by far the most common; others are typhoid (page 231) and amoebiasis (page 16). Other diseases common to the tropics include bilharzia (schistosomiasis, page 200), trypanosomiasis (sleeping sickness, page 208) and cholera (page 59).

Immunization for travellers is outlined on page 239.

Truss

Supportive trusses are designed to press against the abdominal wall to retain hernias. They are used for inguinal hernias and must be carefully fitted because a poorly fitting truss may allow part of the hernia to escape and become trapped between the truss and the abdomen.

Trusses are valuable for the short-term management of hernias, and when a patient's general condition is too poor for surgical repair. It is important that a truss is adjusted and refitted from time to time because stretch and wear of the straps may make it inefficient.

Tuberculosis
(TB)

A bacterial infection prevalent throughout the world but becoming rare in the developed countries, coinciding with improvements in nutrition, better housing and, to a lesser extent, the use of specific antibiotics. The bacterium (*Mycobacterium tuberculosis*) is inhaled from those with active tuberculous pneumonia, or ingested in infected milk.

In the lung, the organism sets up a small pneumonic reaction which heals rapidly—often with no symptoms, if the infected person is healthy and has normal immunity. Otherwise the pneumonia spreads and symptoms of cough with blood-stained sputum and sometimes breathlessness develop. The active organism is coughed into the air, to be inhaled and spread through the community. Spread is common in areas of poor nutrition and housing.

Infected milk from non-TB-tested cattle enters the intestine and infects the wall and its lymph glands. The induced reaction may remain localized and heal if the infected individual is well nourished and

healthy. Otherwise the infection spreads, to involve the other lymph glands and the liver and spleen. If treatment is not started, the infection spreads to the lungs and the brain.

TB is prevented by improved nutrition and housing, and the incidence has fallen dramatically where this has been introduced. Vaccination against the disease is commonly practised in the developed countries and further decreases the chance of infection. The vaccine—BCG—is derived from an original strain from cattle, and is named after its developers (BCG = bacille Calmette–Guérin)

Active infection is diagnosed by identification of the bacterium in sputum, or in infected glands or liver after removal or biopsy of a small specimen of tissue. Anti-TB drugs are very effective but must be taken for at least 9 and sometimes 18 months. Those in common use are isoniazid, rifampicin, ethambutol, streptomycin and para-aminosalicylic acid.

Tumour

The body consists of millions of microscopic cells. In most parts of the body cells are continually dying and being replaced by new cells. For example, the outer layer of the skin (the epidermis) is entirely replaced every 28 days. The control of cell replacement is not completely understood. It is obviously complex, and not surprisingly the control mechanism sometimes becomes disordered. When this happens, an excess of cells may be produced at one site and a visible swelling or tumour is formed.

This excess of cells may cause a simple benign non-spreading tumour or a malignant one. The factors determining the nature of the tumours depend on the nature of the cells produced. Benign tumours are slow growing and are surrounded by a thick fibrous capsule, and contain cells similar to the cells of origin which are of uniform size and appearance. Malignant tumours tend to grow quickly, rarely have a capsule around them and contain cells varying widely in size and shape. They also spread both through adjacent structures and to sites distant from the primary growth. These factors are important when surgical removal is undertaken.

Various factors are believed to promote the formation of malignant tumours. Smoking cigarettes is known to predispose to lung cancer and throat cancer, and to increase the chance of developing bladder cancer. Excessive exposure to sunlight causes skin cancer in a few susceptible individuals. Exposure to certain industrial agents has a known association with the development of cancer; e.g.

asbestos dust may cause a malignant tumour (mesothelioma) in the lungs. The delay between exposure of a cancer-producing agent (carcinogen) and the development of the cancer may be 20 years or more.

The word 'cancer' evokes the fear of an inevitable and unpleasant death. Whilst it is true that some cancers are incurable and have a high mortality, it is equally true that certain cancers are entirely curable. For example, the early detection and treatment of breast, kidney, bowel and laryngeal cancers is often curative, and Hodgkin's disease of the lymph glands (page 126) can now be completely cured.

Twins

The incidence of twin pregnancies is 1 in every 80 normal pregnancies in England and Wales. There are two types of twins. The first and most common are binovular (dizygotic or fraternal) twins, which result from the fertilization of two eggs (ova) shed at the same time from the ovaries, by two sperms. The twins are not identical because they have different genetic constitutions, but they show resemblance as is normally seen between brother and sister. They may or may not be of the same sex.

The second type are monovular (monozygotic or identical) twins. They result from the splitting of one fertilized ovum at early developmental stage. The twins are of the same sex. They develop separately but have virtually identical appearance because they contain identical genetic constituents.

Siamese twins are identical twins who are conjoined at birth.

Twitching eyelids

This is the most common twitch of all. The eyelid may twitch for up to a week or even a few days more, but always stops. There is no known cure for the disorder, which is never serious.

Typhoid

An infection caused by the typhoid bacillus (*Salmonella typhi*). There are more than 1,000 types of Salmonella bacteria, which all cause intestinal infection with acute gastro-enteritis and food poisoning. *Salmonella typhi*, however, causes a specific infection which is more serious; there are about 200 sporadic cases of typhoid occurring in Britain annually and most of these are in travellers who have returned from visits abroad. Epidemics in the past have been spread through contaminated water supplies or food, but the incidence of typhoid has dropped in the developed countries because of better sanitation and hygiene

The source of infection is always human—either a person suffering from typhoid fever or a symptomless carrier of the bacillus. The organisms enter the body in food. The onset of symptoms is slow, and during the first week there is a slow-rising fever, general ill health and abdominal discomfort, constipation and a cough. This is usually followed in the second week by a persistent high temperature with a general worsening in general health. Diarrhoea may develop at this stage.

Treatment consists of intravenous fluid and salt replacement plus an appropriate antibiotic.

Substantial protection against typhoid is achieved with vaccination (*see* TAB) and all persons travelling abroad, except to North America and Northern Europe, are well advised to obtain it.

Typhus

An acute infection occurring throughout the world but rare in Europe. It is spread by the bite of infected fleas (murine typhus), ticks (African and Rocky Mountain spotted fever), mites (scrub typhus) or lice (epidemic typhus and trench fever). The typical features are severe fever with shaking attacks (rigors), severe headache and muscular pains, soon followed by a spotted rash. Typhus responds well to antibiotics if treated early.

Ulcer

An ulcer is a defect in any normal body surface, inside or out, which produces a shallow depression. A skin ulcer on the face which persists or enlarges and shows no sign of healing should be referred to a doctor because it may be a small cancer which is cured by removal (*see* Rodent ulcer).

A common site for skin ulcers is around or above the ankles. These are usually varicose ulcers, which occur because of poor blood flow due to varicose veins (page 239). They are not serious but require regular and expert nursing attention if they are to heal. (*See also* Mouth ulcers *and* Stomach ulcer.)

Ulcerative colitis

An inflammatory disease of the large intestine, which contains multiple small ulcers along the inner lining. It usually occurs in young adults. Characteristically there are periods of normal health and periods of illness. The illness may be severe or mild, depending on the extent of involvement of the colon. In the mildest form the rectum alone is involved (proctitis); there is episodic rectal pain with diarrhoea and bleeding but the outlook is excellent. At the other extreme, the rectum and the entire colon are involved. The illness tends to recur with ill health, weight loss, and persistent abdominal pain, diarrhoea and rectal bleeding.

Treatment varies according to the individual and the severity of illness; high roughage (fibre) diets to reduce constipation and sulphasalazine (Salazopyrin) tablets taken regularly reduce the risk of further attacks. Steroid retention enemas are of value during acute attacks, especially when the inflammation is limited to the rectum. In severe cases, steroid tablets or injections are also used. If treatment does not suppress the symptoms and the illness and general health becomes poor, removal of the inflamed colon offers a complete cure. Motions are them passed through an artificial passage on the front of the abdomen (*see* Ileostomy).

People who have colitis require expert supervision to ensure that relapses are kept to a minimum. The colon seldom has to be removed.

Ulna

The larger of the two forearm bones attached below to the radius by a thin, strong fibrous septum, and forming the elbow joint (with the humerus) above. At the wrist joint it articulates by a modified ball-and-socket joint with the side of the radius (carrying the hand) and thus allows the hand to rotate (*see* diagram, page 267).

Umbilicus
(NAVEL)

The site of attachment of the umbilical cord to the baby before birth.

Umbilical infection may occur in the newborn. This is rarely serious and responds to careful dressing with antiseptic lotions and powder.

An umbilical hernia is a swelling protruding at the umbilicus, due to a small defect in the abdominal wall muscle. Usually this requires no treatment, and in most children resolves spontaneously by the age of 4. Dressings applied to reduce the swelling are of no benefit. An umbilical hernia occurring in later life is usually best left alone, but if large will require surgical correction.

Other problems encountered in children include

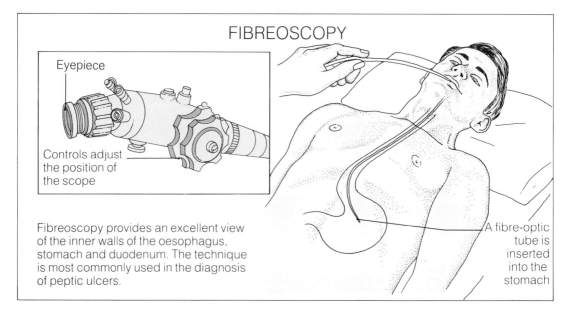

FIBREOSCOPY

Eyepiece

Controls adjust the position of the scope

Fibreoscopy provides an excellent view of the inner walls of the oesophagus, stomach and duodenum. The technique is most commonly used in the diagnosis of peptic ulcers.

A fibre-optic tube is inserted into the stomach

polyps and discharges from the navel. These are very worrying for the parents, and medical advice should be sought for reassurance and to exclude serious disorders—which are very rare.

Undescended testis

Both testes should have descended into the scrotum by the age of 1 year. If they have not appeared by this age then no further spontaneous descent will occur. However, they can be easily pushed well down into the scrotum and no further treatment is required.

Otherwise, a minor operation is required to lower the testis into the scrotum and fix it there (an orchidopexy). This is performed before starting school, at about 4 years of age. If an undescended testis is left, the production of sperm from it will be reduced in later life, and there is also an increased if small chance of cancer developing in it.

Ureter

The muscular tube which carries urine, produced by the kidneys, to the bladder (*see* diagram, page 261).

Urethra

The final outflow tract from the bladder. Infection is common, causing burning on urination (*see* Cystitis) and sometimes a discharge (*see* Venereal diseases *and* Vaginal discharge).

Urethritis

Infection of the urethra—the outflow tract from the kidneys and bladder—causing burning on urination. This may be the only feature of infection within the bladder (cystitis, page 71), but also occurs with venereal infections and is usually associated with a discharge (*see* Gonorrhoea; Syphilis; *and* Vaginal discharge). Investigation is important to identify the causative organism and thus determine the correct treatment. If it is persistent or recurrent, further detailed investigation with cystoscopy and x-rays of the kidneys may be necessary.

Uric acid

A chemical which circulates in the blood. Excess uric acid in the joints tends to form solid crystals which produces the severe joint pain of gout (page 114).

Urticaria
(HIVES; NETTLE RASH)

There are many causes of urticaria but the rash produced is always similar and characterized by itching red hot weals. Nettle stings produce a similar rash, hence the alternative name.

Urticaria occurs in all age groups, but most commonly in the young. Allergy is the main precipitating factor but in over half of the cases no specific cause can be identified. The following may cause urticaria in susceptible people:

Foods: shellfish, strawberries, eggs (and some food additives)
Drugs: penicillin, aspirin and many others
Insect bites: bedbugs, fleas
Temperature: extremes of heat or cold (rare)

Usually an urticarial rash is short lived, provided there is not continued exposure to the precipitating cause. The rash and itch may be reduced by antihistamine tablets or syrup.(*See* chart, page 234.)

Uterus
(LATIN: WOMB)

Part of the female genital tract (page 109) in which the egg (ovum) embeds and develops after fertilization. The inner lining of the uterus, the endometrium, slowly thickens and becomes filled with blood at intervals of 28 days. Unless a fertilized ovum embeds in the wall, this inner lining is shed and seen as a period. This cycle is controlled by hormones from the pituitary gland acting partly via oestrogens from the ovaries. These decrease rapidly 28 days after an ovum is released unless the ovum has been fertilized and is developing safely in the endometrial lining. (*See also* Pregnancy.)

V

Vaccination
(IMMUNIZATION) (LATIN: *VACCINUS*, OF A COW)

In 1796 Edward Jenner realized that milkmaids and cowherds rarely suffered from smallpox. He injected fluid from cowpox into a young boy, who became resistant to smallpox. Jenner's discovery showed that vaccination with a mild form of a disease could protect against a more serious one. This in turn, even if nearly 100 years later, introduced the possibility of vaccinating against disease caused by small infectious agents (i.e. viruses and bacteria) using the same organism after it had been killed or made less toxic and dangerous.

Normally, a child who becomes infected with an infectious organism (e.g. the virus of poliomyelitis or the bacterium of tuberculosis) responds in a number of ways: (1) he may develop no apparent illness whatsoever, but will in response to the infection produce antibodies (page 22) against the infecting agent, which prevents further attacks; (2) the child may develop a mild illness and recover fully, being left perfectly fit and completely immunized; (3) the child may develop serious illness and may die or be left with serious disability

Immunization is recommended by the Department of Health against poliomyelitis, diphtheria, tetanus, tuberculosis, measles and German measles in girls of childbearing age. Immunization against whooping cough is recommended by the Department of Health but there is some difference of opinion about its value to the community when compared to the dangers of the vaccine.

Pertussis vaccination (whooping cough)
The argument against the use of pertussis vaccine is that more deaths from brain damage might be caused than by naturally occurring whooping cough.

The advocates of pertussis vaccination argue that the incidence of brain damage from the vaccine is unknown, particularly because such damage can unfortunately occur in infants for no known cause. Whooping cough is often a very severe illness at all ages and particularly in babies under 3 months who often need to be cared for in hospital because of feeding difficulty during the illness. In addition, the complications can be very serious with widespread pneumonia and brain haemorrhage. At present, the over-all weight of medical evidence and opinion is strongly in favour of vaccination against whooping cough, which should be given as early as possible (3 months of age) because the younger the child the greater the dangers of the disease.

Smallpox vaccination
Smallpox is no longer recommended because the disease has become non-existent following an international vaccine campaign sponsored by the World Health Organization.

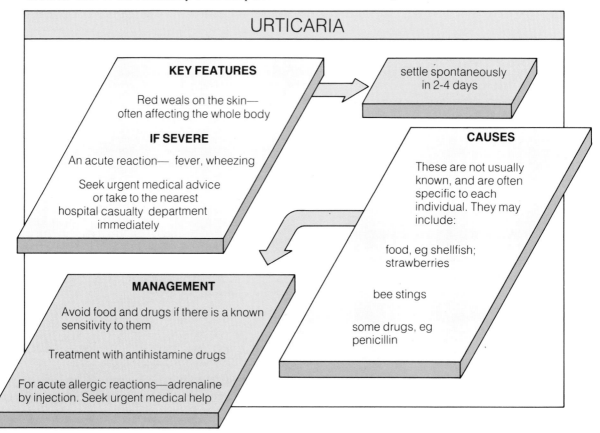

URICARIA

KEY FEATURES

Red weals on the skin— often affecting the whole body

settle spontaneously in 2-4 days

IF SEVERE

An acute reaction— fever, wheezing

Seek urgent medical advice or take to the nearest hospital casualty department immediately

CAUSES

These are not usually known, and are often specific to each individual. They may include:

food, eg shellfish; strawberries

bee stings

some drugs, eg penicillin

MANAGEMENT

Avoid food and drugs if there is a known sensitivity to them

Treatment with antihistamine drugs

For acute allergic reactions—adrenaline by injection. Seek urgent medical help

Skin Disorders

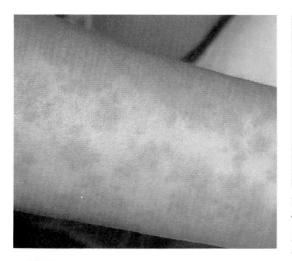

Measles *A dusky red rash begins on the face in patches and spreads from the face to cover the trunk and eventually the whole body. At the same time the patches coalesce and the rash may become confluent. The rash is usually slightly raised.*

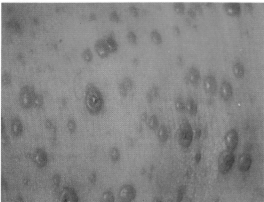

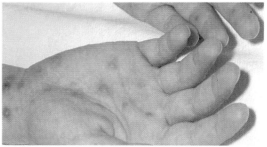

Chickenpox *The rash begins as raised red spots which develop into superficial isolated fluid filled vesicles. Any part of the body can be involved including the mouth, palms and soles. The rash is excruciatingly irritating.*

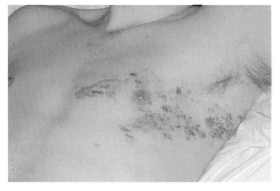

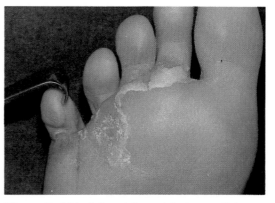

Shingles *The rash is similar to chickenpox–both are caused by the same virus. It follows the line of the nerves, often appearing as a band around the body or down a limb. It is very irritating.*

Tinea pedis *Athlete's foot. A fungus infection usually in adolescents and young adults. It is caught by walking barefoot over infected floors and hence common in athletes.*

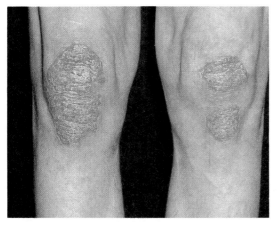

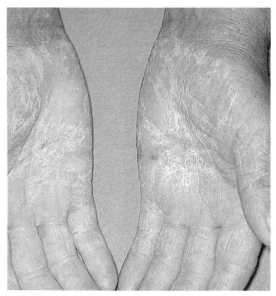

Psoriasis *(above and right) In early psoriasis the affected skin is roughened and red, and covered with fine silvery scales. It is often irritating. Later the lesions become confluent and the skin thickened. The parts commonly affected are the scalp, back, knees, elbows, soles, palms and nails.*

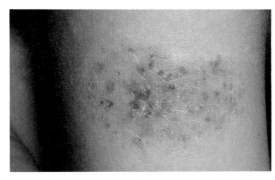

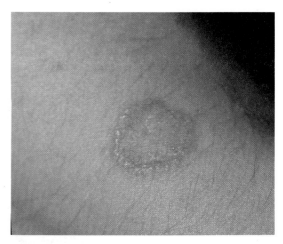

Discoid eczema *A chronic skin rash with a disc-like distribution. It may be intensely irritating and either wet or dry. It commonly occurs on the hands, forearms, thighs and calves.*

Ring worm *(above and left) A fungus infection which can affect any part of the body. Ringworm of the scalp is common in children and appears as an unsightly bald patch. It usually responds well to treatment.*

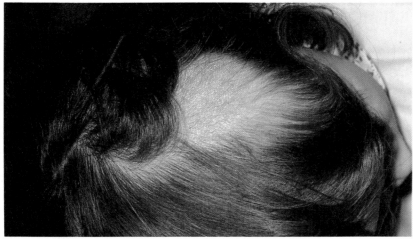

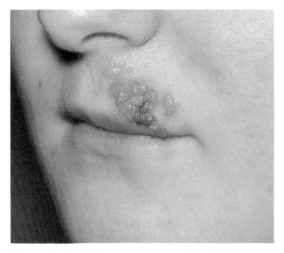

Herpes simplex *Cold sores appear as small painful blisters. The Herpes simplex virus lives in the superficial layers of the skin, and becomes active whenever the subject develops any illness, even a cold. The lips are the most common site.*

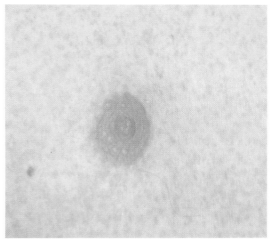

Glandular fever *A rash is uncommon with glandular fever unless the patient has been given antibiotics—which do not affect the disease anyway. The rash is pale pink to red and may affect the whole body.*

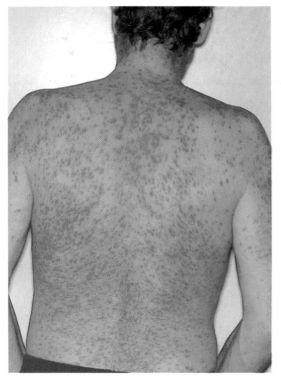

Drug rashes *Almost all drugs can produce a rash in susceptible subjects. The rashes vary from fleeting flat pale pink lesions to highly irritant, raised red wheals. It must be suspected whenever a rash starts soon after a course of drugs is started.*

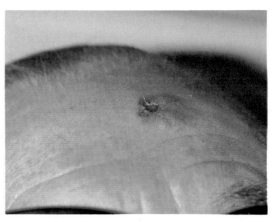

Rodent ulcer *A very slowly growing cancer seen on the skin of the face, commonly the forehead, cheek or eyelid. Early treatment is curative.*

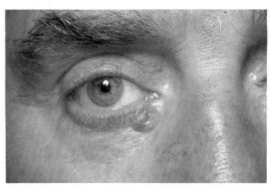

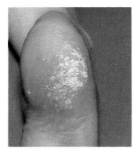

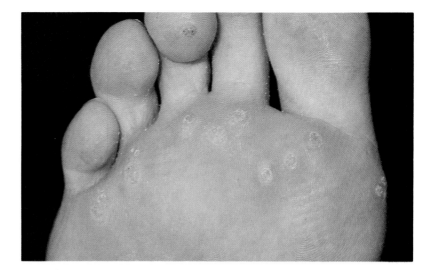

Plantar warts *Warts are caused by viruses. They commonly affect the soles of the feet and toes and are contracted by walking barefoot over wet, infected surfaces such as swimming baths.*

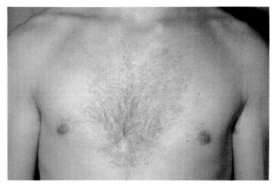

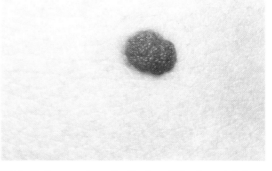

Seborrhoeic dermatitis *A scaly rash which affects hairy areas of the body. It is common on the scalp (dandruff) and often responds to simple treatment with medicated shampoos.*

Pigmented naevus *A small collection of blood vessels below the skin often present from birth. If unsightly or causing anxiety they can be easily removed.*

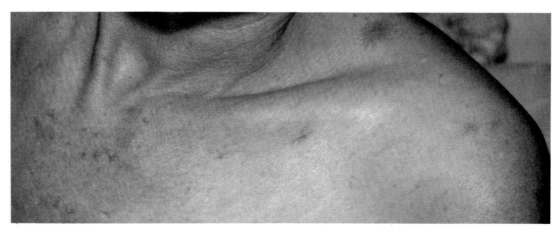

Spider naevi *Small collections of blood vessels in the shape of a spider–the central artery is the body and the capillaries* *assume the position of the legs. They occur on the face, upper chest, arms and hands and are a feature of liver disease–often alcoholic.*

Vaccination for children

3 months	Triple vaccine (diphtheria, tetanus, whooping cough), or diphtheria and tetanus Oral polio
5–6 months	Repeat
10–12 months	Repeat
1–2 years	Measles
School entry	Diphtheria, tetanus, polio
11–13 years	Rubella (German measles) for girls Tuberculosis (the routine need for this is disputed)
School leavers	Polio, tetanus

Vaccination for travellers

Disease	Need for prophylaxis or vaccination
Malaria	Essential for known malarial regions
Yellow fever	Essential for known yellow fever zones
Cholera	Essential for cholera regions
Polio	
Tetanus	
Hepatitis (gamma globulin)	Strongly recommended for tropical regions
Typhoid and paratyphoid (TAB)	

Note The course of injections is best given over 6–12 weeks. Give your family physician plenty of notice that you are planning a tropical journey to allow time to decide what vaccines are necessary and in what order to give them. (Advice may be obtained from specialist centres for tropical diseases.)

Vagina
(LATIN: A SHEATH)

The lowest part of the female genital tract (page 109), which at its upper end sheaths the lower cervix. Infection is common, and causes increased secretion from the lining wall (*see* Vaginal discharge).

Vaginal bleeding after the menopause

Periods (page 169) often become very irregular just before the menopause ('the change'), sometimes with long gaps in between. It is often difficult to know exactly when the menopause occurs. However, if vaginal bleeding occurs a year or more after the last period it is important to seek medical advice.

Usually the bleeding settles spontaneously, but post-menopausal bleeding may be the first sign of a growth in the womb (uterus). For this reason, medical help should be obtained because early diagnosis is important and removal of the uterus (hysterectomy) can be curative.

Vaginal discharge

A common complaint which affects most women at some time in their lives. A slight watery discharge is normal, and this may be increased in pregnancy and by sexual stimulation. When the discharge causes symptoms such as irritation and soreness, or becomes heavy or unpleasant, this suggests infection. Two common causes of infection are *Candida* (thrush) and *Trichomonas*. (*See* chart, page 240.)

Candidiasis is due to a yeast (*Candida albicans*) which is often 'resident' in various parts of the body without causing any problems. If the number of yeasts increases, a thick white irritating discharge develops. This is not serious and treatment is very successful. Two pessaries containing anti-fungal agents (e.g. nystatin) are inserted at night for a week, and a cream may also be applied to the vulva. It may be necessary to treat the male partner with a similar cream. When the infection is recurrent, it is usual to also give nystatin tablets by mouth.

The second common infection is with *Trichomonas*, which is a minute parasite. This infection is spread by sexual contact and produces a green frothy irritating discharge. The male partner is often infected but rarely has symptoms. A course of metronidazole tablets is curative; sometimes pessaries and cream are also used. It is usual to give the male partner a course of tablets at the same time.

Other causes of infection include gonorrhoea (page 114), which may be identified on microscopic examination of the discharge taken from the vagina. It is important to realize that a woman who has gonorrhoea may have no symptoms at all but can still infect her partners.

Varicose veins

Varicose veins in the legs are very common, frequently uncomfortable or even painful, but never serious. Normally blood in the leg is drained by veins leading towards the heart. Blood flows from veins

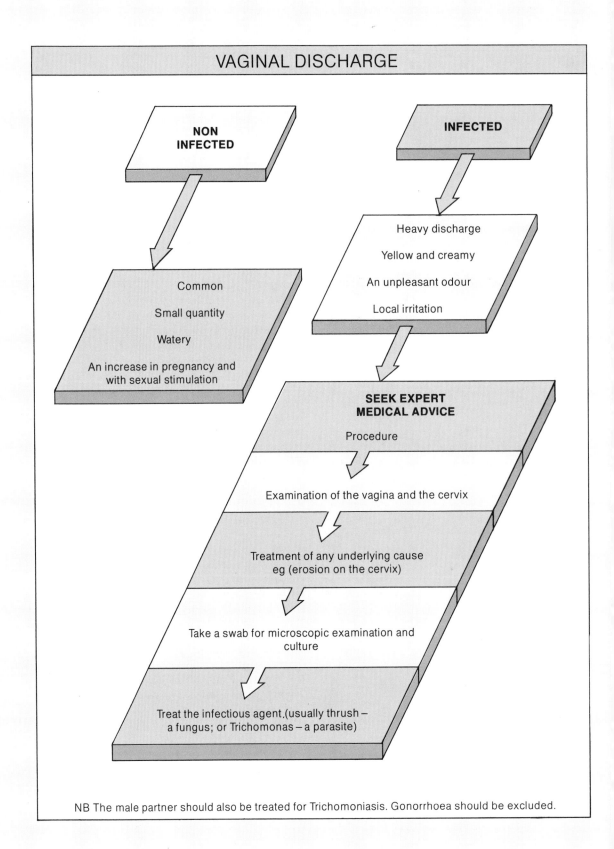

VAGINAL DISCHARGE

NON INFECTED

INFECTED

Heavy discharge

Yellow and creamy

An unpleasant odour

Local irritation

Common

Small quantity

Watery

An increase in pregnancy and with sexual stimulation

SEEK EXPERT MEDICAL ADVICE

Procedure

Examination of the vagina and the cervix

Treatment of any underlying cause eg (erosion on the cervix)

Take a swab for microscopic examination and culture

Treat the infectious agent (usually thrush – a fungus; or Trichomonas – a parasite)

NB The male partner should also be treated for Trichomoniasis. Gonorrhoea should be excluded.

under the skin to deeper veins lying between muscles and these in turn lead to the major veins in the body. The blood normally flows only one way because of non-return valves in the deep veins. Contraction of the calf muscles compresses these veins and, because of the valves, the blood flows 'uphill' towards the heart. Moreover, the pressure of the column of blood extending upwards to the heart from the ankle is broken by the valves. Varicose veins develop when the valves become inefficient and, as a result, the pressure of blood in the ankle veins rises and blood flows the 'wrong way'. The superficial veins become engorged and visible on the surface, to produce the characteristic lumpy appearance.

Varicose veins are unsightly, and this is the most common reason for seeking medical advice. Other common symptoms are itching and a tense discomfort with swelling of the ankles, usually at the end of the day. The skin may ulcerate over the inner side of the ankle.

Treatment varies according to the severity of the varicose veins. There are three ways to improve them: the first is to wear support stockings, the second is to remove the superficial veins surgically, and the third is to inject them. This last method involves a small injection at selected sites along the varicose veins to thrombose or clot them—a tight support bandage must be worn for 6 weeks after the injections.

These methods do not always produce a complete cure and varicose veins can recur. Treatment may prevent less common but more serious complications of leg ulcers, haemorrhage and phlebitis. Varicose ulcers of the legs are uncomfortable and take a long time to heal. If a vein bursts, the haemorrhage is alarming but not serious and is easily stopped by lying down, elevating the leg and pressing on the bleeding point. A tourniquet must *never* be applied above the bleeding veins because this will make the bleeding worse. (*See* chart, page 242.)

Vasectomy

Male sterilization. The tube (vas deferens) along which sperm normally travels is easily accessible through a very small incision at the base of the scrotal skin. The operation involves cutting this tube, removing a small section and tying off the cut ends. The procedure is simple and often performed under local anaesthesia with the patient conscious. It takes 10–15 minutes and there is no need to remain in hospital.

Vasectomy is becoming more popular as a means of contraception, partly as a result of accurate adverse publicity about the oral contraceptive pill in women over the age of 35 years. It is much simpler than female sterilization.

The decision to undergo this operation is an important one and requires careful counselling because vasectomy should be regarded as a permanent, irreversible procedure.

Following vasectomy there is no physical reason why sexual performance should be altered.

Venereal disease

Diseases transmitted by sexual intercourse. These include syphilis (page 219), gonorrhoea (page 114), *Herpes simplex* virus infection (page 124), thrush (page 223), scabies (page 199), venereal warts and Reiter's disease (page 194).

Although there remains a great stigma attached to contracting a venereal disease, it is vital to seek expert medical advice to ensure accurate diagnosis, correct treatment and careful tracing of contacts. This is the only way to prevent further spread. Many attenders at special clinics do not have a venereal disease.

Vertigo

An unpleasant sensation of spinning. It occurs when the balance apparatus (the labyrinth) of the inner ear or its connecting nerves within the brain are damaged (*see also* Ear).

The most common cause of vertigo is acute labyrinthitis, which is a viral infection of the labyrinth. This produces ringing in the ear with fever and vertigo, and frequently with vomiting, lasting for 2–4 days. It may leave a feeling of unsteadiness for 3–4 weeks. It often occurs in minor epidemics. If there is severe vomiting or if the vertigo does not settle within 12–14 hours, further investigation may be required and medical advice should be obtained.

A more persistent or recurrent form of vertigo occurs in Ménière's disease (page 151), which is associated with ringing and impaired hearing in the affected ears.

Vertigo may follow a head injury or an ear infection, and is provoked by movements of the head. Less commonly, vertigo occurs as a result of disorders of the brain (e.g. multiple sclerosis).

Viruses

Small organisms which can be seen only with an electron microscope. They only grow in environments containing living cells.

Virus infections of the respiratory and gastro-intestinal systems are the commonest known to man. Viruses cause all of the common childhood illnesses, including mumps, measles, German measles and poliomyelitis. These are unaffected by antibiotics.

Vitamins

Essential components of a normal diet. They form part of enzyme systems which are necessary for the utilization of the major dietary components—

carbohydrate, fat and protein. Vitamins are not used to provide energy or body building but promote these functions. Much has been discovered about the function of vitamins in deficiency states. The classic example is deficiency of vitamin C, which causes scurvy. Vitamin deficiencies due to an inadequate diet are extremely rare in the developed world but are a cause of much disease in countries where the energy requirements are met by foodstuffs such as polished rice or maize. In the Western world dietary supplements are not normally necessary except in pregnancy and sometimes in the very young or very old.

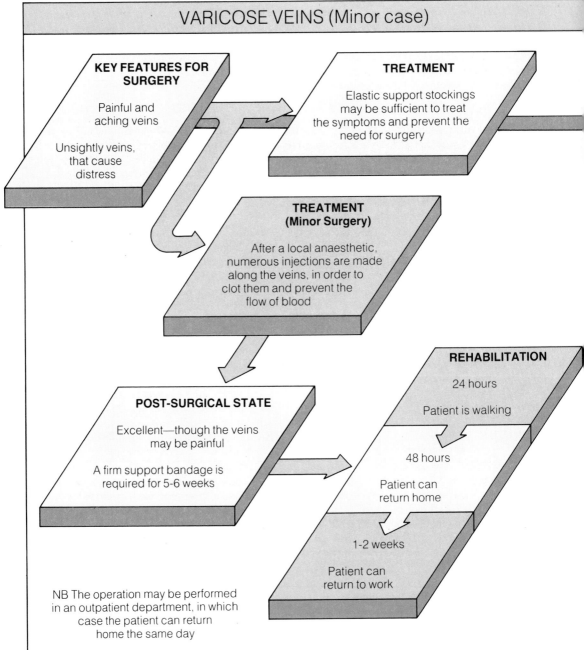

VARICOSE VEINS (Minor case)

KEY FEATURES FOR SURGERY

Painful and aching veins

Unsightly veins, that cause distress

TREATMENT

Elastic support stockings may be sufficient to treat the symptoms and prevent the need for surgery

TREATMENT (Minor Surgery)

After a local anaesthetic, numerous injections are made along the veins, in order to clot them and prevent the flow of blood

POST-SURGICAL STATE

Excellent—though the veins may be painful

A firm support bandage is required for 5-6 weeks

NB The operation may be performed in an outpatient department, in which case the patient can return home the same day

REHABILITATION

24 hours

Patient is walking

48 hours

Patient can return home

1-2 weeks

Patient can return to work

The vitamins are classified as follows:

Vitamin A

Vitamin B complex:

Vitamin B$_1$, aneurine hydrochloride or thiamine hydrochloride	Vitamin B$_6$ or pyridoxine hydrochloride	Vitamin C or ascorbic acid
Vitamin B$_2$ or riboflavine	Nicotinic acid	Vitamin D or calciferol
Vitamin B$_5$ or pantothenic acid	Vitamin B$_{12}$ or cyanocobalamin	Vitamin E
	Folic acid	Vitamin K

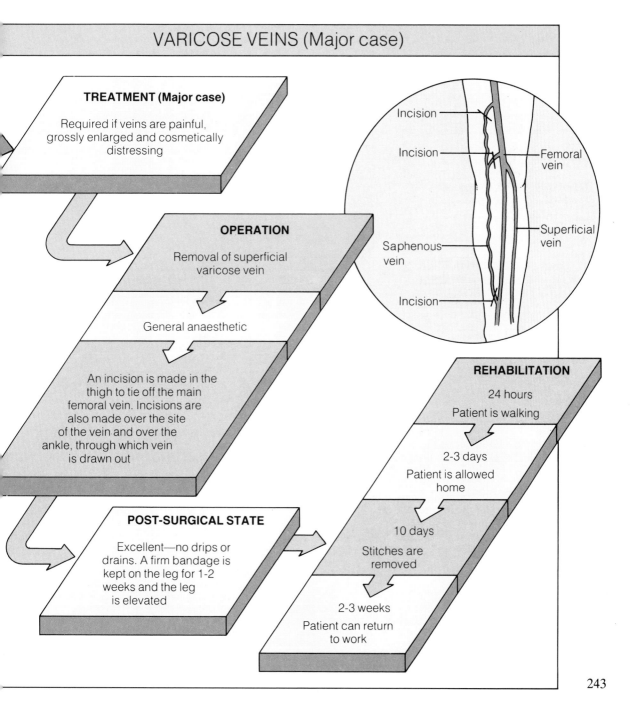

VARICOSE VEINS (Major case)

TREATMENT (Major case)

Required if veins are painful, grossly enlarged and cosmetically distressing

OPERATION

Removal of superficial varicose vein

General anaesthetic

An incision is made in the thigh to tie off the main femoral vein. Incisions are also made over the site of the vein and over the ankle, through which vein is drawn out

Incision
Incision — Femoral vein
Superficial vein
Saphenous vein
Incision

POST-SURGICAL STATE

Excellent—no drips or drains. A firm bandage is kept on the leg for 1-2 weeks and the leg is elevated

REHABILITATION

24 hours
Patient is walking

2-3 days
Patient is allowed home

10 days
Stitches are removed

2-3 weeks
Patient can return to work

243

VITAMIN	SOURCE	REQUIREMENTS (ADULT, DAILY)	FUNCTION/DEFICIENCY
Vitamin A	Milk, butter, egg yolk, fish liver oil. May be converted from beta-carotene in plants; found in many vegetables and fruits	1,000 micrograms retinol	Lack of vitamin A causes: 1 Loss of night vision 2 Dryness of transparent covering of eyes (conjunctiva and cornea) 3 Dry skin
Vitamin B$_1$, thiamine	Husks of cereal, yeast, egg yolk, nuts, liver and leguminous vegetables (e.g. peas and beans)	0–5 milligrams thiamine per intake of 1,000 calories	Deficiency causes beri-beri. 1 Disorder of nerves may cause numbness and tingling in arms and legs and weakness resulting in wrist or foot drop. 2 Muscles may become tender. 3 Heart may enlarge, causing heart failure with associated rapid pulse, swelling of ankles and legs, and shortness of breath. Deficiency may also cause Wernicke's encephalopathy with clouding of consciousness, unsteadiness, squint, confusion. This deficiency, in the Western world, is most commonly seen in alcoholics.
Vitamin B$_2$, riboflavine	Leafy vegetables, meat, fish, eggs	1–2 milligrams	Soreness and later ulcer formation in the tongue, lips, mouth and eyes.
Nicotinic acid	Many foods, including liver, yeast, cheese, milk, eggs and cereals	15–20 milligrams niacin; 1 milligram niacin may be derived from 60 milligrams tryptophan. Niacin is generic term for nicotinic acid and nicotinamide.	Deficiency causes pellagra. This is typically associated with maize (corn) diets which are low in both tryptophan and niacin. Features of pellagra include: 1 Diarrhoea due to inflammation of the lining of the gastro-intestinal tract. 2 Difficulty in swallowing due to severe soreness of the mouth. 3 Dermatitis: scaling, thickening and darkening of skin, especially in sun-exposed areas. Initially may resemble sunburn. 4 Dementia with poor memory, poor attention, disorientation, confusion.
Vitamin B$_5$, pantothenic acid	Many foods especially yeast, liver, eggs, meat and fish	5–10 milligrams	Fatigue, burning, pins and needles in the feet, cramps.

Vitamin B$_6$, pyridoxine	Egg yolk, yeast, peas, soya beans, meat, liver	1–2 milligrams	Deficiency states are rare.
			    Deficiency may occur in children on peculiar artificial diets. The children may present with convulsions and dermatitis.
			    Pyridoxine deficiency may occur in severe vomiting during pregnancy. Some anti-sickness (anti-emetic) preparations contain pyridoxine.
			    Pyridoxine deficiency may occur in some women taking the oral contraceptive pill, and may cause depression. Pyridoxine supplements may help the depression although the evidence is not conclusive.

VITAMIN	SOURCE	REQUIREMENTS (ADULT, DAILY)	FUNCTION/DEFICIENCY
Vitamin B_{12}, cyanocobalamin	Present in low concentration in most animal products, liver. Almost entirely absent in plant products.	3 micrograms	Dietary deficiencies are rare except in certain vegetarian diets (e.g. vegans). Deficiency usually results from faulty absorption despite adequate intake. One cause is pernicious anaemia where the stomach fails to produce a factor which is necessary for vitamin B_{12} to be absorbed from the bowel. Vitamin B_{12} is essential for the production of blood cells, and deficiency causes anaemia. Deficiency in severe cases may affect the nervous system, causing numbness, tingling and weakness in the limbs.
Folic acid	Green leaves, liver, kidney, yeast, milk	400 micrograms	Folic acid dietary deficiency may occur in the elderly with a poor diet or where the vegetables are overcooked. Deficiency may result from faulty absorption, as in coeliac disease. Folic acid deficiency causes an anaemia which resembles that due to B_{12} deficiency.
Vitamin C, ascorbic acid	Fresh fruit, especially blackcurrants, oranges, rose hips, tomatoes, potatoes, green vegetables	45 milligrams	Deficiency causes scurvy: 1 Spontaneous bleeding in the skin. Initially small purplish spots on the front of the thighs, forearms and abdomen. Later more extensive bruising occurs. 2 Gums swell and bleed easily.
Vitamin D, calciferol	Milk, liver, egg yolk, liver oils (particularly fish—halibut, cod)	400 international units	Vitamin D is also produced in the skin on exposure to sunlight. Dietary deficiency is rare in the endogenous British population. Deficiency in children causes rickets. Vitamin D regulates the amount of calcium absorbed from the diet and used for making bones. In adults deficiency causes osteomalacia. This condition is caused by loss of calcium from the bones. In osteomalacia, vitamin D deficiency is usually caused by faulty absorption from the diet as in coeliac disease.
Vitamin E	Wheat germ oil, egg, milk, butter, all seed embryos	15 international units	The role of vitamin E is not entirely clear. In the rat, vitamin E deficiency may lead to sterility or abortion in the pregnant rat. A corresponding deficiency disease does not occur in man.
Vitamin K	Green plants, fishmeal and some animal tissues. Bowel flora.	Very small quantities	Deficiency is very rare because of small quantities required and widespread distribution in foods. Also synthesized by bacteria in bowel. Vitamin K is essential for the production of blood-clotting factors. A newborn baby sometimes lacks vitamin K. This may result in spontaneous bleeding often into the bowel. For this reason many babies are routinely given an injection of vitamin K immediately after birth.

Vocal cords

The two strong fibrous bands which lie from front to back within the supporting cartilage shell of the larynx, and are attached to the walls by the fibrous sheets. From above they have the appearance of the opening to a tent. Their movement is under nervous control, and changes in position alter the pitch of the voice; the closer they are together, the higher the voice. They can become inflamed by over-reaching the voice (an occupational disease of singers) and by infections (see Laryngitis).

Vomiting

A very common symptom and does not necessarily imply that there is anything wrong with the stomach. It occurs during acute and generalized infection, and in children with the common infectious diseases (i.e. measles, mumps, whooping cough).

There are certain patterns and associations which indicate specific diseases. In babies, regurgitation is often confused with vomiting. Babies up to 15 months bring up wind with a small amount of feed and this is normal. However, a few babies have pyloric stenosis (page 191) where the outlet from the stomach to the intestine is constricted by thickened muscle. The vomiting is projectile and the vomitus may travel several feet. More commonly, vomiting in babies is due to a feeding problem—too much, too little, too thick or too thin—and a discussion with the health visitor or family doctor should remedy it.

In adults vomiting is common in acute gastro-enteritis and food poisoning, early pregnancy, migraine, travel sickness, and with certain drugs. Vomiting is not invariable in pregnancy although nausea is frequently experienced in the first 3 months. Likewise in migraine the headache is the predominant feature and is often associated with nausea and sometimes with vomiting. Gastro-enteritis commonly causes vomiting although it is not invariable and diarrhoea may be the only feature.

Vomiting may occur when a stomach ulcer is present, but this is not common as a presenting feature, the usual initial symptoms being indigestion and pain. When vomiting occurs, the pain is often relieved. If vomiting is profuse and associated with

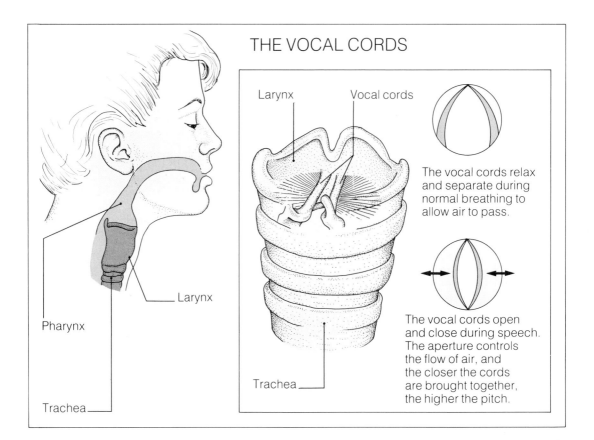

THE VOCAL CORDS

Larynx

Vocal cords

The vocal cords relax and separate during normal breathing to allow air to pass.

The vocal cords open and close during speech. The aperture controls the flow of air, and the closer the cords are brought together, the higher the pitch.

Pharynx

Larynx

Trachea

Trachea

abdominal distension, bowel obstruction may be present. The quantity and frequency of vomiting usually necessitates early treatment and often emergency surgery to relieve the obstruction. When vomiting is associated with headaches, severe migraine is the usual cause.

Nausea and vomiting can be induced by a psychological disturbance. This may be the body's response to a situation which is unpleasant; for instance, some children will be sick to avoid going to school. In extreme cases such as anorexia nervosa (page 21), vomiting may be induced to lose weight.

Vomiting is common and is rarely serious when not prolonged. In children it is frequently associated with feeding problems and with generalized infections such as measles. These will settle as the feeding disturbances are resolved or illness subsides.

If vomiting is severe or persists for more than 24 hours, if it is associated with abdominal pain, or if it occurs with dehydration or drowsiness, medical ★ advice should be obtained. Vomiting in children should always be reported to a doctor, and if the child is drowsy this should be done as a matter of urgency.

Vulva

The external genital organs of the female which surround the opening of the vagina.

Vulval irritation

Vaginal discharge (page 239) is the commonest cause, and the irritation may be cured by treating the cause of the discharge.

It may be associated with burning, frequency or urgency of urination, which suggest a urinary infection. Vulval irritation may be the only symptom present even though the urine is infected, and a sample of urine should be tested for infection and for evidence of diabetes (page 78).

Irritant chemicals (e.g. antiseptics and rubber or chemical contraceptives) may inflame the vulva. Lice (page 159) can be transmitted during intercourse and can produce marked irritation. Persistent scratching may be due to underlying emotional anxiety.

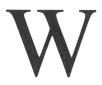

Warts

Caused by a virus, they commonly occur during school age and are spread by direct skin contact; they are not very infectious and many children appear not to be susceptible.

Warts which grow on the sole of the foot are called verrucas or plantar warts (page 238). Warts, however, can occur on any part of the skin surface, most commonly on the fingers and hands where they are unsightly and embarrassing, and a potential source of infection to others.

Warts left untreated usually disappear within 2 years. During that time fresh warts usually grow and it is therefore worthwhile to try to eliminate them. Methods of treatment include ointments, freezing with liquid carbon dioxide or nitrogen, or scraping under local anaesthetic; the choice depends on the number, size and site of the wart.

Warts may also occur on the genitals around the anus and these are usually spread by sexual contact (venereal warts).

Wax

Ear wax is a normal protective substance secreted by glands in the skin of the ear. It normally passes from deep inside the ear to the outside and eventually falls out. Occasionally wax may block the outer ear canal. This is one of the most common causes of temporary deafness and it may even sometimes cause dizziness and ringing (tinnitus) in the ear.

When the wax blocks the ear, medical advice should be sought. The wax can be removed by syringing with warm water. Before this, it is worth trying to soften the wax with warm (not hot) olive oil or proprietary drops left in overnight. The wax may fall out next morning.

It is dangerous to attempt to remove the wax with sticks, even when there is a ball of cotton wool on the end—it is possible to perforate the eardrum and it usually succeeds only in pushing the wax further in.

Before treatment, the ear is carefully examined to ensure that there is no other cause of deafness (see Otitis) and that wax is blocking the channel.

If the eardrum is perforated, syringing should not be used. Instead, the wax is removed with special instruments under direct vision.

Weight loss

When other than by reducing diet, weight loss is always very worrying because it raises the fear of cancer. However, weight loss results from many other treatable disorders, such as anxiety (page 23), depression (page 75), diabetes mellitus (page 78), over-activity of the thyroid gland (thyrotoxicosis, page 224) and anorexia nervosa (page 21).

Anyone who has inexplicably lost his appetite or weight, needs careful medical assessment.

Wheezy bronchitis in children

This common complaint of babies and toddlers is usually caused by a virus infection which starts with a cold. The infection causes inflammation of the larger airways of the lungs, which in turn become swollen and narrowed. This is responsible for the noisy breathing and wheezing. Some children seem particularly prone to wheezy bronchitis every time they catch a cold and they may have asthma. Fortunately, only a minority of children with recurrent wheezy bronchitis develop asthma later in life, but if there is a family history of asthma or of a similar allergic tendency (e.g. hay fever and eczema), the chance of developing asthma is increased.

Wheezy children should be reported to the family physician.

The treatment of wheezy bronchitis depends on the severity of the illness. Most children with bronchitis are not very ill and can be looked after at home. Treatment consists of paracetamol elixir to reduce the fever and a decongestant (e.g. Actifed) to relieve respiratory congestion and to ease the breathing. Antibiotics are required if there is superadded bacterial infection and if there is a complicating ear infection. In children over 18 months of age, an anti-spasmodic such as salbutamol (Ventolin) will relax the muscles in the airways, which in turn relieves the constriction.

Weil's disease
SEE LEPTOSPIROSIS

Whitlow
(PARONYCHIA)

An infection in the skin of the nail fold (the medical term is paronychia). The infection may be caused by either a yeast or fungus (e.g. thrush: *Candida albicans)* or a bacterium. Fungal infection occurs in people whose hands are immersed in water for long periods (e.g. housewives, nurses and cooks), and the infection tends to be chronic. Treatment is by ensuring the hands are kept dry and using rubber gloves when working with water. An anti-fungal cream such as nystatin may be applied.

In bacterial infections, the symptoms are more severe with a sudden onset of redness, swelling and pain around the nail. Treatment is by giving an antibiotic by mouth. It may be necessary to open the abscess surgically or occasionally to remove a nail under anaesthetic to allow the pus to drain.

Whooping cough
(PERTUSSIS)

A common bacterial infection of children affecting the upper respiratory tract. Typically it produces long paroxysms of coughing followed by a 'whoop' on inspiration. The coughs are so close together that the child may be unable to catch his breath and the whoop is the noise made when rapidly breathing in after coughing. Sometimes the child may go blue and vomit after a coughing paroxysm. The whoop is not always present in babies or in older children with milder infection.

In most cases whooping cough is not a serious illness, but the cough can persist for 3 months or more. It is a distressing and tiring illness because the paroxysms of coughing often occur at night and are difficult to suppress. The whole family may be kept awake.

Although antibiotics are frequently used, they probably have little effect on shortening the illness, though they do reduce the period of infectivity and may prevent complicating lung infections. The child is capable of spreading the infection for up to 2 weeks after onset of the cough. The infectious period does not correspond with the duration of the coughing.

Cough linctuses are frequently used. Codeine is the essential ingredient in most linctuses and though it is a good cough suppressant, it can also cause sedation and constipation.

Whooping cough is most serious in the youngest age groups. Babies often have to be admitted to hospital because they are usually very ill and may have feeding difficulties since sucking can trigger a coughing paroxysm. When this happens the baby may have to be tube fed. Most deaths from whooping cough occur in children under 1 year. The younger the child, the greater the risk of death. In view of this, the length of the illness and the seriousness of the complications (which include severe pneumonia and brain haemorrhage), vaccination against whooping cough is recommended by the Department of Health (*see also* Vaccination). As the youngest children are

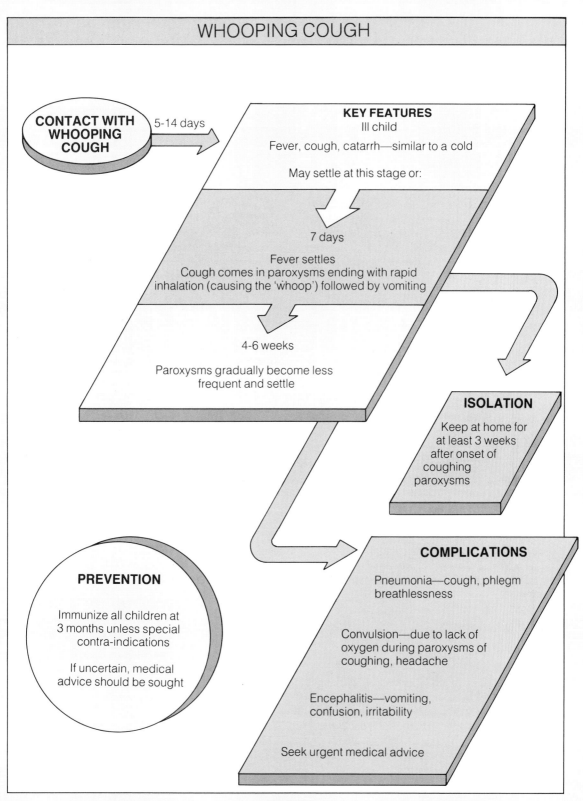

WHOOPING COUGH

CONTACT WITH WHOOPING COUGH

5-14 days

KEY FEATURES
Ill child

Fever, cough, catarrh—similar to a cold

May settle at this stage or:

7 days

Fever settles
Cough comes in paroxysms ending with rapid inhalation (causing the 'whoop') followed by vomiting

4-6 weeks

Paroxysms gradually become less frequent and settle

ISOLATION

Keep at home for at least 3 weeks after onset of coughing paroxysms

PREVENTION

Immunize all children at 3 months unless special contra-indications

If uncertain, medical advice should be sought

COMPLICATIONS

Pneumonia—cough, phlegm breathlessness

Convulsion—due to lack of oxygen during paroxysms of coughing, headache

Encephalitis—vomiting, confusion, irritability

Seek urgent medical advice

most at risk, vaccination should be performed at 3 months.

Windpipe

The major airway to the lungs, comprising the larynx, the trachea and the right and left main bronchi (*see also* Bronchus; *and* diagram, page 255). The larynx has cartilage walls which keep it open (patent), and the other airways are kept patent by a series of incomplete cartilage rings at close intervals along their length.

Wisdom teeth
SEE TOOTHACHE

Worms

Intestinal worms such as threadworms (*Enterobius vermicularis*), hookworms (*Ancylostoma duodenale*), roundworms (*Ascaris lumbricoides*) and tapeworms (*Taenia saginata* and *Taenia solium*) are uncommon in the developed world as a result of better standards of personal and food hygiene. Threadworms are the most common. They cause itching on the skin around the anus and this often disturbs sleep. It is not a serious condition and the worms should first be identified; it is then easily treated with medication taken by mouth. It is best to treat the whole family even when they have no symptoms. This ensures that the person who is the source of infection has been treated.

Medical advice should be obtained to ensure accurate identification of a worm and thus the correct treatment.

Wrist
(ANGLO-SAXON: TO TWIST)

Contains eight small bones arranged in two horizontal groups of four (*see* diagram, page 267). The upper four articulate with the lower end of the radius to form the wrist joint, and the lower four bones articulate with the metacarpal bones of the hand. The wrist joint is a hinge joint, moving mainly backwards and forwards but the position and interplay of the small bones allow some sideways movement. Fractures of the wrist usually occur in the scaphoid bone or the head of the radius.

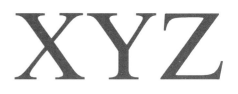

XYZ

Xanthomas

Small deposits of fat and cholesterol in the skin. They may be found on the eyelids, or in the skin of knees, elbows or buttocks, as small yellowish nodules. Similar deposits occur in tendons; e.g. on the back of the hands, or the Achilles tendon. Their presence may occasionally be associated with raised blood cholesterol which itself may be associated with heart disease or under-activity of the thyroid gland.

X-rays

Used for investigation and diagnosis. The principle depends on differing degrees of penetration of the rays through different tissues. The rays then impinge on a photographic plate which records a negative image—i.e. dense tissues and substances such as bone and barium (used in barium meals and enemas to examine the intestines) appear white, and thin tissues (e.g. lung and brain) appear black.

X-rays are also used to treat some cancers (*see* Radiotherapy).

Yellow fever

A viral infection of man, transmitted by mosquitoes, and endemic in the tropical rain forests of Africa and South America. The infection may vary from mild, with 'flu-like symptoms, to severe, with jaundice, internal bleeding and death.

Yellow fever vaccine is a very effective live attenuated (weakened) viral preparation and is available at special centres (*see* Vaccination: for travellers). An international vaccine certificate is valid for 10 years.

Zoster

Herpes zoster (shingles) is a painful skin infection caused by the same virus which causes chickenpox. Chickenpox usually occurs in children and when the disease is over the virus remains latent in the nerves. In later life, especially at times of stress (such as infection), the virus is reactivated and produces shingles. (*See also* Chickenpox *and* Shingles.)

Part 2

Anatomy: The Main Systems and Organs
of the Body

The Heart and Circulation
The Lungs and Respiratory Passages
The Brain and Nervous System
The Skeleton
The Kidneys
The Reproductive System
The Digestive Tract
The Muscles and Joints

The Heart and Circulation

The heart pumps blood from the muscular thick-walled left ventricle into the aorta. At its origin are the two major coronary vessels which supply blood and its contained oxygen and nutrients to the muscles of the heart. Narrowing of these coronary vessels causes heart pain—angina (page 19) and blockage results in death of heart muscle—heart attack (page 120). The aortic valve prevents reflux of blood from the aorta into the ventricle. Blood flows round the arch-shaped aorta and up into the head via the carotid and vertebral arteries. Strokes usually arise from narrowing or occlusion of these arteries or their smaller branches which supply blood to the brain.

From the aorta, blood is supplied to the arms via the subclavian arteries and thence to its branches, the best known being the radial artery where the pulse is easily felt.

The aorta descends on the back wall of the abdomen, supplying blood to the tissues and organs within the abdomen; e.g. the mesenteric arteries to the intestine, the renal arteries to the kidneys, the hepatic artery to the liver. In the abdomen the aorta splits into the iliac arteries to supply the legs. Narrowing or occlusion of these arteries results in a drastic reduction of oxygen to the muscles of the legs, accentuated during exercise and causing severe cramp on walking—intermittent claudication (page 136). This can be relieved by removing the obstruction, or inserting an arterial graft to bypass it.

The Veins

Blood from the toes and feet flows up the legs pumped by the muscles of the calf, and prevented from flowing backward by a system of valves. Incompetence of these valves causes varicose veins (page 239). The blood enters the iliac veins which join to form the large inferior vena cava. This passes upward, collecting blood from the abdomen and lower chest which it carries to the right atrium of the heart where it mixes with blood returning from the head, arms and upper chest via the superior vena cava.

From the right atrium, blood flows to the right ventricle which pumps it through the lungs where it is re-oxygenated. From here it passes to the left atrium and thence to the left ventricle which pumps it round the circulation again.

HOW THE HEART PUMPS THE BLOOD

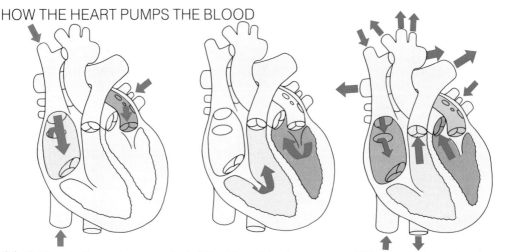

1 As the heart relaxes, deoxygenated blood from the body flows into the right atrium. At the same time, oxygenated blood from the lungs flows into the left atrium.

2 The tricuspid valve opens, allowing deoxygenated blood into the right ventricle, while the mitral valve opens to allow blood from the lungs into the left ventricle.

3 The ventricles contract, forcing open the pulmonary and aortic valves. Oxygenated blood flows through the aorta to the body and deoxygenated blood, to the lungs via the pulmonary artery.

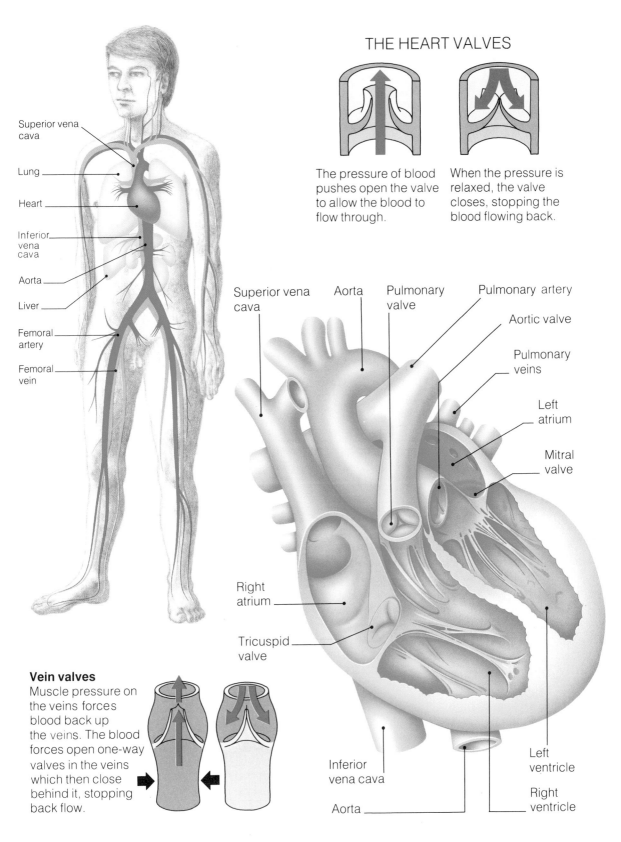

THE HEART VALVES

The pressure of blood pushes open the valve to allow the blood to flow through.

When the pressure is relaxed, the valve closes, stopping the blood flowing back.

Superior vena cava

Lung

Heart

Inferior vena cava

Aorta

Liver

Femoral artery

Femoral vein

Superior vena cava

Aorta

Pulmonary valve

Pulmonary artery

Aortic valve

Pulmonary veins

Left atrium

Mitral valve

Right atrium

Tricuspid valve

Vein valves
Muscle pressure on the veins forces blood back up the veins. The blood forces open one-way valves in the veins which then close behind it, stopping back flow.

Inferior vena cava

Aorta

Left ventricle

Right ventricle

The Lungs and Respiratory Passages

The respiratory tract consists of the larynx, trachea, the major bronchi and the lungs.

Inhaled air passes through the mouth to the pharynx to enter the larynx which is the upper part of the main 'airway'. It has a firm shell of cartilage which keeps it rigid. Two vocal cords run within it from front to back and alter the pitch of the voice—the higher and closer they come together, the higher the pitch.

The larynx is easily felt in the neck and is better known as 'Adam's apple'. Gentle squeezing between the fingers demonstrates its firmness. It is both painful and unwise to squeeze too hard. Just below the larynx the firm rings of cartilage in the trachea can also be felt. These hold the trachea permanently open to allow free passage of air between the larynx above and the lungs. At the level of the upper heart border, about one-third of the way down the sternum (breastbone), the trachea divides into a right and left main bronchus, both of which are held open by rings of cartilage. The bronchi in turn divide into smaller airways which carry air to the lobes of the left and right lungs.

Within each lobe the airways divide into smaller and smaller branches and the smallest ones end in alveoli. These thin-walled sac-like structures are the site of gas exchange between the atmosphere and the blood. Fine blood vessels run over the outer wall of the alveoli carrying blood depleted of oxygen but rich in unwanted carbon dioxide, a by-product of body metabolism. Inspired air is rich in oxygen and contains virtually no carbon dioxide.

Due to the differences in gas concentration oxygen diffuses into the blood for transport to the heart and body tissues and carbon dioxide diffuses out into the alveoli, to be exhaled at the next breath. The large numbers of alveoli create an enormous surface area for this gas diffusion to take place and allows it to remain efficient even if some alveoli are damaged, usually by infection (e.g. pneumonia, bronchitis).

The commonest diseases affecting the respiratory tract are laryngitis and bronchitis. Laryngitis is usually associated with other features of a cold and is caused by viruses. The voice may become gruff or even lost. Sometimes the trachea is also infected (tracheitis) causing soreness on breathing. Acute bronchitis is a disease of the bronchi and causes fever, cough, and phlegm (sputum) which may become yellow or green, i.e. it consists of pus. If smokers fail to stop, bronchitis usually recurs and may become chronic with persistent cough and coloured phlegm, which may be stained with blood. The inner wall of the large bronchi are lined with fine hairs which in health waft the small amount of phlegm normally produced within the lungs up towards the pharynx where it is normally swallowed. In chronic bronchitis the fine hairs or cilia are destroyed. The phlegm can no longer be removed as it is produced, stagnates in the alveoli, becomes infected by bacteria and causes further damage to the delicate tissues which transfer oxygen. Eventually, gas transport is severely reduced.

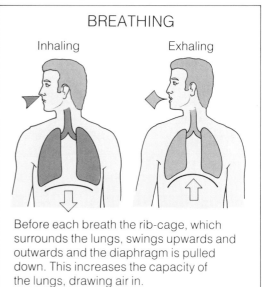

BREATHING

Inhaling   Exhaling

Before each breath the rib-cage, which surrounds the lungs, swings upwards and outwards and the diaphragm is pulled down. This increases the capacity of the lungs, drawing air in.

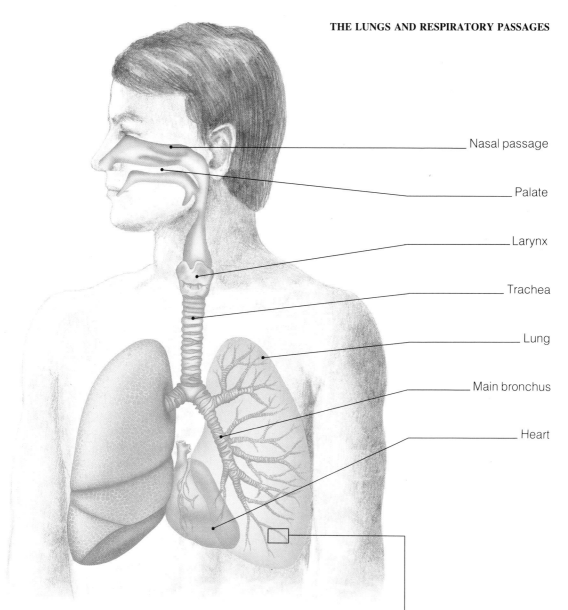

Nasal passage

Palate

Larynx

Trachea

Lung

Main bronchus

Heart

GAS EXCHANGE

Oxygen-rich air is breathed into the lungs, and passes to the alveoli at the end of the small bronchi. Here oxygen from the air dissolves in the lining of the alveoli and passes into the blood vessels that surround them. Carbon dioxide from the blood passes into the alveoli and is breathed out.

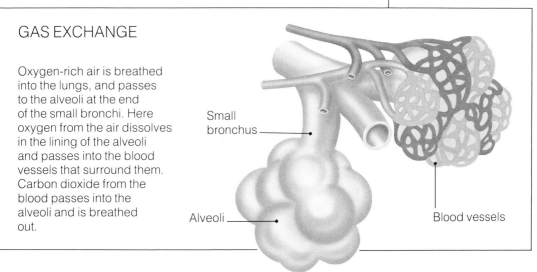

Small bronchus

Alveoli

Blood vessels

The Brain and Nervous System

The nervous system consists of the brain, the spinal cord and the nerves. It has three major functions: (a) control of consciousness, emotion and memory; (b) initiation and control of movement through the muscles; (c) receipt and integration of sensations and stimuli from both within and outside the body.

The *brain* sits within the protective bony skull. It is divided into a large cerebrum and a smaller cerebellum. The cerebral surface is convoluted and furrowed. This allows a greater number of brain cells within the space limited by the volume of the skull. Different areas of the cerebrum control different functions; e.g. the frontal lobes control emotion and social responsibility, the parietal lobes are the major centres receiving sensory impulses and controlling muscle movement and power, vision is perceived in the occipital lobes and smell in the olfactory lobes. All the brain cells are interconnected and the healthy brain acts as an integrated unit. Damage to one region may produce predictable dysfunction—e.g. a cerebral haemorrhage (a stroke) into one parietal region results in weakness of the arm and leg of the side of the body controlled by that parietal lobe; damage to the frontal lobes from haemorrhage, infection or malignant tumours can result in poor memory and detachment from reality.

The *cerebellum* controls and integrates the muscle power and movement required for fine complex actions and balance. The cerebellum connects with the cells of the rest of the brain via the brain stem. Within the brain stem are groups of nerve cells which control vital non-voluntary functions, such as the maintenance of normal blood pressure and initiation and control of breathing.

There are four major blood vessels supplying the brain. The two largest, the internal carotid arteries, arise from the aorta and form a network of vessels below the brain with the two vertebral arteries, named because of their position just in front of the vertebrae.

From this network arise three important arteries, the anterior cerebral artery which curves around the front and over the top of the brain, the middle cerebral artery which supplies the bulk of the brain, and the posterior cerebral artery which runs backward on the base of the brain to supply the occipital lobes involved principally with vision.

Strokes usually result from bleeding (cerebral haemorrhage) or clotting (cerebral thrombosis) within these arteries, the middle cerebral being the most commonly affected. They are much more common in those with high blood pressure and the risk of stroke is greatly reduced if their blood pressure is returned to normal.

The *nerves* receive information from all the tissues of the body such as the legs, heart and skin; electrical impulses are relayed along the nerves to the *spinal cord*. The impulses ascend to reach the brain, which assesses these messages, with other stimuli from the eyes and ears, in the light of its stored memory. If necessary it can initiate a response by passing impulses back down the spinal cord. Certain responses can take effect in the spine, without reference to the brain—the response to touching a very hot object, for example.

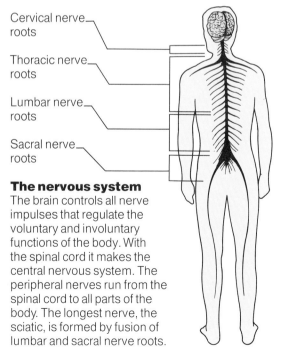

Cervical nerve roots

Thoracic nerve roots

Lumbar nerve roots

Sacral nerve roots

The nervous system
The brain controls all nerve impulses that regulate the voluntary and involuntary functions of the body. With the spinal cord it makes the central nervous system. The peripheral nerves run from the spinal cord to all parts of the body. The longest nerve, the sciatic, is formed by fusion of lumbar and sacral nerve roots.

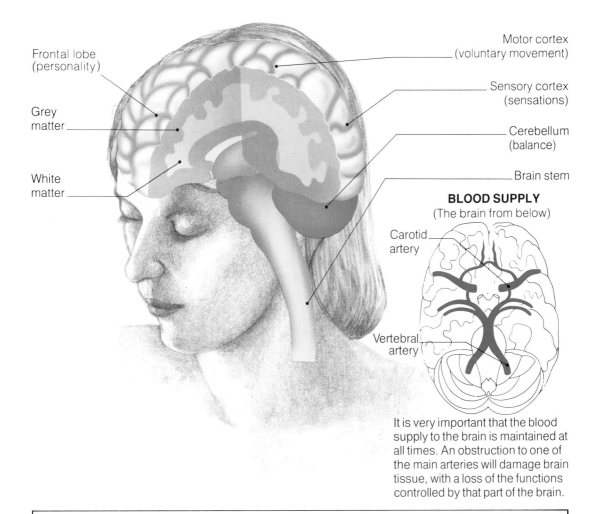

Frontal lobe (personality)

Grey matter

White matter

Motor cortex (voluntary movement)

Sensory cortex (sensations)

Cerebellum (balance)

Brain stem

BLOOD SUPPLY
(The brain from below)

Carotid artery

Vertebral artery

It is very important that the blood supply to the brain is maintained at all times. An obstruction to one of the main arteries will damage brain tissue, with a loss of the functions controlled by that part of the brain.

The spinal cord

The spinal cord is the route for nerve signals travelling to and from the body and the brain. The cord is protected by the vertebrae of the spine and emerges as two roots from the gaps between each vertebra. These join to form the peripheral nerves. Damage to the spine can impair the function of a nerve and the tissues that nerve controls.

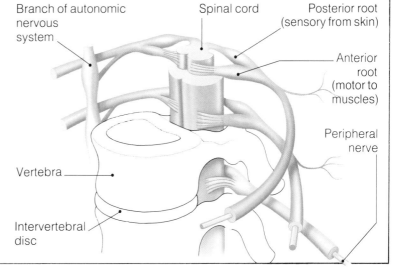

Branch of autonomic nervous system

Spinal cord

Posterior root (sensory from skin)

Anterior root (motor to muscles)

Peripheral nerve

Vertebra

Intervertebral disc

257

The Skeleton

The skeleton is composed of all the bones in the body. It has three main functions. It maintains the erect posture, protects the most important body tissues (i.e. the brain within the skull, the spinal cord within the vertebrae and the heart and lungs within the rib cage), and it is the body's reserve pool of calcium required for bone growth and repair.

Bones are very light for their strength. This gives optimum protection whilst maintaining posture and also allows ease of movement. This compares with animals with a strong external skeleton—e.g. the crab family, which though well protected can move only very slowly.

Fractures are very common and invariably caused by trauma, often multiple and severe following road traffic accidents. The commonest fractures following accidents are to the long bones of the limbs, the skull and the ribs. The pelvis is very strong and less commonly damaged. The elderly are more prone to falls and fractures.

Other than in road accidents, bones commonly fractured include the clavicle following falls onto the shoulder, the lower end of the radius from falls onto the outstretched hand and very common in winter with icy pavements, and fractures of the ankle when both the lower tibia and fibula can break following a fall or severe twisting injury—common in skiers.

Because of the thickness and strength of the skull bones, severe trauma is usually needed to cause skull fracture. Damage to the brain depends upon the degree of trauma and whether the fracture has damaged blood vessels or the brain surface.

Several nerves run very close to or over bones and are in danger of damage from pressure or trauma if the bones are diseased or fractured. Common sites are: the median nerve at the wrist which produces weakness, numbness, and pins and needles in the hand and fingers (see Carpal tunnel syndrome); the radial nerve at the elbow which causes wrist drop—inability to raise the hand when arms are outstretched; the popliteal nerve where it runs over the top of the fibula which causes foot

THE SKULL

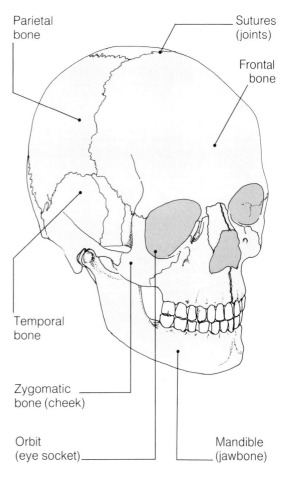

drop. Sciatica (page 203) is caused by pressure on nerves as they leave the spine and produces a severe sharp pain which shoots down the leg along the course of the affected nerve.

In malnutrition bones may lose their calcium and become thin, soft and fragile. This may produce rickets (page 197) or osteomalacia due to low calcium and vitamin D in the diet. It is very common worldwide. In developed countries these conditions are more often due to poor absorption of vitamin D from the gut. The bones bend easily producing marked deformities and are liable to fracture. The disease is preventable by adequate diet and supplements of vitamin D.

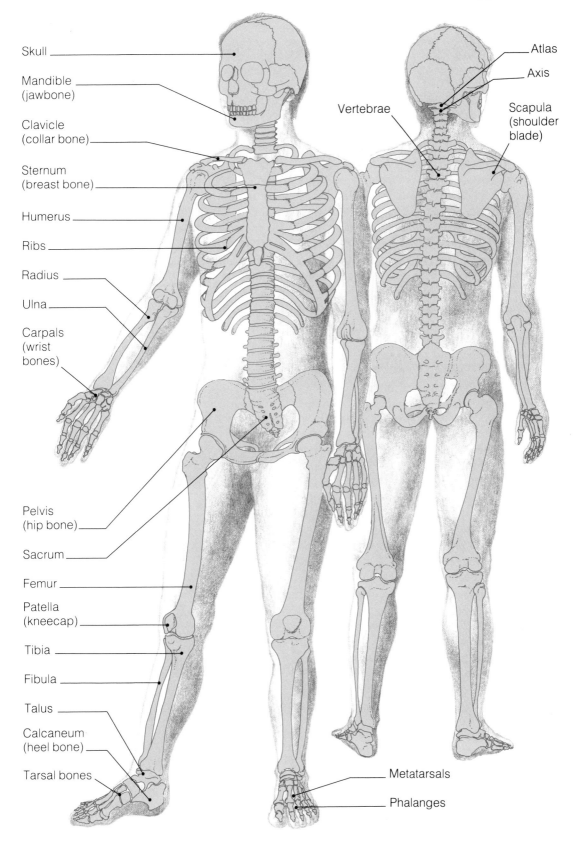

Skull

Mandible
(jawbone)

Clavicle
(collar bone)

Sternum
(breast bone)

Humerus

Ribs

Radius

Ulna

Carpals
(wrist
bones)

Pelvis
(hip bone)

Sacrum

Femur

Patella
(kneecap)

Tibia

Fibula

Talus

Calcaneum
(heel bone)

Tarsal bones

Atlas

Axis

Vertebrae

Scapula
(shoulder
blade)

Metatarsals

Phalanges

The Kidneys

The renal system consists of the kidneys, ureters and the bladder in which urine is stored until excreted from the body through the urethra.

The kidneys sit high up in the back of the abdomen, protected by the bony spine, lower ribs and the bulky muscles of the back. The kidneys receive arterial blood containing waste products, particularly urea, formed during metabolism in all body cells. The blood is filtered by millions of convoluted glomeruli, leaving the remaining blood to pass back into the circulation via the veins of the kidney. The watery filtered fluid, rich in salt, passes from the glomeruli through fine tubules where water and salt are reabsorbed, leaving concentrated urine to flow down the ureters to the bladder. This reabsorptive system is the body's main method of balancing water and salt output with intake. Waste products of metabolism (such as urea) are normally excreted in the urine, but in kidney disease may accumulate in the body (uraemia).

The urine is passed down the ureters by a series of regular slow contractions of the ureteric wall into the bladder. This muscular walled bag stores urine until distension signals the need to urinate. This is normally under the control of the brain which retains control of the muscular sphincter at the base of the bladder. At a convenient time urine is voided by relaxation of the sphincter and simultaneous contraction of the bladder wall. Urine is voided through the urethra. This is short in the female but in men it passes through the middle of the prostate gland where it can be obstructed easily, and thence along the length of the penis.

The kidneys are so efficient that normal renal function is possible with only one kidney, as occurs when kidneys are removed for tumours or following road accidents. If both kidneys are damaged or seriously diseased their function can be replaced by haemodialysis (i.e. dialysing the blood across a membrane as a substitute for the glomerular filter which allows removal of waste products) or, if possible, by transplanting a healthy kidney from a donor.

The commonest disorders of the renal system are cystitis and urethritis due to infection, occasionally caused by venereal diseases. Prostatic enlargement in elderly men is very common, and because the prostate surrounds the urethra it will produce varying degrees of blockage. At first this is noticed as delay in micturition with a narrow stream of poor force. If enlargement increases, the urethra may be completely obstructed. If not relieved surgically, pressure increases in the bladder, the ureters and the kidneys; permanent damage can result.

Stones may occur both in the kidney and in the bladder and produce pain behind the kidney which spreads to the groin—renal colic—or over the bladder in the lower abdomen. Infection around the stone is common and this with damage caused by the stone results in pain on micturition and blood in the urine.

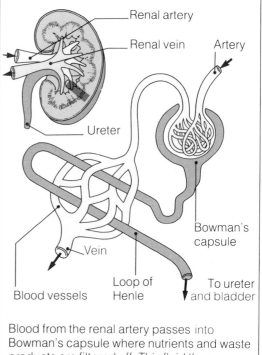

Blood from the renal artery passes into Bowman's capsule where nutrients and waste products are filtered off. This fluid then moves through thin tubes (the loop of Henle) where the nutrients are reabsorbed by the surrounding blood vessels. The waste products are carried on to the ureter, then to the bladder.

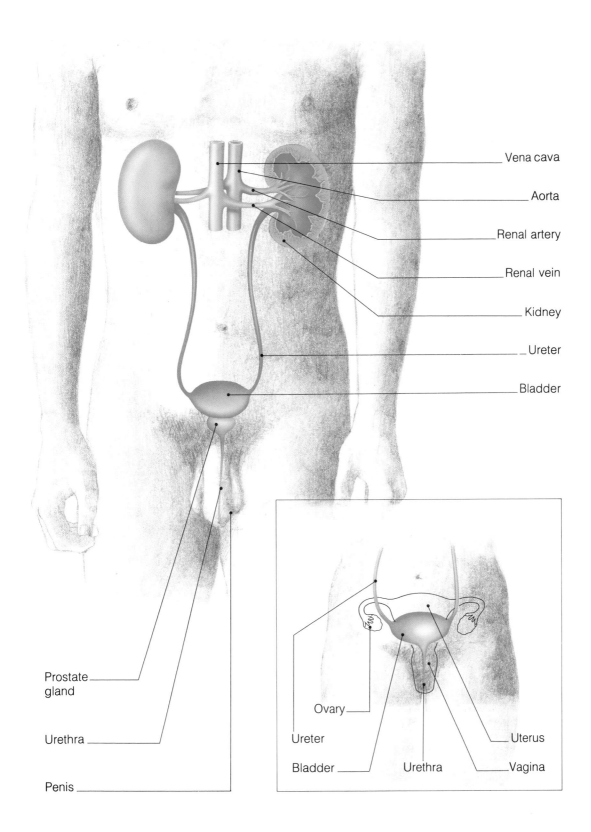

Vena cava

Aorta

Renal artery

Renal vein

Kidney

Ureter

Bladder

Prostate gland

Urethra

Penis

Ovary

Ureter

Bladder

Urethra

Uterus

Vagina

The Reproductive System

The genital system of the female is composed of the ovaries, the uterus and the vagina and in the male, the testes, the vasa deferentia and the penis.

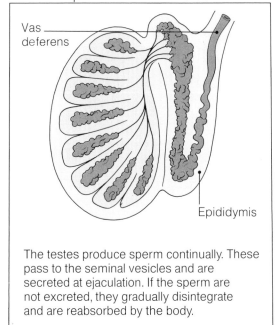

Bladder

Vas deferens

Penis

Urethra

Testicle

Scrotum

Seminal vesicle

Prostate gland

Epididymis

Vas deferens

Epididymis

The testes produce sperm continually. These pass to the seminal vesicles and are secreted at ejaculation. If the sperm are not excreted, they gradually disintegrate and are reabsorbed by the body.

The *male* genital system is designed to produce sperm and deliver them to the unfertilized ovum. Sperm are produced in the testes, and in response to sexual stimulation are ejected via the urethra of the erect penis into the vault of the vagina. From here they can pass through the cervix and into the uterus to fertilize the ovum.

Male infertility results usually from impotence or a low sperm count often for reasons which cannot be explained. This is detected by microscopic examination of ejaculate to determine sperm numbers and their activity.

Mumps can infect the testes to cause severe pain and swelling and occasionally results in infertility if contracted in adolescence. Due to the anatomical system of suspending the testes in the scrotum, twisting can occur and obstruct the blood supply. The testis then becomes swollen and very tender, and if not untwisted quickly the testis may be irreparably damaged.

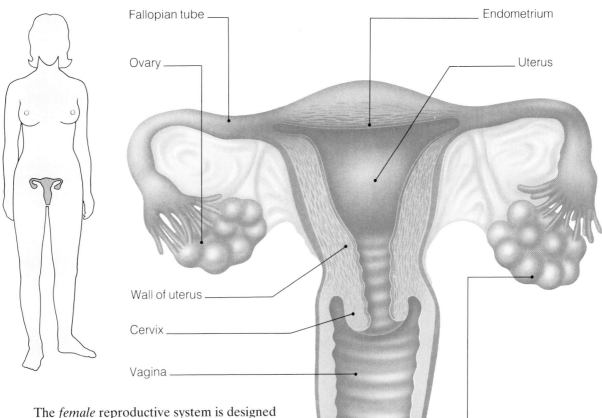

Fallopian tube

Ovary

Endometrium

Uterus

Wall of uterus

Cervix

Vagina

The *female* reproductive system is designed to bring the egg (ovum) from the ovary to the womb (uterus) for fertilization. Ova are produced every month within the ovary about mid-way between periods and are wafted along the Fallopian tubes to the uterus. At the same time the inner wall of the uterus develops an increased blood supply to allow a fertilized ovum to embed and receive adequate nutrition and oxygen. If the ovum is implanted in the uterus, it develops into a fetus which grows there until birth.

If the ovum is not fertilized, it does not develop, and the blood-filled inner lining of the uterus disintegrates resulting in a period.

Infertility may result from damage to the ovaries or Fallopian tubes, sometimes from tuberculosis or gonorrhoea. The uterus is a site of cancer in women over the age of 40. The cervix of the uterus is the commonest site and this can be detected early when still curable by regular cervical smears when a small number of cells are removed from the cervix for microscopic examination.

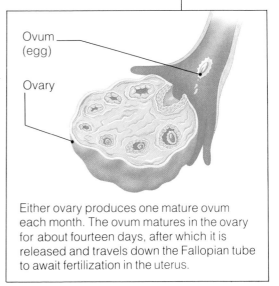

Ovum (egg)

Ovary

Either ovary produces one mature ovum each month. The ovum matures in the ovary for about fourteen days, after which it is released and travels down the Fallopian tube to await fertilization in the uterus.

The Digestive Tract

The gastro-intestinal tract with the liver and pancreas act to digest food and absorb the digested components for use as energy and for growth and replacement of damaged tissues.

Digestion begins in the mouth where food is chewed and subject to enzymes in saliva secreted by the parotid and submandibular glands. The food is swallowed and passes down the oesophagus to the stomach. Difficulty in swallowing often occurs with infections of the throat and tonsillitis, and settles as the acute illness subsides. In the absence of throat infection, swallowing difficulty may result from anxiety but suggests obstruction in the oesophagus. Sometimes a bone has lodged in the gullet but the problem should always be taken seriously and medical advice obtained.

In the stomach the food is churned and broken down by gastric acid and enzymes and then passed into the duodenum of the small intestine. Both the stomach and duodenum are common sites for peptic ulcers. The duodenum is the major site for digestion and receives enzymes in bile from the liver and juices from the pancreas. Here fats and proteins are metabolized or broken down into their component parts which are moved along by waves of muscular contraction in the intestinal wall and absorbed across the small intestinal wall into the blood stream. Water, sodium, calcium and other essential food constituents are also absorbed here.

Damage to the cells lining the inner wall of the small intestine results in inability to absorb food and particularly fats. A well recognized disorder is coeliac disease (page 62) caused by sensitivity to gluten, a major constituent of most grains. Deficient absorption results in excess fat passing into the large intestine and diarrhoea with fatty stools and weight loss. The disease is controlled with a gluten-free diet.

All undigested food remaining in the small intestine passes into the large intestine or colon for excretion.

The commonest disorders affecting the tract are constipation, acute appendicitis, piles which cause pain and rectal bleeding, acute gastroenteritis, usually caused by viruses and producing one or more of nausea, vomiting, abdominal colic and diarrhoea, and viral hepatitis. Another disease commonly seen is cholecystitis—inflammation of the gall bladder.

ABSORPTION

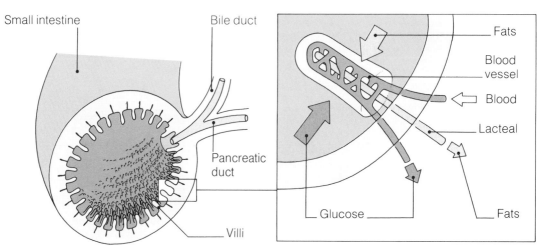

The inner surface of the small intestine is covered with small, finger-like projections called villi. Minerals, sugars and vitamins are absorbed into the blood capillaries to be taken to the liver, while fats diffuse into the lacteals and enter the bloodstream via the lymph system.

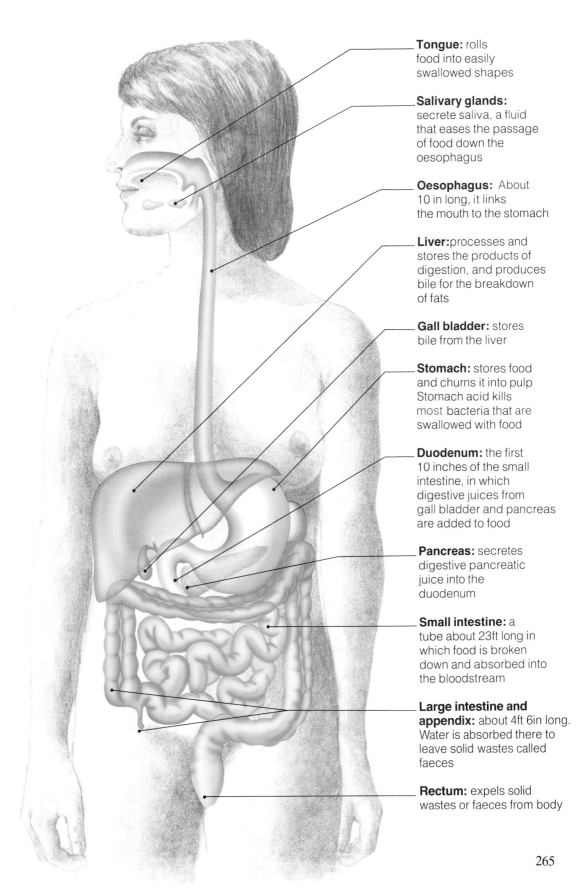

Tongue: rolls food into easily swallowed shapes

Salivary glands: secrete saliva, a fluid that eases the passage of food down the oesophagus

Oesophagus: About 10 in long, it links the mouth to the stomach

Liver: processes and stores the products of digestion, and produces bile for the breakdown of fats

Gall bladder: stores bile from the liver

Stomach: stores food and churns it into pulp Stomach acid kills most bacteria that are swallowed with food

Duodenum: the first 10 inches of the small intestine, in which digestive juices from gall bladder and pancreas are added to food

Pancreas: secretes digestive pancreatic juice into the duodenum

Small intestine: a tube about 23ft long in which food is broken down and absorbed into the bloodstream

Large intestine and appendix: about 4ft 6in long. Water is absorbed there to leave solid wastes called faeces

Rectum: expels solid wastes or faeces from body

The Muscles and Joints

The muscles constitute 40 per cent of the body's bulk and use more than half of its total energy supply during normal activity. The heat produced by this activity is most important in maintaining normal body temperature. Their function is to move the body and they are arranged in groups around the joints so that each movement can be reversed. The muscle groups work in conjunction, e.g. when the elbow bends by contraction of the biceps muscle, the triceps muscle relaxes at the same time. The action of both muscles is carefully monitored and regulated by the nerves which supply them allowing smooth controlled movement.

Muscle contraction is initiated in the cortex of the brain either in response to a voluntary need, or in response to an outside stimulus such as pain on touching a hot object, or the visual stimulus of a moving object as in ball games. A nervous impulse begins in large nerve cells within the brain, and passes down the spinal cord. From here nerves transmit impulses to the muscles which move the limbs and the body in response to the stimulus or desire. Nervous impulses move at phenomenal speed—up to 120 metres per second—and the response to any stimulus is almost instantaneous.

Each muscle group is controlled by a different region of the brain, and damage to any part of the brain will prevent the nervous response which initiates movement in those muscles. This is commonly seen following a stroke which is usually caused by haemorrhage into the brain tissue controlling the nerve supply to the muscles of the face and the limbs. Weakness may occur in one leg, one arm or the face on the same side. If the haemorrhage is extensive all may be affected. Single muscle groups can be immobilized if their nerves are damaged or cut. This is now rare but occurs in poliomyelitis, a virus infection of the spinal cord. It may also result in foot drop if the nerve controlling the muscle which lifts the foot is stretched or bruised as it passes around the top of the fibula just below the knee, or wrist drop if the ulnar nerve which passes behind the elbow is damaged when the elbow is dislocated or fractured.

The commonest disorders of muscle result from strains and tears, often the result of sports injury and common in the unfit. The tears are followed by swelling and bruising which takes 3 to 4 weeks to settle. They tend to recur if exercise is started too quickly. Serious and life-threatening muscle diseases are rare (*see* Muscular dystrophy *and* Myasthenia gravis).

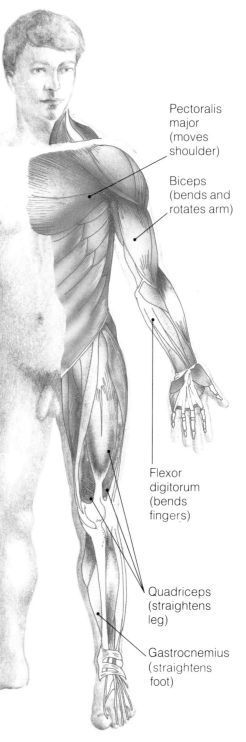

Pectoralis major (moves shoulder)

Biceps (bends and rotates arm)

Flexor digitorum (bends fingers)

Quadriceps (straightens leg)

Gastrocnemius (straightens foot)

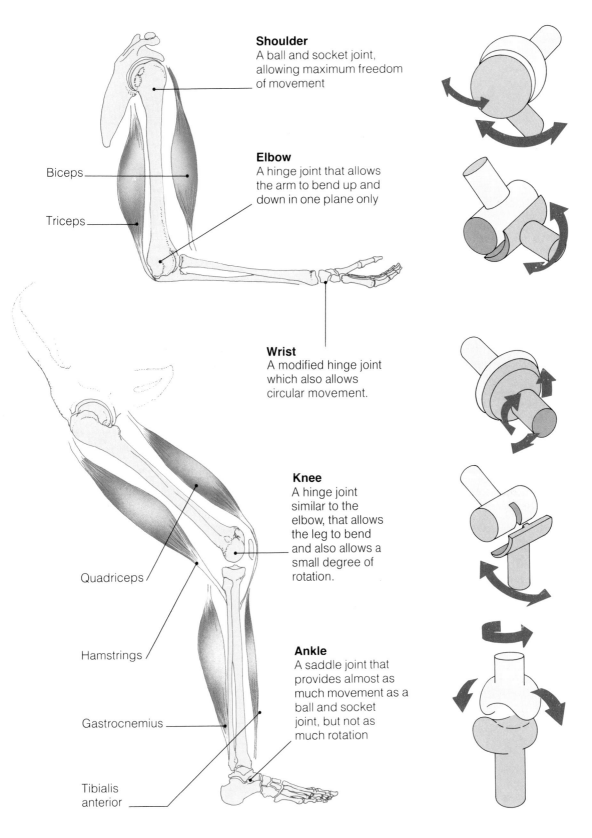

Shoulder
A ball and socket joint, allowing maximum freedom of movement

Elbow
A hinge joint that allows the arm to bend up and down in one plane only

Biceps

Triceps

Wrist
A modified hinge joint which also allows circular movement.

Knee
A hinge joint similar to the elbow, that allows the leg to bend and also allows a small degree of rotation.

Quadriceps

Hamstrings

Ankle
A saddle joint that provides almost as much movement as a ball and socket joint, but not as much rotation

Gastrocnemius

Tibialis anterior

Part 3

Special Topics

First Aid

Shock

This is usually the result of severe bleeding, often following road accidents. The patient is pale and cold, with rapid breathing and a fast shallow pulse. The blood pressure is low and the flow of blood to the brain, kidneys and other vital organs seriously diminished. This may cause confusion or unconsciousness. Immediately, get someone to send for an ambulance or emergency medical help and at the same time look for *bleeding*. Compression over the bleeding point will often control the loss (*see below*). Do not warm the patient or give alcohol; these are very dangerous because they open up the blood vessels and cause an even greater fall in blood pressure and increase the severity of shock.

The *mouth* and airways can be blocked by food or false teeth, which should be removed gently. It may be dangerous to move the injured because there may be fractures of the bones which are not obvious. In spinal injury there is a risk of increasing damage to the spinal cord. If possible, it is best to await the arrival of properly trained experts.

Bleeding

Visible bleeding

Arteries contain bright red blood at high pressure which spurts out. It can usually be stopped by very firm pressure with the thumb or thumbs over the site of bleeding. This is very tiring and it is often necessary for bystanders to take turns until medical help arrives. Rarely, local pressure is unsuccessful, and as a second resort pressure over the artery above the bleeding point (where it is close to a bone) can be tried. Tourniquets are rarely required and may be dangerous because nearby nerves may be crushed, resulting in paralysis or gangrene of the limb. However, if a reasonable attempt at local pressure has failed, a tourniquet can be applied to the mid-forearm or mid-thigh.

Bleeding from a vein causes dark blood to ooze from the site. The pressure inside veins is very low and easily stopped by elevating the limb above the level of the heart, with light pressure applied with a clean handkerchief over the bleeding site. This type of bleeding takes place from superficial cuts to the wrists and from varicose veins.

Bleeding points
Nose bleeds
These are usually from small veins high up on the central wall of the nostril. Although they may appear serious, they rarely are and can usually be stopped by firmly pressing the outside of the nose against the central wall. There is a natural tendency to stop pressure too soon, but pressure must be maintained for at least 5 minutes. It is better to hold the head forward than back, to stop blood running down the back of the throat. It is best to breathe slowly and steadily, keeping the mouth open wide. If local

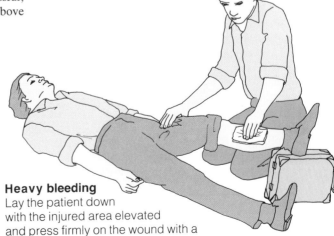

Light bleeding
Press firmly on the area of the wound with a clean pad, until the bleeding stops.

Heavy bleeding
Lay the patient down with the injured area elevated and press firmly on the wound with a clean pad. If the bleeding continues apply firm pressure to the main artery.

pressure for 5 minutes is unsuccessful, it should be tried for a further 10 minutes. If bleeding continues, medical advice should be sought. Rarely, the nose has to be packed with lint under direct vision. This requires skill and should be left to experienced practitioners. The age old remedy of putting a cold coin down the back inside the clothing is probably effective only if the nose bleed is minor.

Abdominal bleeds

Laceration of the abdominal organs, particularly the spleen and liver, can cause severe shock. Surgery to stop the bleeding is essential, and there is little that can be done immediately to stop the bleeding. Rapid action in calling for an ambulance may be life-saving; it is vital to comfort the patient, who can be reassured that most people with internal injuries and bleeding can be treated in good time. Many ambulances and family practitioners carry blood plasma, which may be required to relieve shock and maintain the blood pressure before reaching hospital.

Rectum

The commonest cause of rectal bleeding is haemorrhoids (piles, page 175), which usually leave a few streaks of bright red blood in the pan or on the stool or paper. Severe bleeding from the rectum is very uncommon, though it can occur during dysentery. Other causes of bleeding include diverticular disease (page 85) and intestinal tumours, although these are much rarer than piles.

Everyone with rectal bleeding needs careful clinical assessment and some will require more detailed investigation, including sigmoidoscopy (page 207) and a barium enema (page 36).

Stomach

Bleeding from a peptic ulcer is usually small but the blood is mixed with food and stomach fluids and the total volume of fluid vomited may be very large. When vomited, it has the appearance of brown coffee grounds in water. When blood is passed in the faeces, they tend to become tarry black (melaena); but remember that iron preparations taken by mouth also turn the faeces black. Sudden bleeding may be sufficiently severe to cause shock. When bleeding causes shock, the emergency medical service or ambulance should be called immediately.

Lungs

Bleeding from the lungs is almost invariably small. Bright red blood is coughed up mixed with sputum. There is nothing which can be done outside hospital to stop the bleeding but medical advice should be sought immediately, and the patient reasssured that there is no need for hurry and that there is no immediate danger.

Burns

There is little difference between burns from a naked flame and scalds from hot and boiling fluids. Most burns are small and usually affect the fingers. Holding the burnt area under running cold water will usually relieve the pain but you may need to do this for 10 minutes. Such burns may be very painful but are not serious, although they can become infected. If a blister forms, it should be left alone.

Severe burns affecting large areas of the body cause shock and widespread infection. If clothes or hair are on fire, they should be smothered in a blanket or large cloth. The emergency medical or ambulance service should be called immediately and they will treat pain and give plasma for shock. Severe burns in children are often caused by pulling cooking pots from the stove onto their heads; these can be avoided by using guards on the front of cookers and by turning the handles away from the front. Boiling fat will spurt if water is poured onto it and fat fires should be smothered (e.g. with a plate or fire cloth) rather than extinguished. Do not attempt to carry a burning pan outside. Fat must be allowed to cool before frying-pans are cleaned. Fat scalds on the face and hands are extremely painful, and may be deep and occasionally disfiguring.

Electrical injury

This may cause shock and severe burns and cardiac arrest (*see below*). If a cable or terminal is gripped, muscle spasm may prevent release while the current is flowing. *Turn off the current* or disconnect the appliance if possible. If onlookers attempt to pull the sufferer away, they may also receive the shock unless they are protected by wearing rubber boots and gloves, or standing on an insulating rubber mat.

The best protection is care in handling all electrical appliances. Only those who really know what they are doing should work with equipment using mains voltage—including wiring plugs.

Cardiac arrest

If the sufferer's heart has stopped—as noted by their loss of consciousness, stillness, pallor and absent

Child Development

All children should develop the same physical and mental attributes at various times, over the first two years of their life. These pages illustrate the stages of development they go through and the approximate age of the child when these features should become apparent, though the age will vary from child to child. However, if your baby fails to show any particular feature of its development over two to three months after it should, seek medical advice from your family doctor.

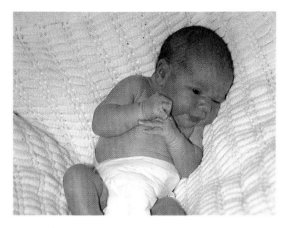

At birth *Baby lies supine (flat) with flexed limbs (arms folded back and legs bent).*

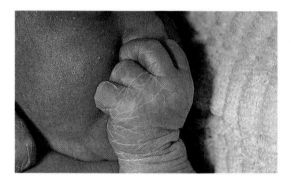

At birth *White lines are normally found on hands and feet of an overdue baby, as well as milk spots on the cheeks.*

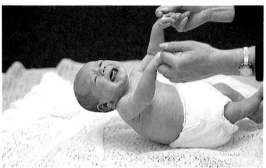

6 Weeks *Baby holds its head up when pulled upward.*

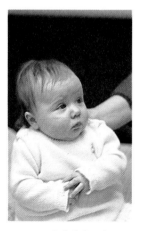

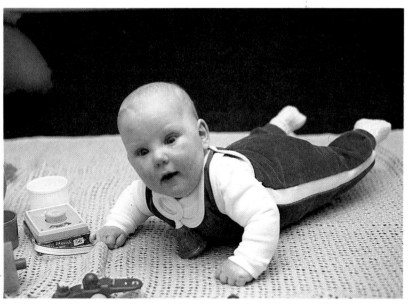

3 Months *Baby's hands are held loosely open (above) and when placed on its tummy on the floor, the baby will hold its chin and shoulders off the floor.*

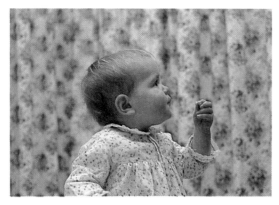

9-10 Months *Finger and thumb apposition. This means the child can manipulate its thumb and fingers to touch each other enabling it to grip objects firmly.*

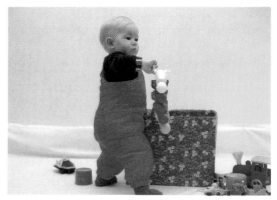

One Year *The child will sit and pivot around and begins to walk on hands and feet like a bear. Begins to throw objects to floor and offer toys to mother.*

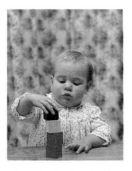

15-18 Months *Can build a tower comprising of two to four toy bricks.*

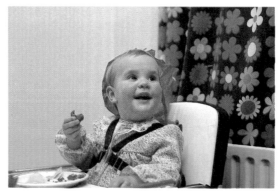

16 Months *The child begins to feed itself.*

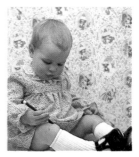

16 Months *The child starts to pick up and grip a pencil or crayon and will begin scribbling.*

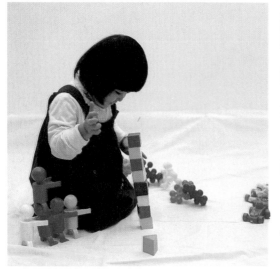

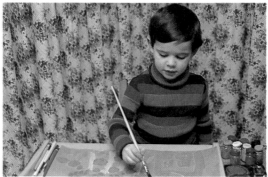

Two Years *In general will run, pick up object from the floor without overbalancing and can climb stairs. Can build tower of six or seven cubes.*

Four Years *The child will by now be painting or drawing easily recognizable pictures.*

wrist or neck pulse—cardiac resuscitation should be started. Initially a *sharp blow to the centre of the chest* may start the heart beating again. If not, press firmly with the heel of the hands applied to the lower end of the breastbone so that it is obviously depressed, at a rate of 60 per minute. Mouth-to-mouth respiration should be started when the airway has been cleared. The assistant takes a deep breath and then breathes out forcefully with his mouth over the patient's open mouth. The patient's nose should be pinched and his jaw held firmly forward during this. The chest should be seen to rise and fall. This is repeated once every 10 chest beats. Alternatively, a small plastic airway can be used if available. The emergency medical or ambulance service must be called. These manoeuvres sound difficult but can be learned easily in one or two sessions of first-aid training.

Choking

Food caught in the throat usually causes a severe bout of coughing which dislodges the food particle. The patient should be calmed. Children sometimes do not chew food well and a large piece of meat may stick in the back of the throat. If possible remove it with the fingers or a pair of tweezers. If unsuccessful,

Choking
If coughing does not clear the obstruction, grasp the sufferer from behind, clasp one hand over the other and pull hard, inwards and upwards against the bottom of the breastbone.

With a child, sit with it face down across your knee, and thump gently with the heel of the hand, between the shoulder blades.

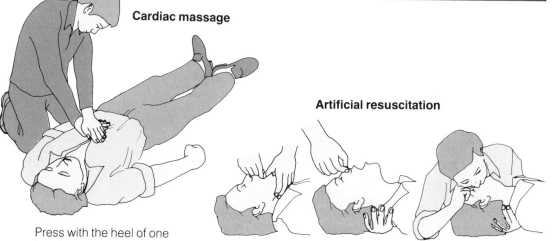

Cardiac massage

Press with the heel of one hand, covering it with the other, on the lower end of the breast bone. Rock backwards and forwards to apply and release pressure, 50-60 times a minute.

Artificial resuscitation

1 Remove any obstruction from the mouth, such as false teeth.

2 Bend the head well back, supporting it with the hand under the neck and close the nostrils.

3 Take a deep breath and blow into the patient's mouth, keeping the nose closed by pinching the nostrils. Repeat 6-8 times per minute.

turn the child upside down, and shake him. This usually dislodges the food.

A serious problem may arise in restaurants when customers, after taking considerable alcohol, inhale large pieces of food which stick in the upper end of the larynx and pharynx. Some restaurants keep long-armed tweezers to pull the food out. If these are not available, the patient should be grasped round the upper abdomen from behind, with a fist in the angle in the rib cage. A sharp and rapid bear-hug is given. This suddenly increases the pressure in the chest and forces the food out. The same principle can be used in children.

Drowning

At the outset, call for the emergency medical service. After removing the patient from the water, he should be laid on his back and false teeth, seaweed and all other objects removed from the mouth. Check if the patient is breathing and the heart is going. If so, roll the patient onto his side in the 'coma position'. If the heart is going but there is no spontaneous breathing, start mouth-to-mouth resuscitation:

1 Breathe in fully.
2 Pinch the patient's nose and hold his jaw forwards.
3 Breath out fully into the patient's open mouth and repeat 6–8 times per minute.

If the heart has stopped (no pulse), start external cardiac massage (*see* diagram, page 273) by pressing firmly on the lower end of the sternum at a rate of about 60 times per minute. After each 10 beats wait for an assistant to apply mouth-to-mouth resuscitation. Older methods of artificial respiration such as the Holger–Nielsen and the Silvester methods are much less effective than mouth-to-mouth respiration.

Sprains and fractures

Sprains

These are very common and follow sudden and unexpected movements (page 215). The ankles, knees and elbows are commonly sprained. A firm bandage will support the joint and partially relieve the pain but it is important not to tie it so tightly that it stops the flow of blood in the veins. The joint should be used as soon as the pain settles, but if the pain persists, medical advice should be sought to ensure that there is no fracture. If the pain prevents sleep even when the joint is rested, there may be an underlying fracture. In any case, a warm bottle applied to the joint and simple pain-killers such as two aspirin tablets can relieve the pain.

Fractures

These usually follow traumatic accidents, and the severity of the pain and odd angulation of the limbs make the diagnosis obvious. Nevertheless, some minor fractures which do not completely break the bones, may not be very painful and heal spontaneously without ever being recognized.

If bones are obviously fractured, they should not be moved except under expert guidance because the

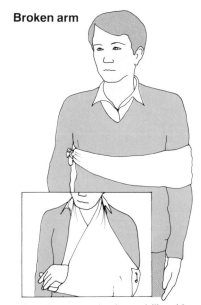

Broken arm

An injured arm can be immobilized by binding it firmly to the side of the chest with a broad bandage. The injured arm can be further protected by placing it in a sling.

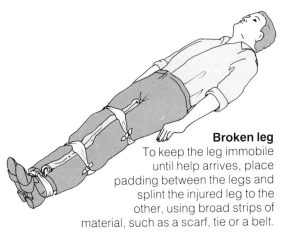

Broken leg
To keep the leg immobile until help arrives, place padding between the legs and splint the injured leg to the other, using broad strips of material, such as a scarf, tie or a belt.

bones may become more difficult to realign and more painful. If no advice is available, the affected limb should be immobilized before the patient is moved. This will reduce pain and stop the fracture becoming worse or damaging adjacent tissues such as arteries and nerves. Fractured arms can be immobilized by bandaging them to the body. A fractured leg can be firmly but not tightly bound to the other leg. Alternatively, the limb can be bound to lengths of wood which should be long enough to extend beyond the joints above and below the fractured bone.

Fractures of the ribs may follow severe crushing injuries, or falls. The pain can be very severe. Occasionally, a fractured rib punctures the lung and causes a pneumothorax (page 179). Rib fractures should not be bound because this restricts expansion of the lungs and causes pneumonia.

If fractures of the skull, neck and spine or pelvis are suspected, it is imperative not to move the patient except under expert guidance, because permanent brain damage, paralysis of the legs or severe bleeding may result.

Eyes

Foreign bodies

If in doubt, seek medical help. Incorrect or rough handling may cause permanent damage. The common problem is due to an eyelash in the eye. This can be removed by pulling the upper lid over the lower eyelashes. This acts as a brush and, when released, it frequently carries the lash with it; the natural movement of the tears will carry the lash to the inner corner of the eye where it falls away.

Other small foreign bodies such as flecks of dust can be removed in the same way. If this is not successful, washing the eye with water with an 'eye bath' may remove superficial grit or a lash.

Small pieces of metal or wood may penetrate the front of the eye—usually during metal or wood working—and may cause superficial ulcers or go deeper. In either case, expert medical advice must be

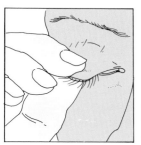

Foreign bodies
Pull the upper lid down over the eye, to cover the lower eyelashes. On releasing the eyelid, any foreign body will be brushed out of the way. Tears will then carry it to the edge of the eye, where it will fall out.

sought because incorrect treatment may result in permanent damage.

Chemical burns
Industrial or home cleansing agents may be splashed into the eye and cause severe pain. The eye should be washed immediately with large quantities of cold water either with an eye bath or, if not available, by very gently pouring cold water over the front of the eyeball. The patient should then be taken without delay to the nearest hospital.

Animals and insects

Dog bites
Dog bites tend to be irregular and dirty, and they are prone to infection. There is no rabies in the domestic or wild animals of the United Kingdom—the last rabid fox was killed in Scotland at the end of the last century. However, the danger of rabies is very real elsewhere.

Dog bites *in the UK* can be treated simply:
1 Clean the wound with an antiseptic such as cetrimide or iodine.
2 Stop excessive bleeding by local pressure applied over a clean and preferably sterile pack.
3 Give anti-tetanus serum (Humotet) or tetanus toxoid as appropriate.

Serious wounds may require stitching and even minor lacerations may become infected. This will be obvious from the swelling, redness and tenderness of the wound and the patient will need medical advice.

If a dog bite has occurred *abroad*, serious consideration must be given to the possibility of rabies. Medical advice must be sought immediately the danger becomes apparent, even if the bite has occurred some time before whilst travelling, and appears to have healed completely. If the attack by the dog was unprovoked, rabies vaccination is usually recommended.

Snake bites
The adder or viper is the only poisonous snake found in the British Isles and the bite is recognized by its characteristic 'V' pattern. Viper bites in adults are virtually never fatal, but small children are at greater risk.

Emergency treatment of snake bites is:
1 Prevent the poison entering the blood stream by tying a ligature or handkerchief firmly around the limb to isolate the wound and close the veins but not the arteries. This should be released for 1 minute every half hour. Immobilize the limb with a splint to stop spread of the venom.

2 Clean the poison from the surface of the wound with water—do not open or disturb the wound as this may increase absorption of the poison and produce greater tissue damage.
3 Reassure the patient (who is usually terrified) that death from snake bites is very rare and most unlikely.
4 Try to identify the snake.

Medical advice should be sought immediately and the patient carried to hospital, taking great care not to disturb the bitten limb. Specific anti-venoms are available but are not generally required for adder bites. Treatment to prevent tetanus and other infections may be given.

Bee stings

These are usually more painful than dangerous. The sting should be removed if possible and the patient strongly reassured that all will be well. The stings are alkaline, and the pain may be relieved by applying a weak acid solution such as vinegar or lemon juice. Ice packs applied to the sting sometimes give marked relief. Very occasionally, in people who are specifically sensitive to them, the sting may cause swelling of the face and larynx and difficulty with breathing. Medical help must be sought immediately, and adrenaline given by injection to reverse the swelling. Most family practitioners carry adrenaline in their emergency bag for this purpose.

Wasp stings

Wasps do not usually leave their sting behind. The stings are acid and the pain may be relieved by a weak alkaline solution such as bicarbonate of soda.

Poisoning

Common poisons	Effects	Immediate action
Antidepressants (*e.g. Tofranil, Tryptizol*)	Abnormal heart rhythms	Hospital, to monitor and treat abnormal heart rhythms
Aspirin	Nausea, vomiting, blurred vision, ringing in the ears	Hospital—the patient may look well initially but may become unconscious later
Berries (*e.g. deadly nightshade*)	Red, hot, dry skin; slow heart	Induce vomiting, and then hospital
Corrosives	Damage to pharynx, gullet and stomach	Milk, and then hospital. DO NOT INDUCE VOMITING
Iron	Nausea, vomiting, abdominal pain, shock	Induce vomiting in children; hospital in case of later need for resuscitation
Paraquat (*weed killer*)	Slow destruction of lungs	Hospital, for immediate dialysis
Toadstools and fungi	Vomiting and shock	Induce vomiting, and then hospital
Tranquillizers (*e.g. Librium, Valium*) **and barbiturates**	Depressed respiration Coma	Hospital, as (rarely) artificial respiration is required

Notes
1 Almost all who take poisons should be taken to hospital.
2 Almost all will require a stomach wash-out (but NOT for corrosives).
3 Never induce vomiting in the unconscious, as they may then inhale gastric contents into the lungs.
4 Do not use salt water to induce vomiting especially in young children, as it may seriously disturb the salt and water balance. A finger down the throat should be sufficient.

The recovery position

1 Place one arm straight out behind the patient's head and lay the other across the chest. Raise one knee and cross it over the other leg.

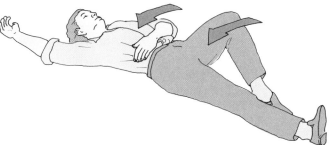

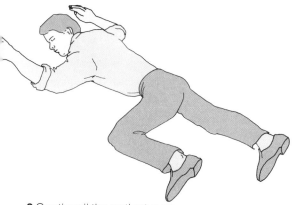

2 Gently roll the patient over onto his front, protecting the face with your hand as you do so. Move the upper arm out to lay at right angles to the body and do the same with the thigh. Tilt the head well back, with the chin jutting forward to allow a clear breathing passage.

Care of the unconscious patient

Loss of consciousness usually follows a head injury with concussion (page 64), a stroke or cerebral haemorrhage (page 217), an epileptic fit (page 93) or drug overdose. Other causes are rare (*see* Blackout).

Whatever the cause, the important steps are to:
1. Remove false teeth, food or anything else in the mouth to ensure that the airway is clear.
2. Gently roll the patient onto one side into the coma position (*see* diagrams) to prevent inhalation of vomit, which could cause severe pneumonia.
3. Call the emergency or ambulance service.

Further help requires expert assessment to determine the degree of damage to bones or internal organs and/or the cause of the unconsciousness.

Home first-aid kit

Scissors
Tweezers
Safety pins
Eye bath
Dettol or cetrimide
Burnol
Plastic skin

Sterile dressing
Sticking plasters
Crêpe bandage
Paraffin gauze for burns
Fire extinguisher
Paracetamol or aspirin

Car first-aid kit

As for the home *plus*
Flashing lamp
Reflector triangle
Torch

Essential first aid

Shock
1. Clear the mouth and airway (e.g. false teeth)
2. Stop the bleeding; press firmly on bleeding site
3. Don't warm, or give alcohol
4. Do not move unless imperative
5. Send for an ambulance
6. Warn oncoming traffic (road accident)

Prevent accidents in the home

1. Lock drugs and chemicals away from children
2. Use cooker guards
3. Keep sharp implements out of reach
4. Turn off appliances
5. Don't pour water onto boiling fat
6. Don't leave wires trailing
7. Don't leave toys on the stairs
8. Mats and floors should be non-slip

Going to Hospital

People are admitted to hospital either as in-patients or attend clinics as out-patients. They attend for medical advice and nursing care. In Britain they are usually referred by their family (or primary-care) doctor. If there has been an accident, and in countries where no system of family practitioners exists, people go direct to the hospital.

Accidents—minor and major injuries

Accidents range from minor mishaps, such as sprained joints, insect bites and small cuts, to major life-threatening situations such as accidental poisoning, traffic accidents, occupational injuries and falls. The hospital Accident and Emergency Departments are usually divided into two working areas, for minor or major problems. All patients with minor accidents are seen by a doctor or senior nurse who will assess the injury, decide whether further tests and x-rays are required and then start treatment. If there is an open wound, particularly after cuts which may be contaminated by dirt (e.g. road accidents, open-air sports and gardening), anti-tetanus serum will be recommended for immediate protection and the patient advised to start a full course of immunization against tetanus (page 222).

Major accidents require immediate attention, and if many people are involved the entire medical and nursing staff may be transferred from the minor injuries section. In these circumstances, other staff of the hospital are frequently called upon. Most hospitals have a MAJAX (major accident) plan ready to put into action when necessary. This mobilizes a large proportion of the hospital staff. Road accidents may result in considerable loss of blood and transfusion is frequently required urgently, even before surgery. Another life-saving measure sometimes urgently required in the Accident and Emergency Department is to ensure that breathing is not obstructed by the tongue falling backward. This occurs when unconscious people lie on their backs. Any food remaining in the mouth is removed to stop it entering the lungs when the patient breathes in. After these life-saving procedures, a thorough assessment can be made of other injuries. Fractures of the bones are common, as are head injuries—though both are becoming less frequent in countries where drivers and passengers use safety-belts, which prevent them being thrown forward at collision.

Fractures of the ribs are commonly caused when car drivers are thrown forward onto the steering wheel. At the same time they may fracture their femurs (page 101) on the lower edge of the dashboard and cut the face on the driving mirror.

Motorcyclists are at great risk because even minor collisions can throw them off, sometimes into the path of oncoming traffic. When travelling at high speeds they hit the ground with great velocity. If the cyclist is not killed outright, he frequently sustains brain damage, though crash helmets reduce the severity of head injury. They also have severe and complicated fractures, crushed chest injuries with multiple rib fractures and rupture of the abdominal organs such as the spleen and liver.

Accidents on the road
(approximate figures)

Annual number of road traffic accidents in UK	250,000
Number killed	6,000
Seriously injured	80,000
Slightly injured	240,000
Annual number of people injured and killed in UK	326,000

Accidents involving motorcycles
and two-wheeled vehicles

Annual number in UK	63,000
	(1 in 4 of all road accidents)
People killed	1,000
	(1 in 6 of all road deaths)
People seriously injured	20,000
	(1 in 4 of all serious road injuries)

Accidents in the home
(approximate figures)

Annual number in UK	76,000
Number in those aged less than 10 years	25,000

Number in those aged
over 70 years   7,000

Note Almost half occur in the very young and very old and the majority are caused by falls.

Acute illnesses other than accidents

Most people who have acute illnesses, such as bronchitis, tonsillitis, etc., are best cared for at home. More serious illnesses (e.g. pneumonia, acute appendicitis, miscarriage, ectopic pregnancy) make hospital care essential. The very old and the very young can be seriously affected by illnesses which are relatively minor at other ages, and are more likely to need hospital treatment.

In the UK, patients are usually seen at home by the family doctor and sent by ambulance or taken by relatives to the hospital Emergency Department. They are seen by a nurse who assesses the problem and decides if a medical opinion is required. A doctor will attend to make a diagnosis or to give treatment immediately. A blood transfusion can be given if life-threatening loss of blood has occurred, as from a bleeding stomach ulcer or severe injury.

Depending upon the diagnosis, the patient may be admitted to a hospital ward under the care of a surgeon, a physician (internist) or obstetrician/gynaecologist, or other specialist. In some hospitals a patient may be looked after throughout by his own family doctor if he is on the staff of the local hospital. He will call in other specialists if the patient's illness is outside his expertise.

Within the hospital ward the patient is nursed by the ward sister and nurses, and a team of doctors consisting of the houseman or senior house officer (junior resident), a registrar (senior resident) and a consultant specialist. In the UK, the care of the patient is the responsibility of the consultant, and the residents (junior doctors) are directly responsible to him. In some hospitals in other countries the senior resident is responsible for the patient's day-to-day care though he is frequently guided by specialists.

If the diagnosis is not immediately obvious, investigations such as blood tests and x-rays may be required to confirm or exclude likely diseases, and when complete the patient can be reassured, or treatment started. This may be with drugs supplied from the pharmacy, or a surgical operation, or x-ray treatment (radiotherapy), or physical treatment in a Physiotherapy Department. Physiotherapists, occupational therapists and speech therapists are specially trained lay members of the clinical team, particularly useful in the care of the elderly and following strokes. Physiotherapists are also intimately involved in pre- and post-operative care.

Out-patient department
Most people who attend hospital are not acutely ill and are able to attend the out-patient clinics. Here they see consultant specialists and members of the specialist's medical staff. Usually the family practitioner has decided what might be wrong and refers him to the clinic either because he requires a second opinion to confirm his views or because he wants specialist advice on management, treatment or prognosis. Occasionally, the patient needs specialized treatment which can only be given under the guidance of clinicians with special expertise (e.g. radiotherapy, leukaemia therapy).

Specialists deal with three groups of diseases which are classified as Surgery, Obstetrics and Gynaecology, and Medicine. After talking with the patient ('taking a history') and examining him, the specialist may know what is wrong and be able to reassure the patient that there is no serious illness. He may make a diagnosis and start treatment with drugs, or recommend surgery if necessary. If investigations are required to confirm the diagnosis, they are usually performed on the patient's blood. These are carried out and interpreted by specialists in Pathology who examine for disorders of the chemicals within the blood (biochemists) or for disorders of the blood cells (haematologists). Bacteria present in discharges may be taken to the laboratory on swabs (cotton wool on a stick) where they can be grown and identified (bacteriologists). Occasionally, diseased tissues may be removed (a biopsy) and a small piece sent for examination under the microscope (histologists). If x-rays are required, these are interpreted by specialist radiologists.

Once the diagnosis is confirmed, treatment can be recommended. Most patients can then return to the care of their family doctor, though many with complicated disorders or those needing specialist treatment or supervision may need to attend the hospital out-patients department for months or years. Special out-patient facilities (day hospitals) exist for the elderly, who can spend hours with physiotherapists, occupational and speech therapists whilst still living at home.

Having an operation
Operations may be performed for acute illnesses (e.g. appendicitis, ruptured spleen or perforated stomach ulcer), but most operations are planned.

Patients are generally physically fit but require removal of a diseased tissue or organ (e.g. removal of gall bladder for stones, varicose veins or correction of a hernia). Patients with cancer do not usually require urgent operation and can be treated prior to surgery so that they are in the optimum possible physical condition. Patients should stop smoking as soon as surgery is planned because smokers are more prone to chest infections immediately after surgery.

The use of modern anaesthetics and muscle-relaxing drugs and the better understanding of the way they work in the human body have made modern surgery and post-operative management skilled and safe. The immediate outcome of surgery can be expected to be very good. The final outcome will depend upon the seriousness of the underlying disease and the strength of the heart and lungs.

Before operation, the surgeon will explain what he intends to do, and the patient's general health will be assessed by the anaesthetist to ensure that he is fit and has no unexpected heart or lung abnormalities. If there is a previous history of lung disease (e.g. bronchitis), physiotherapy will be given 1–2 days before surgery to teach the patient how to breathe properly and how to clear his lungs. If necessary, his blood may be tested to exclude anaemia; if the operation might result in blood loss, his blood group will be determined and blood cross-matched and held in reserve for the day of operation. On that day the patient will be fasted to ensure that there is no food in the stomach which could be inhaled into the lungs while unconscious.

About 1 hour before surgery, pre-medication is given with a sedative drug and a drug to clear up respiratory secretions. Just before surgery, the patient will be taken to the anaesthetics room next to the operating theatre. Here he will meet the anaesthetist again, though he may later remember little of this because of the effect of the sedative. The anaesthetist will give an injection into the patient's arm vein and he will rapidly fall asleep in a matter of 5–15 seconds. He is kept asleep by a combination of anaesthetic injections and gases. A tube is placed in the windpipe and connected to the machine which delivers controlled amounts of anaesthetic gases and oxygen.

Throughout surgery the anaesthetist carefully monitors the actions of the heart and lungs to ensure that they remain satisfactory. Soon after surgery the patient will slowly awake either in the recovery room next to the theatre or in the ward.

Physiotherapy and breathing exercises are intensified for 2–3 days or more before and immediately after surgery if there is a previous history of lung disease—usually chronic bronchitis in smokers. Within 1–2 days the patient is got out of bed and slowly but progressively mobilized by the nurses or physiotherapists to regain strength rapidly and to ensure that no blood clots develop in his legs. The latter used to be a common complication when patients were kept in bed for days and weeks following surgery—and still is more common in women on the contraceptive pill after surgery unless special precautions are taken.

Care of the Elderly

Accidents in the home

Most accidents in the elderly occur either in the kitchen or on the stairs. Anyone with responsibility for the care of an elderly man or woman, particularly if they are living on their own or with no young companions, should check the following items:

1   Electrical appliances, for these are often very old and unsafe because of obsolete design. The flexes leading to them may have decayed rubber insulation, and may not be safely fixed to the terminals either inside the appliance or at the plug. It should be checked that the flex does not trail where it might trip someone up.
2   Check all heat sources for these can be hazards for other reasons than their heat. Particularly check coal fires where live coals can fall onto the carpet, oil stoves which can be knocked over, and gas appliances (cookers and fires) which may give poisonous fumes if the flues are blocked or explode if not properly ignited.
3   Check worn carpets and edges, slippery mats, slippery flooring, loose stair carpets and stair rods. Check all insecure and rickety structures which may have to support weight such as balustrades, rails and furniture. Check that rubbish, particularly food matter, is disposed of properly because vermin and houseflies may be attracted, together with disease and there may be a fire hazard if there are piles of newspapers.

4 Check all dark corners especially corridors and where there may be a step or two between rooms. Older generations grew up with poor levels of illumination and light, but dimming eye sight makes this potentially dangerous.

Illness in the home

1 If the elderly patient is in bed, try if at all possible to get them to sit out at least twice a day. The elderly may easily become bed-fast because their muscles weaken and joints stiffen so quickly.

2 If the patient is immobile in bed then it is exceedingly important to prevent bed sores. They should be turned from one side to the back, and to the other side at least every two hours. It is a good idea to put a soft cushion under the heels and a pillow between the legs where they cross each other with the patient lying on his side.

3 Ensure a good fluid intake, 3-5 pints (2-3 litres) per day, but do not give too much of preparations which contain too much sugar or glucose (e.g. fizzy yellow 'health' drinks and lemonade) or those which contain too much salt (meat and yeast extracts). Leakage of urine (urinary incontinence) is often due to immobility or, less often, to forgetfulness in those who are mildly confused. For some patients it is necessary to ask frequently whether they feel the need to pass urine; in those even less well, the patient may need to be taken to the lavatory regularly, say every two hours.

4 Leakage of motions (faecal incontinence) may be due to confusion or muscular weakness. It is much more likely to happen in those who have diarrhoea. Remember that those who are severely constipated—another risk of staying in bed—may leak faecal-coloured fluid.

5 Try to understand the medicines supplied. Some will have to be taken regularly, for instance antibiotics to treat an infection, and some will only need to be taken to relieve symptoms. Do not continue an old supply of tablets when a new kind is supplied unless you are sure that your doctor intended them to be taken in addition.

Help for certain disabilities

Your doctor should be able to put you in contact with a trained occupational therapist who can give professional advice on these matters.

Deafness Some skill at lip reading can be learnt at any age. Modern ear trumpets with flexible tubing can be very helpful. A microphone, small amplifier and earphones can help some people for whom a conventional hearing aid is insufficient.

Blindness Seek professional aid from the Royal National Institute for the Blind. Make sure that landmarks are not changed and that walkways are always kept free, even of the smallest objects on the floor and the stairs.

Incontinence Use commodes by the bed rather than bedpans and if possible adjust the height. A commode with one arm can help the patient get on and off. The male urinal can be very helpful.

Baths Getting in and out can be helped by a seat at rim height across the bath and another in the bath raised about a foot from the bottom. Side grips on the bath or nearby and a pole are helpful. A bath stool at the side is helpful for resting on. There should be a non-slip mat at the base. A shower with a chair in it can avoid many of these problems.

Kitchen Kettle or teapot cradles which pour when swung can avoid dangerous spillage of hot water. Tap extension levers help turning on and off taps. Padded cutlery handles, high-sided plates and non-slip mats help at meal times.

Dressing and personal hygiene Lazy tongs help with picking objects up from the floor. Long handles on objects such as combs, shoe horns can be very helpful. Nail clippers are often easier to use than scissors. Clothing is easier to manage with Velcro fastening than with zips or buttons.

Walking Walking sticks or tripods and even frames should not be despised, though they will often only be needed on rare occasions. Firm rails down corridors, up stairs and in the w.c. can save many falls. All floor coverings should be secure and non-slip.

Sitting Seats should not be too low and occasionally ejection seats can help weakened limbs in rising from the sitting position. Seat heights are usually best between 18 and 26 inches (45-65 cm). Good strong arms to the chair are essential and a high back with not too deep a seat will help posture.

Sleeping The bed should be firm, particularly at the edges so that it does not give way when the patient is getting into or out of bed; the height should be such that the patient does not either drop out of bed onto the feet (as with many old beds) or have to lever himself up (as from a divan). A back rest behind the pillows helps with posture and a rope fitted to the foot of the bed with a good handle for the patient can help with moving around. The pressure of the bed clothes can be taken off the feet with a bed cradle—a chair put on its side will often do temporarily. A standard cantilever bed table helps with meal times and reading. Conventional electric underblankets should not be used because they may be electrically unsafe, especially with incontinence and spilling drinks. Special underblankets can be obtained and most overblankets are satisfactory.

Special problems

Isolation Make sure the patient can call for help with a telephone, alarm bell or window card. Arrange for visitors to call regularly and make sure that milkmen, dustmen and postmen are aware.

Mobility It is very important that all old people keep on the move if at all possible; if there is much pain from osteoarthritis in the legs, sufficient tablets should be taken to reduce the pain to tolerable levels. Obesity, when present, is a terrible problem with increasing age and it is a common observation that there are very few old people who are fat. Particular attention should be paid to foot care and appropriate shoes which fit well and give firm support without pinching. Permanent wearing of slippers should be strongly discouraged. Regular chiropody may help mobility.

Perspective The elderly sometimes develop a feeling of pointlessness at their further existence which can amount to severe depression. This is worse following the death of spouse or friends, and made worse when they are unhappy about their children or grandchildren. It is absolutely true that the elderly can be just as happy and fulfilled as younger people, and have much to contribute to those who are their juniors or actively trying to cope with the day-to-day problems of holding down a job and bringing up a family.

Cold The elderly are not as good as the young at keeping their body temperature normal in a cold environment, and they may not be aware of the cold to the same degree as a younger person. It is better to keep an elderly person warm by heating the room than by heating the patient.

Shopping Reduced mobility and a fear of slipping in cold weather can make shopping a considerable problem, and unless helped many elderly people will go hungry. Good neighbours will frequently do the shopping whilst they are doing their own.

Tolerance It is a paradox that tolerance should be a problem, but the elderly will frequently tolerate unpleasant symptoms because they think it is natural for the elderly to have them. They will also often feel that it is not worth bothering a younger relative and neighbour nor the doctor or nurse. Apart from unnecessary suffering this may also mean that a disease may become severe enough to require admission to hospital, when earlier attention could have helped quite easily.

Strokes Remember that even when speech is severely affected or absent, understanding is often not impaired and the hearing almost invariably unaltered. It is therefore important to continue to talk normally even if the patient cannot answer in his usual manner. Early physiotherapy can often help mobility considerably, especially after moderately severe strokes. The limbs should be moved through their full range of movement regularly.

Calls for help

Medical
1 General practitioner
2 Hospital doctor (via the general practitioner)
He may (a) admit the patient; (b) arrange for a consultant to visit at the patient's home to give advice; (c) arrange a visit to a local day hospital which will provide hospital investigation and treatment in the day time, though the patient returns home at tea time.

Nursing The practice nurse (contacted through the general practitioner) or the community nurse will visit for nursing procedures. The health visitor, who is a qualified nurse, and often specialized in geriatric care, will call to give advice.

Rehabilitation These services are contacted via the general practitioner, hospital or social services. A physiotherapist will advise on mobility; an occupational therapist on altering environment to make life easier and on the use of aids.

Social services Can be contacted directly at the local authority, or via the hospital, general practitioner, health visitor, nurse or friend. A medical social worker will call to give advice on facilities, funds available through supplementary benefit and possible future accommodation in warden-controlled flats or old peoples' homes. A home help will call primarily to keep the house clean but performs many other functions around the house in the way that a good friend would. Meals on Wheels is a service which will call at lunch time to provide hot food. Local authorities vary greatly in what they can provide and how frequently. Day centres are different from day hospitals for they are primarily there to provide social contacts and social environments. Laundry service can be made available for the incontinent. Chiropody is extremely important for the elderly for, even if they can reach their feet and possess a pair of good scissors which they can work, the nails are frequently too tough for anything but specialist management. If you are not happy with the service obtained through the above agencies, the Citizens Advice Bureaux can often give advice and put you in touch with various local voluntary schemes. Age Concern may have a local office and another charity, Help the Aged, can give general advice and local contacts.

General principles

1 Keep out of bed.
2 Walk hourly: if an assistant is necessary, he should be at the side or back, not at the front.
3 Self-help is important even when the going is slow, difficult and painful.
4 Ensure a balanced diet (*see* page 291).
5 Slowness at absorbing new information progresses from middle age onwards, so it becomes increasingly important to speak slowly, clearly, possibly loudly and to be prepared to repeat the information without offence.

Home Nursing for Common Symptoms

The commonest medical problems are the consequences of the common cold, coughs, sore throats and runny noses, and stomach upsets with either vomiting or diarrhoea or both.

Runny nose

This is occasionally due to hay fever or related disorder and your doctor will give advice on specific treatment. If the runny nose is due to a cold, two tablets of soluble aspirin (or paracetamol if you cannot take aspirin) taken 4 to 6 hourly will help. Take plenty of fluids of any kind. Alcohol may sometimes make the symptoms worse but at the same time make you less concerned about them. Some people find steam inhalations with or without the addition of menthol crystals or similar preparation helpful. Pour boiling water into a bowl, lean over it and put a large towel over the head and bowl. Five to ten minutes three or four times a day is adaquate. Various commercial preparations contain special compounds to shrink the swollen membranes of the nose (pseudoephedrine hydrochloride or phenylpropranolamine hydrochloride). These have few side-effects as long as you are taking no other medicines. They can, however, react badly with certain drugs such as antidepressant tablets and you should check with the chemist or doctor that they will mix satisfactorily with whatever medications you are already taking. Babies and very small children with colds should be laid on the side so the secretions can run out because there is a danger of breathing them back in again or choking on them. With a baby as ill as this, it is necessary to call your doctor anyway.

Coughs

Dry coughs can be very wearing and interfere with sleep. Most cough medicines from the chemist will remove satisfactorily the worst of the distress. Remember that some of the compound cough mixtures contain potent medicines which can interfere with other treatment, and you should check with the chemist that there is no problem. If you have a cough producing sputum (phlegm), this should not be suppressed by a sedative cough linctus. When a cough produces yellow or green phlegm and if you feel unusually ill you should consult your doctor because this may indicate acute bronchitis which needs antibiotic treatment. If the cough persists, or if you produce blood or have associated pain or breathlessness, consult your doctor.

Sore throat

Sore throats are usually caused by virus infection, and antibiotics are not effective against viruses. Children may often get swollen sore tonsils with white blebs on them and the lymph glands in the neck may swell. This can be quite normal in children because it is part of their defence against new infections. Small doses of soluble aspirin gargled before swallowing can be helpful. From 5 to 8 years half a standard soluble aspirin tablet is suitable and from 8 to 14 one whole tablet. Adults usually take two whole tablets. If there is a high fever or earache it is best to consult your doctor.

Vomiting and diarrhoea

Vomiting
This is usually caused by a virus infection and may occur in epidemics, particularly in children. If it occurs in a whole group of people who have had a prepared meal it may be due to food poisoning and is often so severe that medical advice is needed urgently. Less severe vomiting usually stops within 24 hours without treatment. It may well be associated with diarrhoea. Some people, particularly children, will vomit when they have infections such as tonsillitis, ear infection or infection of the urine. If the vomiting is associated with stomach pain or persists for longer than 24 hours or is associated with fever, the doctor should be consulted. Treatment at home involves having nothing to eat and taking small quantities of clear fluid frequently. When the vomiting is over, the patient will often be very thirsty rather than hungry and should be allowed to consume clear fluids freely or milky fluids more slowly.

Diarrhoea
This is usually caused by a virus. It is often accompanied by colicky cramp pain in the abdomen just before passing a motion and relieved by it. It is commonest in the summer when the housefly transmits infection and on travel abroad. A doctor should be consulted for babies up to a year old and for older children if it is severe and persists through to the next morning. It would also be a good idea to consult the doctor if it continues for more than 24 hours, if it is associated with the passage of blood or if it comes on after a visit abroad, especially to the Mediterranean or tropics. If two or three attacks occur within a period of months, consult your doctor in case some other treatment is needed to prevent further episodes. Treatment at home involves bed rest, no food and only clear fluids (e.g. squashes or fruit juices). Various kaolin preparations can be bought at the chemist which will often give quick relief.

Commonly Used Drugs

For each drug mentioned, the official name will be given first and then the proprietary names given to each drug by a drug company will be placed in brackets. The name in brackets is often the name by which a drug is best known in the UK.

Heart and circulation

Blood pressure
The most commonly used treatments are 'beta blockers' and 'diuretics'. The official names of beta blockers all end '-olol'. Commonly used beta blockers are:
propranolol (Inderal)
acebutolol (Sectral)
atenolol (Tenormin)
labetalol (Trandate)
metoprolol (Lopresor, Betaloc)
oxprenolol (Trasicor)
timolol (Blocadren)

Commonly used diuretics in blood pressure control are:
bendrofluazide (Aprinox, Centyl, Neo-NaClex)
chlorthalidone (Hygroton)
cyclopenthiazide (Navidrex)
mefruside (Baycaron)
xipamide (Diurexan)

Diuretics are often prescribed with potassium either separately (Slow K, Sando K), or altogether in the one tablet (Neo-NaClex K, Navidrex K).

Diuretics and beta blockers are often combined in one tablet with names that sound like the parent trade name for the beta blockers. Diuretics are often combined with 'potassium-sparing diuretics' (Moduretic, Dyazide, Aldactide).

Other preparations commonly used to treat blood pressure include:
hydralazine (Apresoline)
prazosin (Hypovase)
methyl dopa (Aldomet, Dopamet)
indoramin (Baratol)

Angina

There are three main groups of drugs, each group acting in different ways with side-effects in common. First, vasodilators: these include glyceryl trinitrate, usually taken as a tablet under the tongue but occasionally swallowed as a tablet (Sustac, Nitrocontin) or rubbed into the skin (Percutol); isosorbide (Sorbitrate, Cedocard), isordil is similar. Beta blockers are frequently used (*see above*). Calcium antagonists are now often used. These include nifedipine (Adalat), verapamil (Cordilox).

Drugs to strengthen the heart beat

Digitalis is usually used as digoxin (Lanoxin). Even slightly too high a dose may result in loss of appetite or upset bowel. Diuretics mentioned under Blood pressure are also frequently used including more powerful diuretics such as frusemide (Lasix, Frusid) and bumetanide (Burinex).

Drugs to regulate the heart beat

These include the beta blockers, digoxin and calcium antagonists already mentioned with a few others such as disopyramide (Rythmodan, Norpace, Dirythmin), amiodarone (Cordarone X), tocainide (Tonocard).

Drugs to improve circulation to the legs or brain

This group includes cyclandelate (Cyclospasmol), isoxsuprine (Duvadilan, Defencin), co-dergocrine (Hydergine), nicotinic acid (Bradilan, Hexopal).

Anticoagulants

On the whole only one drug is used in this country unless it proves unsatisfactory—warfarin (Marevan). It reduces the power of the blood to clot and is used often after heart attacks and almost always after operations inside the heart. There are also several other occasions in which it is used such as clotting in the veins of the legs. The level of its effect on the clotting powers of the blood has to be checked frequently so that the dose, which may vary from time to time, is kept accurate. Those on anticoagulants have to observe certain precautions in their diet.

Stomach and bowels

Stomach and duodenal ulcers, and hiatus hernia

Antacids usually taste of peppermint and are a white mixture. The usual preparations include Asilone, Aludrox, Gaviscon, Rennie, Settlers, Bisodol, Dijex, Gelusil. Magnesium trisilicate mixture is the commonest non-proprietary preparation. There are two H2 blockers called cimetidine (Tagamet) and ranitidine (Zantac) which stop acid forming in the stomach and when taken for several weeks will allow ulcers to heal. Some drugs work by protecting the lining of the stomach; e.g. Biogastrone, De-nol, Pyrogastrone.

Drugs which dissolve gallstones

There are two: chenodeoxycholic acid (CDCA, Chendol) and ursodeoxycholic acid (Destolit).

Constipation

It is best to take enough roughage in the diet together with fluids as fruit, vegetables, high bran cereals and wholemeal bread. Bulking agents can also be given as drugs; e.g. Millers bran 2 dessertspoonfuls daily, Fybranta, Proctofibe,

Normacol, Isogel, Fybogel. The liquid lactulose (Duphalac) is similar. Many drugs act by stimulating the bowel; e.g. Senokot, Dulcolax, Dorbanex, Normax.

Large bowel disorders

Treatment of diarrhoea is usually based on kaolin preparations. Doctors may prescribe diphenoxylate, with atropine (Lomotil), loperamide (Imodium) or codeine phosphate.

Ulcerative colitis

This is treated with sulphasalazine (Salazopyrine) by mouth (or steroids by enema).

Travel sickness

These are very effective if taken quarter to half an hour before the journey. They include hyoscine (Sea-legs, Kwells), cinnarizine (Stugera), cyclizine (Marzine) and promethazine (Avomine).

Appetite suppressants

These drugs do no more than help you to refuse food and have no other way of working, so that if you do not reduce the calorie intake you will not lose weight despite taking the tablets. The commonest are diethylpropion (Tenuate, Apisate) and phentermine (Ionamin, Duromine).

Lungs and Respiratory Passages

Asthma

There are two major groups of preparations to be taken by mouth. Aminophylline preparations include Phyllocontin, Nuelin, Choledyl. The other group includes salbutamol (Ventolin) and terbutaline (Bricanyl). These latter are also given as inhaled preparations usually in little pressurized canisters delivering short puffs of measured amounts of drugs. It is essential that the patient breathe in fully at precisely the right time to inhale the cloud of fine particles which the aerosol delivers. Two kinds of drugs are dispensed in pressurized metered aerosols: one which acts immediately for the relief of asthma and the other which instead builds up background resistance. The first kind includes terbutaline, salbutamol, fenoterol (Berotec) and ipratropium (Atrovent). The second group, which should not be taken for immediate treatment of wheeze, includes the steroids beclamethasone (Becotide) and betamethasone (Bextasol), and the membrane stabilizer sodium cromoglycate (Intal).

Emotional problems

Tranquillizers

The minor tranquillizers include many well known names such as chlordiazepoxide (Librium, Tropium), diazepam (Valium, Atensine), lorazepam (Ativan), hydrozyzine (Atarax), clorazepate (Tranxene). The major tranquillizers include chlorpromazine (Largactil), promazine (Sparine), thioridazine (Melleril), and haloperidol (Serenace).

Antidepressants

The commoner ones include imipramine (Tofranil), amitriptyline (Tryptizol, Lentizol), clomipramine (Anafranil), dothiepin (Prothiaden), mianserin (Bolvidon), nomifensine (Merital). Specialist psychiatrists may use other preparations which are often reserved for patients in whom conventional treatment has not been fully effective. Monoamine oxidase inhibitors (MAOI) are drugs such as phenelzine (Nardil) and tranylcypromine (Parnate). These may react very adversely with fermented food such as cheese, pickles, savoury spreads, strong red wine, some yoghurt and with broad beans. They also interact with many of the antidepressants mentioned above. Lithium (Priadel, Camcolit) has to have its concentration in the blood very carefully controlled. High levels over a period of time can give rise to unsteadiness. In schizophrenia some long-acting drugs are given every 2–3 weeks, by injection; e.g. fluphenazine (Modecate).

Sleeplessness
These are usually temazepam (Euhypnos, Normison), nitrazepam (Mogadon) or flurazepam (Dalmane).

Pain

Mild analgesics
Includes paracetamol (Panadol, and many other preparations over the chemist's counter), dihydrocodeine (DF118), paracetamol with proproxyphene (Distalgesic, Cosalgesic) and mefenamic acid (Ponstan).

Mild analgesics with anti-inflammatory effect
These drugs are often used for arthritis and can irritate the stomach lining. They include soluble aspirin (acetylsalicylic acid), naproxen (Naprosyn), ibuprofen (Brufen), ketoprofen (Orudis, Alrheumat), flurbiprofen (Froben), piroxicam (Feldene) and indomethacin (Indocid).

Powerful analgesics
These are related to morphia but some of them only distantly. Most are addictive. They include morphine and heroin but additionally methadone (Physeptone), dipipanone (Diconal), pethidine and buprenorphine (Temgesic).

Brain and nervous system

Epilepsy and fits
The commonest drug nowadays is phenytoin (Epanutin) with carbamazepine (Tegretol) and valproate (Epilim) also commonly used. The doses, particularly of phenytoin, have to be accurately judged and adhered to.

Migraine
Ordinary mild analgesics such as paracetamol and aspirin, if taken early enough, may be very effective. Commercial preparations, such as Migraleve, Migravess, Paramax, suit some people better especially if there is a problem with vomiting. Ergotamine-containing preparations (Migril, Cafergot) are best for some patients; do not exeed the stated maximum dose. Different preparations are sometimes taken to ward off attacks; these include clonidine (Dixarit) and pizotifen (Sanomigran).

Parkinson's disease
There are three main groups of drugs for treating this condition. The first includes various compounds containing levodopa usually nowadays in combination with another drug (Sinemet, Madopar), but also on its own (Brocadopa, Larodopa). They can give rise to loss of appetite and nausea

and in high dose may give rise to involuntary movements of the tongue and lips and also mild confusion. All of these can be reversed by reducing the dose a little. The anticholinergic drugs act in a different way and may be complicated by blurred vision, constipation and trouble passing water as well as nausea. In low dosage, however, they have very few side-effects. This second group includes benzhexol (Artane), benztropine (Cogentin), orphenadrine (Disipal) and methixene (Tremonil). The third group contains amantadine (Symmetrel); there is also bromocriptine (Parlodel), which has to be taken initially in a very low dosage and gradually worked up because it easily gives rise to nausea.

Ear

Ear wax
If the simple home remedy of a few drops of olive oil does not work, various wax-softening preparations may be used. These include sodium bicarbonate ear drops, Waxsol and Exterol. Occasionally the ears have to be syringed.

Irritation of outer ear (otitis externa)
There is usually an infection with some inflammation. Ear drops with various constituents are used such as Otosporin, Audicort, Predsol N and Locorten-Vioform.

Mouth and throat

Sore throat
Sore throats are usually due to a virus infection so ordinary antibiotics cannot really help except in relieving secondary bacterial infection. Many satisfactory preparations can be bought over the chemist's counter.

Mouth ulcers
Some preparations are based on steroids such as hydrocortisone (Corlan) and triamcinolone (Adcortyl A in Orabase) and others on different principles (e.g. Bonjela, Bioral). If initial treatment is unsuccessful, obtain medical or dental advice.

Eye

Infection
Eye infections can be treated with local antibiotics either with eye drops or ointment (*see* page 103). Chloramphenicol (Chloromycetin) is often used for bacterial infections and idoxuridine also known as IDU (Dendrid, Kerecid) for some viral infections.

Glaucoma
Glaucoma is often treated with drugs that make the pupil smaller such as physostigmine or pilocarpine. Timolol (Timoptol) is now more frequently used and tablets of acetazolamide (Diamox) taken by mouth.

Skin

Many conditions are satisfactorily treated with steroid preparations. There are many of these including hydrocortisone (Efcortelan, Cortril), beclamethasone (Propaderm), betamethasone (Betnovate), clobetasol (Dermovate), flucinolone (Synalar, Synandone), fluocinonide (Metosyn) and triamcinolone (Ledercort). Many of these steroid preparations are marketed with various antibacterial preparations included. These can be recognized frequently by capital letters after the main name such as N for neomycin and C for clioquinol. Fungus infections of the skin are treated with preparations such as clotrimazole (Canesten), miconazole (Dermonistat), nystatin (Nystan) and amphoteracin (Fungilin).

Vagina

Apart from venereal disease, most vaginal infections are due to monilia, a kind of yeast. Pessaries (a special kind of tablet for vaginal use) or creams are usually given with much the same range as the fungal infection of the skin (*see above*). Infection with trichomonas is treated with metronidazole (Flagyl). With many vaginal infections it is also necessary to treat the male sexual partner. A few women after the menopause may develop trouble which is treated with a local hormone preparation containing oestrogens (e.g. Hormofemin, Premarin).

Glands and Metabolism

Over-active thyroid gland (thyrotoxicosis), hyperthyroidism
Carbimazole (Neo-mercazole) is used to quieten down an over-active thyroid, usually for a period of 9–18 months. Approximately half the people treated in this way will not become over-active again when the treatment is stopped. Many are instead treated with small doses of radioactive iodine which is very safe. It has been used for over 30 years and seems to have no serious long-term consequences.

Under-active thyroid (myxoedema), hypothyroidism
The natural thyroid hormone can be given as a pure chemical compound—thyroxine (Eltroxin). Once the right dose is established the drug is usually continued for life.

Gout
The excess chemical present in the body in this condition (uric acid) can be made to leak out in the urine with the use of substances such as allopurinol (Zyloric) and sulphinpyrazone (Anturan) or probenecid (Benemid). The inflammation of an acute attack can be stopped with drugs such as indomethacin (Indocid) or a short course of phenylbutazone (Butazolidin) or steroids.

Anaemia

There are three main causes of anaemia, the most common being a shortage of iron either because not enough iron is being absorbed or because the patient has been losing more blood than can be replaced—usually from a stomach ulcer or a woman's periods. It is usually given in the form of tablets containing ferrous sulphate but various other preparations, some of them 'slow releasing', are available such as Feo-span, Ferrogradumet and Slow-Fe. During pregnancy the mother and baby may require not only iron but a little more folic acid than is usually found in the diet and this is added to iron in standard preparations which are then called Slow-Fe Folic, Fefol and other names usually with *fli*.

A few people are deficient in folic acid, usually because the bowels are not absorbing properly, and relatively large doses by mouth are then given.

Pernicious anaemia is treated with injections of hydroxocobalamin (Neo-cytamen) or cyanocobalamin (Cytamen), a reddish fluid injected every 6 weeks or so. Treatment is continued for life.

Vitamins

In ordinary life with ordinary health and diet no vitamin supplements are required. Most can do no harm even in large quantities though poisoning with vitamin D occurs occasionally and overdose with vitamin A is possible.

Infections

At the moment there are few satisfactory ways of treating most virus infections, e.g. the common cold, influenza, shingles, chickenpox, measles, cold sores. Treatment of bacterial infections is usually with an antibiotic. Most commonly used are the penicillins, all related chemically to the original penicillin discovered by Fleming. The commoner penicillins are amoxycillin (Amoxil), ampicillin (Penbritin, Amfipen), cloxacillin (Orbenin), flucloxacillin (Floxapen) and penicillin V. Other groups are the cephalosporins, including cephalexin (Ceporex, Keflex), cephaloridine (Ceporin) and cephradine (Velosef). The tetracycline group includes tetracycline itself (Achromycin), chlortetracycline (Aureomycin) and oxytetracycline (Terramycin). Most of the other commonly used drugs do not fit easily into groups. These are co-trimoxazole (Septrin, Bactrim), sodium fusidate (Fucidin), trimethoprim (Ipral, Monotrim, Syraprim), nalidixic acid (Mictral, Negram) and nitrofurantoin (Furadantin, Macrodantin). The latter two are used chiefly for urinary infections.

Notes for those taking medicines (drugs)

1   Do not take more than one kind of tablet at a time unless your doctor tells you that it is safe to do so.
2   There are very few drugs which are known to be safe in early pregnancy, and nursing mothers should be careful.
3   The commoner drug side-effects include headaches and drowsiness, nausea, loss of appetite, bowel upset and skin rashes. With almost all drugs you should stop taking them forthwith and report to your doctor for further instructions. Often he will use alternative therapy.
4   All medications have to include the constituents usually in very small type on the box and all bottles. Many of the names will be on the lists given above.
5   Remember that aspirin (acetylsalicylic acid) is an excellent drug in many circumstances, but some people are very sensitive to it and others may bleed from the stomach.

Part 4

Useful Information

Infant Feeding
Children
  Development
  Eruption of teeth
  Weight, height
  Common infectious diseases and
  exclusion from school
Diet and Health
  Reducing diets
  Ideal weights
  Calorie value of foodstuffs
Weights and Measures
Care Organizations

Infant feeding

One of the major problems confronting a new mother is whether she should bottle or breast feed. Unfortunately the problem is confused by professionals and experts who within the last 10 years have moved confidently from one to the other—some have even returned to their original position with equal confidence and certainty.

It is a relief to realize that probably an equal number of bottle-fed and breast-fed children grow perfectly normally. There is evidence that breast feeding has some advantages including convenience and a reduced incidence of infant diarrhoea but in the developed countries these advantages are marginal (and it is probably more important to regard the wishes of the mother as paramount).

Medical opinion currently favours breast feeding but not to such a degree that it overrides the mother's feelings. If in any doubt discussion with the family physician, midwife or health visitor may help to resolve any problems.

During pregnancy, most maternity hospitals offer advice on preparation for breast feeding. Immediately after delivery and before leaving hospital nursing advice will be given about techniques of breast feeding. If breast feeding is not possible or bottle feeding is preferred, advice is available about types of milk, length of feeding and winding. After returning home, the midwife or health visitor will visit the mother.

Common problems

1 Many women with small breasts fear that they will not be able to breast feed. This is untrue as breast size gives no indication of milk production.
2 Shallow or inverted nipples do not prevent breast feeding but expert advice should be obtained. It may be necessary to wear nipple shields to make them more prominent.
3 Breast milk when first produced is creamy but as milk production increases it becomes thinner. After 7 or 8 days it looks watery. This is normal and does not indicate that it is weak.
4 Painful and lumpy breasts, and sore nipples make breast feeding difficult. Advice should be sought to determine the cause and eliminate the problem. Breast feeding can usually be restarted. Sprays for use prior to feeding may prevent cracking.
5 Most women are easily tired after returning home.

This is to be expected but may make feeding exhausting. It is very important to rest during the day for the first few weeks after delivery.
6 During breast feeding ensure an adequate intake of fluids and calories otherwise breast milk may not be produced in sufficient quantity. Do not diet until breast feeding is stopped. Do not take any medicines—ask your doctor first.
7 Bottle-fed children and their parents are no less loved or loving than breast-fed children.
8 Bottle feeding: ordinary milk must not be used for newborn babies. A number of cow's milk preparations are available and suitable for newborn infants. They are all carefully prepared and it is very important to follow the maker's instructions exactly. In particular:
a Wash your hands and sterilize bottles, teats, jugs and other equipment in a chemical solution (e.g. Milton) before feeding.
b Do not 'pack' the scoop of measure. Use only the scoop supplied with its own powder. It cannot be used for other makes or for measuring water.
c Measure the water in a measuring jug—not by eye.
d Do not add an 'extra scoop for luck'.
e Pour a little onto the back of the hand to ensure that it is not too hot.
f Store made-up milk in the fridge but not elsewhere as the temperature will encourage the growth of bacteria. Do not use milk that has stood for more than 24 hours.
g Wash the bottles and teats out thoroughly immediately after use.

There is great individual variation between children and they soon find their own pattern. Initially it is best to feed them 'on demand' and allow them about 10 minutes on each breast or about 15 minutes with a bottle (this ranges from about 5 to 20 minutes depending on the mother and child). Babies soon settle to feeding about 3 to 5 hourly and will take as much as they need. As long as they are content and putting on weight normally they are probably feeding properly.

Recommended reading
New Baby. Health Visitors Association. B. Edsall & Co., London.
Feeding Your Baby. Family Doctor Publications. BMA House, London.

Children

Development chart (average) for first year of life *SEE ALSO* PAGES 271–72

Age		
6	weeks	Smiles in response to mother
8	weeks	Smiles and coos
12	weeks	Turns head to follow mother and objects
		Holds rattle
16	weeks	Responds to sounds
		Excited by sight of food
		Takes weight on forearms
24	weeks	Takes weight on hands
		Rolls over from front to back
		Holds head up steadily
26	weeks	Chews semi-solids and solids
		Sits with hands forward for support
28	weeks	Rolls over from back to front
		Stands with support
36	weeks	Stands holding onto nearby object
40	weeks	Crawls
		Waves goodbye
44	weeks	One word—begins speaking
48	weeks	Walks holding onto furniture
1	year	Speaks—a few words only
		Plays simple games

Note   Children develop at widely differing speeds and there is little correlation between their speed of development and later intelligence.

Eruption of teeth (average time)

Milk teeth (total = 20)

Central lower incisors	6–10 months
Lateral and upper central incisors	8–12 months
Lateral lower incisors and first molars	12–18 months
Canines	18–24 months
Second molars	20–30 months

Permanent teeth (total = 32)

First molars	6 years
Central incisors	7 years
Lateral incisors	8 years

Weight, height (average)

Age	Weight		Height	
	kg	*lb*	*cm*	*in*
Birth	3.4	7.5	51	20
3 months	5.72	12.6	60	24
6 months	7.58	16.7	66	26
9 months	9.07	20.0	71	28
1 year	10.07	22.2	75	30
2 years	12.56	27.7	87	34
3 years	14.61	32.2	96	38
4 years	16.51	36.4	103	41
5 years	18.89	41.7	110	43
6 years	21.91	48.3	117	46
7 years	24.54	54.1	124	49
8 years	27.26	60.1	130	51
9 years	29.44	66.0	135	53
10 years	32.61	71.9	140	55
11 years	35.29	77.6	144	57
12 years	38.28	84.4	145	59

Note   Measurements are for boys and are slightly smaller for girls.

Common infectious diseases and exclusion from school

Disease	Exclusion period
Chickenpox	14 days from appearance of rash
German measles	7 days from appearance of rash
Influenza	Until recovery
Infectious hepatitis	Until recovery
Measles	10 days from appearance of rash
Meningitis	Until recovery
Mumps	7 days after enlargement of glands has subsided
Rubella	*See* German measles
Tuberculosis	Until no longer excreting organism, e.g. in sputum
Typhoid and	Until clinical recovery (but insist

| paratyphoid | on meticulous hand-washing after toilet as bacteria is excreted in stools after clinical recovery) |
| Whooping cough | 10 days after illness begins unless coughing attacks persist |

Note Well children who have been in contact with an infectious disease may go to school, but:

1 Inform the school first; some children who have been in contact with typhoid or meningitis may be excluded by the school health officer.

2 Contacts of whooping cough should stay away for 21 days following contact.

Diet and Health

General hints for a healthy diet

1 Eat less processed and package food.
2 Eat more vegetable produce and less animal produce.
3 Eat more roughage.
4 Eat less fat of all kinds, especially animal fat.
5 Eat less salt.
Remember we are tempted to eat more of the wrong items such as savoury (salt), sweet (sugar), and dairy (fat) foods than is generally good for us.

Hints for losing weight

1 Ask yourself why you want to lose weight and then build on your own motivation. The reasons may be cosmetic, general health, or doctor's orders—for instance to help reduce blood pressure.
2 Calorie count everything without cheating. Refer to the chart on page 296 and prepare a list, totting it up at the end of the day. Aim at 800–1000 calories a day, but check with the doctor first.
3 You are probably aiming at a change in eating habits for the rest of your life. Crash diets only provide temporary solutions.
4 The only real authority on whether you are eating too much is your weighing machine. Generally speaking, if you are not losing weight you are eating too much. Again, it is wise to check with your doctor.
5 Reduce fat intake. For instance, use skimmed milk rather than whole milk and avoid all cream. Take little fatty meat and concentrate on the low-fat meat in chickens and turkeys. Try making a quarter pound (250 g) packet of butter or margarine last a fortnight.
6 Reduce the meat content of your diet (except for fowl).
7 Increase the vegetable content of your diet. This will provide more roughage.

Average energy requirements (adults)

Age (years)	Occupation	Men (calories)	Women (calories)
20–40	Clerical	2500–2800	2000–2200
	Heavy manual	3500–3800	2400–2600
40–60	Clerical	2400–2600	2000–2200
	Heavy manual	3500–3800	2400–2600
60–80		2100–2500	1800–2100

Note The requirements are higher during pregnancy and breast feeding.

Average energy requirements during growth

Age (years)	Boys (calories)	Girls (calories)
1	800	800
1–2	1100–1300	1100–1300
2–4	1300–1500	1300–1500
4–6	1500–1700	1500–1700
6–8	1700–1900	1700–1900
8–10	1900–2200	1900–2200
10–12	2200–2600	2200–2600
12–18	2600–3600	2400–3400

Note There is considerable individual variation in requirements throughout growth.

Reducing diets

The following 800 calorie and 1000 calorie reducing diets are reproduced by kind permission of the Department of Dietetics, Addenbrooke's Hospital, Cambridge. The following general rules apply.

Allowed without restriction

Salt, mustard, vinegar, pepper, herbs and spices

'Low calorie' squashes, diabetic squash, and 'Slimline' drinks

Tea and coffee (not bottled)

Clear soups, meat and yeast extracts, stock cubes, meat and fish paste

Salad vegetables

Vegetables (except potatoes, parsnips, dried pulses, avocado pear)

Saccharin and saccharin sweeteners

Ideal weights (dressed)

MEN

Height in feet and inches, and centimetres; weight in pounds and kilograms

Height	Small frame	Medium frame	Large frame
5′ 2″	112–120	118–129	126–141
157.5	50.8–54.4	53.5–58.5	57.2–64
5′ 3″	115–123	121–133	129–144
160	52.2–55.8	54.9–60.3	58.5–65.3
5′ 4″	118–126	124–136	132–148
162.6	53.3–57.2	56.2–61.7	59.9–67.1
5′ 5″	121–129	127–139	135–148
165.1	54.9–58.5	57.6–63	61.2–68.9
5′ 6″	124–133	130–143	138–156
167.6	56.2–60.3	59–64.9	62.6–70.8
5′ 7″	128–137	134–147	142–166
170.2	58.1–62.1	60.8–66.7	64.4–73
5′ 8″	132–141	138–152	147–166
172.7	59.9–64	62.6–68.9	66.7–75.3
5′ 9″	136–145	142–156	151–170
175.3	61.7–65.8	64.4–70.8	68.5–77.1
5′ 10″	140–150	146–160	155–174
177.8	63.5–68	66.2–72.6	70.3–78.9
5′ 11″	144–154	150–165	159–179
180.3	65.3–69.9	68–74.8	72.1–81.2
6′	148–158	154–170	164–184
182.9	67.1–71.7	69.9–77.1	74.4–83.5
6′ 1″	152–162	158–175	168–189
185.4	68.9–73.5	71.7–79.4	76.2–85.7
6′ 2″	156–167	162–180	173–194
188	70.8–75.7	73.5–81.6	78.5–88
6′ 3″	160–171	167–185	178–199
190.5	72.6–77.6	75.7–83.5	80.7–90.3
6′ 4″	164–175	172–190	182–204
193	74.4–79.4	78.1–86.2	82.7–92.5

Allowed with restriction

Milk—200 millilitres (⅓ pint) of whole milk or 400 millilitres (⅔ pint) of skimmed milk

Butter or margarine—15 grams or ½ ounce

Bread—90 grams or 3 bread exchanges (*see below*)

Fruit—up to 4 portions (unsweetened, fresh, stewed, baked, or juice)

Exchanges for one thin slice of bread (30 grams)

1   2 crispbreads or 3 'low calorie' crispbreads
2   2 plain biscuits
3   1 small portion of unsugared cereal
4   3 tablespoons of boiled rice
5   1 small potato

Allowed in moderation

Protein foods are essential to good health but they are high in energy (calories)—so strike a balance.

Lean meat   up to 100 grams per serving (3 oz)

Ideal weights (dressed)

WOMEN

Height in feet and inches, and centimetres; weight in pounds and kilograms

Height	Small frame	Medium frame	Large frame
4' 10" 147.3	92–98 41.7–44.5	96–107 43.5–48.5	104–119 47.2–54
4' 11" 149.9	94–101 42.6–45.8	98–110 44.5–49.9	106–122 48.1–55.3
5' 152.4	96–104 43.5–47.2	101–113 45.8–51.3	109–125 49.4–56.7
5' 1" 154.9	99–107 44.8–48.5	104–116 47.2–52.6	112–128 50.8–58.1
5' 2" 157.5	102–110 46.3–49.9	107–119 48.5–54	115–131 52.2–59.4
5' 3" 160	105–113 47.6–51.3	110–122 49.9–55.3	118–134 53.5–60.8
5' 4" 162.6	108–116 49–52.6	113–126 51.3–57.2	121–128 54.9–62.6
5' 5" 165.1	111–119 50.3–54	116–130 52.6–59	125–142 56.7–64.4
5' 6" 167.6	114–123 51.7–55.8	120–135 54.4–61.2	129–146 58.5–66.2
5' 7" 170.2	118–127 53.5–57.6	124–139 56.2–63	133–150 60.3–68
5' 8" 172.7	122–131 55.3–59.4	128–143 58.1–64.9	137–154 62.1–69.9
5' 9" 175.3	126–135 57.2–61.2	132–147 59.9–66.7	141–158 64–71.7
5' 10" 177.8	130–140 59–63.5	136–151 61.7–68.5	145–163 65.8–73.9
5' 11" 180.3	134–144 60.8–65.3	140–155 63.5–70.3	149–168 67.6–76.2
6' 182.9	138–148 62.6–67.1	144–159 65.3–72.1	153–173 69.4–78.5

White fish	up to 150 grams per serving (4–6 ounces)	

Fatty fish may be taken once a week if desired—drain off oil if canned.

Eggs	2 at main course, 1 at breakfast
Hard cheese	up to 50 grams at main course (1–2 ounces)
Cottage cheese	up to 120 grams per serving (4 ounces)

The following vegetables are higher in energy (calories) than others and servings should not exceed 50 grams (1-2 ounces) per day.

Peas	Sweetcorn	Swede
Broad beans	Beetroot	

The following fruits are lower in energy (calories) than others and servings of up to 100 grams (3 ounces) may be taken in addition to your fruit allowance.

Lemons	Melon	Blackcurrants
Gooseberries	Rhubarb	Loganberries
Grapefruit		

Forbidden
Foods with a high fat content:

Lard, suet, dripping

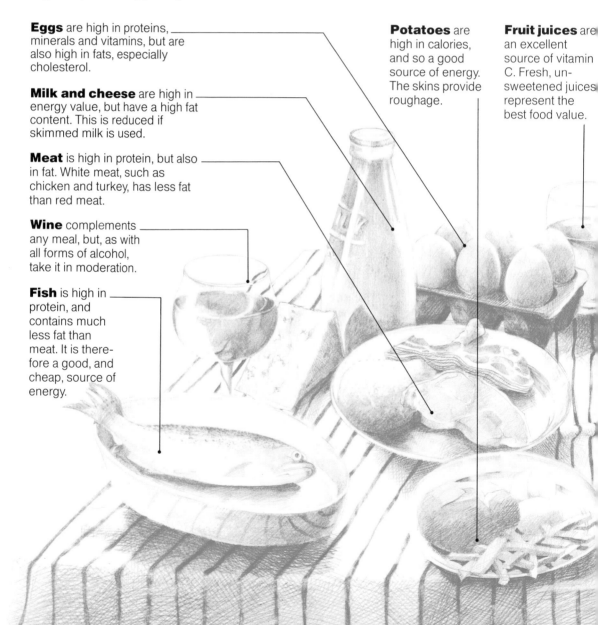

Eggs are high in proteins, minerals and vitamins, but are also high in fats, especially cholesterol.

Milk and cheese are high in energy value, but have a high fat content. This is reduced if skimmed milk is used.

Meat is high in protein, but also in fat. White meat, such as chicken and turkey, has less fat than red meat.

Wine complements any meal, but, as with all forms of alcohol, take it in moderation.

Fish is high in protein, and contains much less fat than meat. It is therefore a good, and cheap, source of energy.

Potatoes are high in calories, and so a good source of energy. The skins provide roughage.

Fruit juices are an excellent source of vitamin C. Fresh, un-sweetened juices represent the best food value.

Fatty meat and fried foods
Oil, salad dressings, mayonnaise and salad cream
Cream and evaporated milk
Cream cheese
Foods with a high carbohydrate content:
Sugar, Sorbitol, glucose, sweets and chocolate
Puddings of all descriptions
Sweetened tinned fruit and fruit juices
Grapes and dried fruits
Cocoa, bottled coffee (e.g. Camp), proprietary
bed-time drinks (e.g. Ovaltine, Horlicks)
Custard powder, flour and cornflour

Pasta
Jam, honey, marmalade, syrup, treacle
Diabetic foods
Parsnips and dried pulses (e.g lentils)
Alcoholic beverages of all descriptions including
diabetic beers and lagers

A balanced, sensible diet is vital for good health. The illustration below shows a variety of everyday foods, and gives an indication of the nutritive value of each.

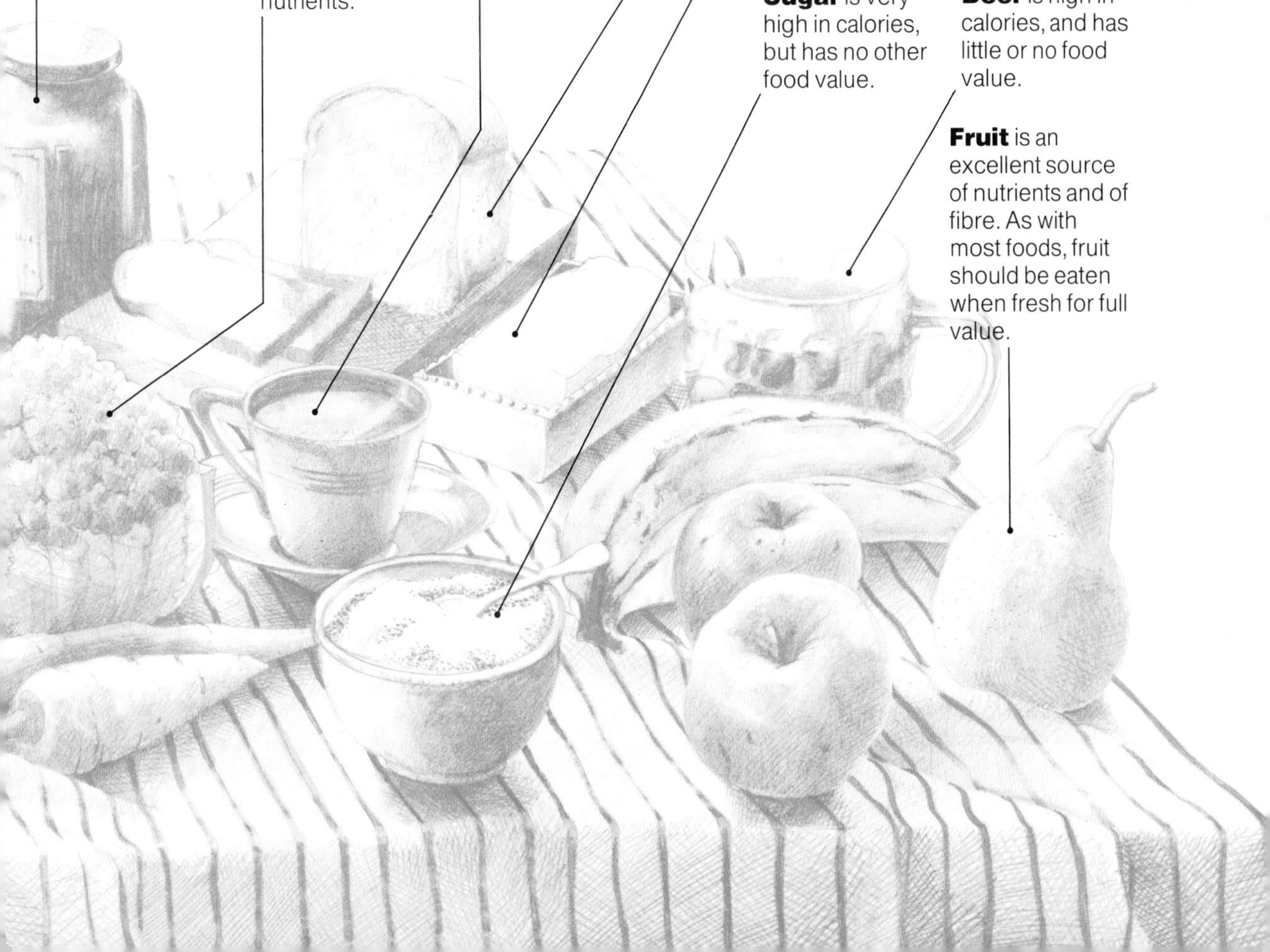

Preserves add variety to the diet, but often have a high sugar content. They are often partly cooked, which destroys some of the nutrients.

Vegetables are an excellent food, providing roughage and essential vitamins. However, over-cooking destroys valuable nutrients.

Tea and coffee have little or no food value. Taken in excess, they may cause palpitations.

Bread is a good source of calories and vitamins. Brown bread is much better than white, as it contains more roughage.

Butter is high in calories and fats. Margarine contains less animal fat, and fewer calories.

Sugar is very high in calories, but has no other food value.

Beer is high in calories, and has little or no food value.

Fruit is an excellent source of nutrients and of fibre. As with most foods, fruit should be eaten when fresh for full value.

Reducing diet—3.5 MJ or 800 calories

Meal plan

Breakfast
Small glass of unsweetened fruit juice
Milk from allowance in tea or coffee
Boiled or poached egg or/
1 rasher lean grilled bacon
1 large thin slice of bread
Mid-morning
Milk from allowance in tea or coffee
Lunch
Milk from allowance in tea or coffee
Lean meat, fish, egg or cheese
Green vegetables or salad
1 boiled potato or/
1 large thin slice of bread
1 portion of fruit (e.g. apple or orange)
Mid-afternoon
Milk from allowance in tea or coffee
Evening meal
Milk from allowance in tea or coffee
As lunch but no bread except if bread exchange has been taken at lunch
Bed time
Milk from allowance in tea or coffee

Reducing diet—4 MJ or 1000 calories

Meal plan

Breakfast
Small glass of unsweetened fruit juice
Milk from allowance in tea or coffee
Boiled or poached egg or/lean grilled bacon
1 large thin slice of bread
Mid-morning
Milk from allowance in tea or coffee
Lunch
Milk from allowance in tea or coffee
Lean meat, fish, eggs or cottage cheese
Green vegetables or salad
1 small boiled potato
1 portion of fruit (e.g. apple or orange)
Mid-afternoon
Milk from allowance in tea or coffee
Evening meal
Milk from allowance in tea or coffee
As lunch
1 small boiled potato may be exchanged for 1 large thin slice of bread with butter from allowance
Bed time
Milk from allowance in tea or coffee

Calorie value of foodstuffs

Value per ounce

Less than 5 calories

Artichokes	Onions
Asparagus	Salad vegetables
Beans (French)	Turnips
Broccoli	Black coffee
Brussels sprouts	Lemon juice
Cabbage (cooked)	Low-calorie drinks
Cauliflower (cooked)	Bouillon
Egg plant	Clear soup
Marrow	Tea
Mushrooms	Tomato juice

5–15 calories

Apples	Peaches	Broad beans
Apricots	Pears	Carrots
Blackberries	Pineapple	Leeks
Cherries	Plums	Cabbage (raw)
Gooseberries	Raspberries	Cauliflower (raw)
Melons	Strawberries	Spinach
Oranges	Beetroot	Beer, cider

Jellies made with low-calorie squash and gelatine
Malted milk made without milk
Milk (skimmed)
Ovaltine made without milk
Stout
Yoghurt

15–30 calories

Brain	Avocados	Parsnips
Heart	Bananas	Peas
Tripe	Grapes	Potatoes
Cod	Figs	Cottage cheese
Haddock	Prunes	Champagne
Oysters	Baked beans	Jellies
Prawns	Corn (sweet)	Milk
Sole	Olives	Wines

30–70 calories

Chicken	Herring	Dumplings
Goose	Kippers	Eggs
Ham (lean)	Lobster	Fruit gums
Kidneys	Mackerel	Ice cream
Rabbit	Pilchards	Macaroni
Turkey	Salmon	Milk (evaporated)
Veal		Milk puddings
		Blancmange
Sherry	Potatoes (roast)	Cream (thin)
Spirits		Yorkshire pudding
Squashes (neat)		

70–120 calories

Bacon	Sultanas
Beef	
Duck	Potatoes (chipped)
Ham (lean and fat)	Bread
Lamb	Breakfast cereals
Liver	Cheese (Camembert,
Mutton	Edam, Danish Blue)
Sausages	Jam
	Milk (sweetened,
Eels	condensed)
Sardines	Sponge cakes
	Sugar, sweets
Dates	Suet puddings
Raisins	Syrup

Source *The Composition of Foods*, R.A. McCance and E.M. Widdowson, HMSO, London, 1967.

Weights and measures

1 fluid ounce (oz)	= 30 millilitres (ml)
20 fluid ounces	= 1 pint
1 litre (l)	= 1000 millilitres
1 pint	= 560 millilitres
1 metre (m)	= 39 inches
	= 100 centimetres (cm)
	= 1000 millimetres (mm)
1 kilogram (kg)	= 1000 grams (g)
	= 2.2 pounds (lb)
Teaspoon	= 3.5 millilitres
Dessertspoon	= 7 millilitres
Tablespoon	= 15 millilitres (½ oz)
Teacup	= 150 millilitres (5 oz)

Note If a measure or dropper is supplied with a drug it is essential to use it and not rely on approximate measurements.

Care Organizations

The following include most national organizations where helpful information may be obtained. For other specific problems and local groups consult your family physician.

Action against Allergy Association
43 The Downs, London SW 20

Action on Smoking and Health (ASH)
27/35 Mortimer Street, London W1N 7RJ

AFASIC (Association for All Speech Impaired Children)
347 Central Markets, Smithfield, London EC1A 9HN

Age Concern England
National Old People's Welfare Council
Bernard Sunley House, 60 Pitcairn Road, Mitcham, Surrey CR4 3LL

Age Concern Northern Ireland
Northern Ireland Old People's Welfare Council, 2 Annadale Avenue, Belfast BT7 3JR

Age Concern Scotland
Scottish Old People's Welfare Council, 33 Castle Street, Edinburth EH2 3DW

Age Concern Wales
1 Park Green, Cardiff CF1 3BJ

Alcohol Education Centre Ltd
The Maudsley Hospital, 99 Denmark Hill, London SE5 8AZ

Alcoholics Anonymous
England and Wales

General Service Office: 11 Redcliffe Gardens, London SW10 9BG

Alzheimer Disease Society
c/o Cora Phillips SRN, Flat 6, Bromley College, London Road, Bromley, Kent

Anorexic Aid
Gravel House, Copthall Corner, Chalfont St Peter, Buckinghamshire

Arthritis Care
6 Grosvenor Crescent, London SW1X 7ER

The Association for Children with Heart Disorders
44 Sutton Avenue, Burnley, Lancashire BB10 2NS

Association for Spina Bifida and Hydrocephalus
Tavistock House North, Tavistock Square, London WC1H 9HJ

The Association for the Education and Welfare of the Visually Handicapped
East Anglian School, Church Road, Gorleston on Sea, Norfolk NR31 6LP

Association for the Treatment of Brain Damaged Children
21 Rowington Close, Coventry CV6 1PR

Association of Parents of Vaccine Damaged Children
2 Church Street, Shipston on Stour, Warwickshire

Association to Combat Huntington's Chorea
Lyndhurst, Lower Hampton Road, Sunbury on Thames, Middlesex TW16 5PR

Back Pain Association
31/33 Park Road, Teddington, Middlesex TW11 OAB

British Anti-Smoking Education Society (Bases)
78 Langley Road, Watford, Hertfordshire WD1 3PL

British Association for the Retarded
117 Golden Lane, London EC1Y ORT

British Association of the Hard of Hearing
7/11 Armstrong Road, London W3 7JL

British Deaf Association
38 Victoria Place, Carlisle CA1 1HU

British Diabetic Association
10 Queen Anne Street, London WIM OBD

British Dyslexia Association
4 Hobart Place, London SW1 0HU

British Epilepsy Association
Crowthorne House, Bigshotte, New Wokingham Road, Wokingham, Berkshire RG11 3AY

British Homoeopathic Association
27a Devonshire Street, London W1N IRJ

British Institute of Mental Handicap
Information and Resource Centre, Wolverhampton Road, Kidderminster, Worcestershire DY10 3PP

British Kidney Patient Association
Oakhanger Place, Bordon, Hampshire

British Migraine Association
178a High Road, Byfleet, Weybridge, Surrey KT14 7ED

British Pregnancy Advisory Service
Head Office: Austy Manor, Wootton Wawen, Solihull, West Midlands B95 6BX

Cancer Aftercare and Rehabilitation Society (CARE)
Lodge Cottage, Church Lane, Timsbury, Bath, Avon BA3 1LF

Cancer Information Association
2nd Floor Marygold House, Carfax, Oxford OX1 1EF

Church Army
Independents Road, Blackheath, London SE3 9LG

Coeliac Society of the UK
PO Box 181, London NW2 2QY

Colostomy Welfare Group
38-39 Eccleston Square, London SW1V 1PB

Cripples Help Society (Manchester, Salford and North-West England) (Inc)
26 Blackfriars Street, Manchester M3 5BE

Cystic Fibrosis Research Trust
5 Blyth Road, Bromley, Kent BR1 3RS

Depressives Associated
19 Merleys Way, Wimborne Minster, Dorset BH21 1QN

Disabled Living Foundation
346 Kensington High Street, London W14 8NS

Disabled Persons Information Centre
45 Park Place, Cardiff

Down's Children's Association
Quinborne Community Centre, Ridgacre Road, Birmingham B32 2TW

Dyslexia Institute
133 Gresham Road, Staines, Middlesex

Family Planning Association
ENGLAND
North of Thames:
38b St Peter's Street, Bedford MK40 2NN
South East:
13a Western Road, Hove, East Sussex
South West:
53a Bridge Street, Taunton, Somerset
Eastern:
20a Bridewell Alley, Norwich NR2 1SY
Midlands:
7 York Road, Birmingham B16 9HX
North West:
9 Gambier Terrace, Liverpool
Yorkshire and North East:
17 North Church Street, Sheffield S1 2DH
London:
160 Shepherd's Bush Road, London W6
WALES
6 Windsor Place, Cardiff
SCOTLAND
4 Clifton Street, Glasgow G3 7LA
NORTHERN IRELAND
47 Botanic Avenue, Belfast BT7 1JL

Five-Day Plan to Stop Smoking
Stanborough Park, Watford, Hertfordshire

Food Allergy Association

Depsad, 27 Ferringham Lane, Ferring by Sea, Worthing, West Sussex

Friedreich's Ataxia Group
12c Worplesdon Road, Guildford, Surrey GU2 6RW

Greater London Red Cross Blood Transfusion Service
4 Collingham Gardens, London SW5

Guide Dogs for the Blind Association
Alexandra House, 9-11 Park Street, Windsor, Berkshire SL4 13R

Haemophilia Society
PO Box 9, 15 Trinity Street, London SE1 1DE

Help the Aged
32 Dover Street, London W1A 2AP

Ileostomy Association of Great Britain and Northern Ireland
Central Office, Amblehurst House, Chobham, Woking, Surrey GU24 3PL

Invalid Children's Aid Association
Room 55, 126 Buckingham Palace Road, London SW1W 9SB

Invalids-at-Home
23 Farm Avenue, London NW2 2BJ

Leukaemia Society
c/o Mrs Janet Pankhurst, Secretary, Hamlyn's View, St Andrews Road, Exeter, Devon EX4 2AF

London Association for the Blind
14-16 Verney Road, London SE16 3DZ

Mastectomy Advisory Service
40 Eglantine Avenue, Belfast, Northern Ireland BT9 6OX

Mastectomy Association
25 Brighton Road, South Croydon Surrey CR2 6EA

Medic-Alert Foundation
9 Hanover Street, London W1R 9HF

Mental After Care Association
110 Jermyn Street, London SW1Y 6HB

Migraine Trust
45 Great Ormond Street, London WC1N 3HD

MIND (National Association for Mental Health)
22 Harley Street, London W1N 2ED

Motor Neurone Disease Association
245 Popes Lane, London W5

Multiple Sclerosis Society of Great Britain and Northern Ireland
286 Munster Road, Fulham, London SW66AP

Muscular Dystrophy Group of Great Britain
Nattrass House, 35 Macaulay Road, Clapham, London SW4 OPQ

National Advisory Centre on the Battered Child
Denver House, The Drive, Bounds Green Road, London N11

National Ankylosing Spondylitis Society
c/o The Royal National Hospital for Rheumatic Diseases, Upper Borough Walls, Bath, Avon BA1 IRL

National Association for Deaf-Blind and Rubella Handicapped
164 Cromwell Lane, Coventry CV4 8AP

National Association for Maternal and Child Welfare
1 South Audley Street, London W1Y 6JS

National Association for Remedial Education
77 Chignall Road, Chelmsford, Essex CM1 2JA

National Association of Laryngectomy Clubs
Michael Sobell House, 30 Dorset Square, London NW1 6QL

National Childbirth Trust
Queensborough Terrace, London W2 3TB

National Council of Voluntary Child Care Organisations
40 Brunswick Square, London WC1

National Deaf Children's Society
45 Hereford Road, London W2 5AH

National Eczema Society
Tavistock House North, Tavistock Square, London WC1H 9SR

National League of the Blind and Disabled
2 Tenterden Road, Tottenham, London N17 8BE

National Library for the Blind
Cromwell Road, Bredbury, Stockport, SK6 2SG

National Listening Library (Talking Books for the Handicapped)
49 Great Cumberland Place, London W1H 7LH

National Marriage Guidance Council
Herbert Gray College, Little Church Street, Rugby, Warwickshire CV21 3AP

National Schizophrenia Fellowship
79 Victoria Road, Surbiton, Surrey KT6 4NS

National Society for Autistic Children
1A Golders Green Road, London NW11 8EA

National Society for Cancer Relief
Michael Sobell House, 30 Dorset Square, London NW1 6QL

National Society for Epilepsy
Chalfont Centre for Epilepsy, Chalfont St Peter, Buckinghamshire SL9 ORJ

National Society for Phenylketonuria and Allied Disorders
c/o Dr J Noble-Nesbitt, 14 Newfound Drive, Cringleford, Norwich, Norfolk

National Society for the Prevention of Cruelty to Children (NSPCC)
1 Riding House Street, London W1P 8AA

National Society of Non-Smokers
Latimer House, 40/48 Hanson Street, London W1P 7DE

Parkinson's Disease Society of the United Kingdom
81 Queens Road, London SW19 8NR

Partially Sighted Society
40 Wordsworth Street, Hove, West Sussex BN3 5BH

Patients Association
11 Dartmouth Street, London SW1H 9BN

PHAB (Physically Handicapped and Able Bodied)
42 Devonshire Street, London W1N 1LN

Phobic Society
4 Cheltenham Road, Chorlton-cum-Hardy, Manchester M21 1QN

Psoriasis Association
7 Milton Street, Northampton NN2 7JG

Psychiatric Rehabilitation Association
21A Kingsland High Street, London E8

Rape Crisis Centre
PO Box 42, London N6 5BU

Riding for the Disabled Association
Avenue R, National Agricultural Centre, Kenilworth, Warwickshire CV8 2LY

Royal Association for Disability and Rehabilitation (RADAR)
23-25 Mortimer Street, London W1N 8AB

Royal Association in Aid of the Deaf and Dumb
27 Old Oak Road, Acton, London W3 7AN

Royal British Legion Headquarters
49 Pall Mall, London SW1Y 5JY

The Royal London Society for the Blind
105/109 Salisbury Road, London NW6 6RH

Royal National Institute for the Blind
224 Great Portland Street, London W1N 6AA

Royal National Institute for the Deaf
105 Gower Street, London WC1E 6AH

Royal Scottish Society for the Prevention of Cruelty to Children
Nelville House, 41 Polworth Terrace, Edinburgh EH11 INU

INDEX

Main entry in italic, illustration in parentheses